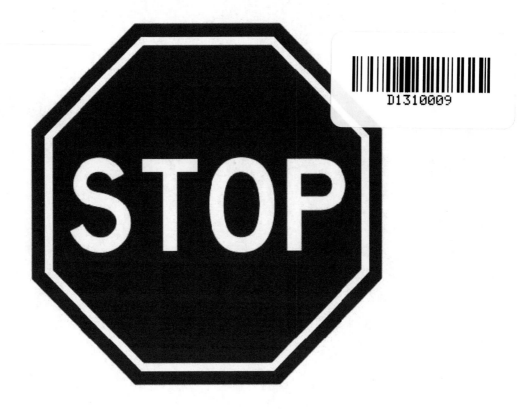

D1310009

FREE Test Taking Tips DVD Offer

To help us better serve you, we have developed a Test Taking Tips DVD that we would like to give you for FREE. **This DVD covers world-class test taking tips that you can use to be even more successful when you are taking your test.**

All that we ask is that you email us your feedback about your study guide. Please let us know what you thought about it – whether that is good, bad or indifferent.

To get your **FREE Test Taking Tips DVD**, email freedvd@studyguideteam.com with "FREE DVD" in the subject line and the following information in the body of the email:

    a. The title of your study guide.

    b. Your product rating on a scale of 1-5, with 5 being the highest rating.

    c. Your feedback about the study guide. What did you think of it?

    d. Your full name and shipping address to send your free DVD.

If you have any questions or concerns, please don't hesitate to contact us at freedvd@studyguideteam.com.

Thanks again!

PAX Study Guide Book 2019 & 2020

PAX RN & PN Study Book and Practice Test Questions for the NLN Pre Admission RN & PN Exam

Test Prep Books

Copyright © 2019 Test Prep Books

All Rights Reserved.

Table of Contents

Quick Overview

As you draw closer to taking your exam, effective preparation becomes more and more important. Thankfully, you have this study guide to help you get ready. Use this guide to help keep your studying on track and refer to it often.

This study guide contains several key sections that will help you be successful on your exam. The guide contains tips for what you should do the night before and the day of the test. Also included are test-taking tips. Knowing the right information is not always enough. Many well-prepared test takers struggle with exams. These tips will help equip you to accurately read, assess, and answer test questions.

A large part of the guide is devoted to showing you what content to expect on the exam and to helping you better understand that content. In this guide are practice test questions so that you can see how well you have grasped the content. Then, answer explanations are provided so that you can understand why you missed certain questions.

Don't try to cram the night before you take your exam. This is not a wise strategy for a few reasons. First, your retention of the information will be low. Your time would be better used by reviewing information you already know rather than trying to learn a lot of new information. Second, you will likely become stressed as you try to gain a large amount of knowledge in a short amount of time. Third, you will be depriving yourself of sleep. So be sure to go to bed at a reasonable time the night before. Being well-rested helps you focus and remain calm.

Be sure to eat a substantial breakfast the morning of the exam. If you are taking the exam in the afternoon, be sure to have a good lunch as well. Being hungry is distracting and can make it difficult to focus. You have hopefully spent lots of time preparing for the exam. Don't let an empty stomach get in the way of success!

When travelling to the testing center, leave earlier than needed. That way, you have a buffer in case you experience any delays. This will help you remain calm and will keep you from missing your appointment time at the testing center.

Be sure to pace yourself during the exam. Don't try to rush through the exam. There is no need to risk performing poorly on the exam just so you can leave the testing center early. Allow yourself to use all of the allotted time if needed.

Remain positive while taking the exam even if you feel like you are performing poorly. Thinking about the content you should have mastered will not help you perform better on the exam.

Once the exam is complete, take some time to relax. Even if you feel that you need to take the exam again, you will be well served by some down time before you begin studying again. It's often easier to convince yourself to study if you know that it will come with a reward!

Test-Taking Strategies

1. Predicting the Answer

When you feel confident in your preparation for a multiple-choice test, try predicting the answer before reading the answer choices. This is especially useful on questions that test objective factual knowledge. By predicting the answer before reading the available choices, you eliminate the possibility that you will be distracted or led astray by an incorrect answer choice. You will feel more confident in your selection if you read the question, predict the answer, and then find your prediction among the answer choices. After using this strategy, be sure to still read all of the answer choices carefully and completely. If you feel unprepared, you should not attempt to predict the answers. This would be a waste of time and an opportunity for your mind to wander in the wrong direction.

2. Reading the Whole Question

Too often, test takers scan a multiple-choice question, recognize a few familiar words, and immediately jump to the answer choices. Test authors are aware of this common impatience, and they will sometimes prey upon it. For instance, a test author might subtly turn the question into a negative, or he or she might redirect the focus of the question right at the end. The only way to avoid falling into these traps is to read the entirety of the question carefully before reading the answer choices.

3. Looking for Wrong Answers

Long and complicated multiple-choice questions can be intimidating. One way to simplify a difficult multiple-choice question is to eliminate all of the answer choices that are clearly wrong. In most sets of answers, there will be at least one selection that can be dismissed right away. If the test is administered on paper, the test taker could draw a line through it to indicate that it may be ignored; otherwise, the test taker will have to perform this operation mentally or on scratch paper. In either case, once the obviously incorrect answers have been eliminated, the remaining choices may be considered. Sometimes identifying the clearly wrong answers will give the test taker some information about the correct answer. For instance, if one of the remaining answer choices is a direct opposite of one of the eliminated answer choices, it may well be the correct answer. The opposite of obviously wrong is obviously right! Of course, this is not always the case. Some answers are obviously incorrect simply because they are irrelevant to the question being asked. Still, identifying and eliminating some incorrect answer choices is a good way to simplify a multiple-choice question.

4. Don't Overanalyze

Anxious test takers often overanalyze questions. When you are nervous, your brain will often run wild, causing you to make associations and discover clues that don't actually exist. If you feel that this may be a problem for you, do whatever you can to slow down during the test. Try taking a deep breath or counting to ten. As you read and consider the question, restrict yourself to the particular words used by the author. Avoid thought tangents about what the author *really* meant, or what he or she was *trying* to say. The only things that matter on a multiple-choice test are the words that are actually in the question. You must avoid reading too much into a multiple-choice question, or supposing that the writer meant something other than what he or she wrote.

5. No Need for Panic

It is wise to learn as many strategies as possible before taking a multiple-choice test, but it is likely that you will come across a few questions for which you simply don't know the answer. In this situation, avoid panicking. Because most multiple-choice tests include dozens of questions, the relative value of a single wrong answer is small. As much as possible, you should compartmentalize each question on a multiple-choice test. In other words, you should not allow your feelings about one question to affect your success on the others. When you find a question that you either don't understand or don't know how to answer, just take a deep breath and do your best. Read the entire question slowly and carefully. Try rephrasing the question a couple of different ways. Then, read all of the answer choices carefully. After eliminating obviously wrong answers, make a selection and move on to the next question.

6. Confusing Answer Choices

When working on a difficult multiple-choice question, there may be a tendency to focus on the answer choices that are the easiest to understand. Many people, whether consciously or not, gravitate to the answer choices that require the least concentration, knowledge, and memory. This is a mistake. When you come across an answer choice that is confusing, you should give it extra attention. A question might be confusing because you do not know the subject matter to which it refers. If this is the case, don't eliminate the answer before you have affirmatively settled on another. When you come across an answer choice of this type, set it aside as you look at the remaining choices. If you can confidently assert that one of the other choices is correct, you can leave the confusing answer aside. Otherwise, you will need to take a moment to try to better understand the confusing answer choice. Rephrasing is one way to tease out the sense of a confusing answer choice.

7. Your First Instinct

Many people struggle with multiple-choice tests because they overthink the questions. If you have studied sufficiently for the test, you should be prepared to trust your first instinct once you have carefully and completely read the question and all of the answer choices. There is a great deal of research suggesting that the mind can come to the correct conclusion very quickly once it has obtained all of the relevant information. At times, it may seem to you as if your intuition is working faster even than your reasoning mind. This may in fact be true. The knowledge you obtain while studying may be retrieved from your subconscious before you have a chance to work out the associations that support it. Verify your instinct by working out the reasons that it should be trusted.

8. Key Words

Many test takers struggle with multiple-choice questions because they have poor reading comprehension skills. Quickly reading and understanding a multiple-choice question requires a mixture of skill and experience. To help with this, try jotting down a few key words and phrases on a piece of scrap paper. Doing this concentrates the process of reading and forces the mind to weigh the relative importance of the question's parts. In selecting words and phrases to write down, the test taker thinks about the question more deeply and carefully. This is especially true for multiple-choice questions that are preceded by a long prompt.

9. Subtle Negatives

One of the oldest tricks in the multiple-choice test writer's book is to subtly reverse the meaning of a question with a word like *not* or *except*. If you are not paying attention to each word in the question, you can easily be led astray by this trick. For instance, a common question format is, "Which of the following is…?" Obviously, if the question instead is, "Which of the following is not…?," then the answer will be quite different. Even worse, the test makers are aware of the potential for this mistake and will include one answer choice that would be correct if the question were not negated or reversed. A test taker who misses the reversal will find what he or she believes to be a correct answer and will be so confident that he or she will fail to reread the question and discover the original error. The only way to avoid this is to practice a wide variety of multiple-choice questions and to pay close attention to each and every word.

10. Reading Every Answer Choice

It may seem obvious, but you should always read every one of the answer choices! Too many test takers fall into the habit of scanning the question and assuming that they understand the question because they recognize a few key words. From there, they pick the first answer choice that answers the question they believe they have read. Test takers who read all of the answer choices might discover that one of the latter answer choices is actually *more* correct. Moreover, reading all of the answer choices can remind you of facts related to the question that can help you arrive at the correct answer. Sometimes, a misstatement or incorrect detail in one of the latter answer choices will trigger your memory of the subject and will enable you to find the right answer. Failing to read all of the answer choices is like not reading all of the items on a restaurant menu: you might miss out on the perfect choice.

11. Spot the Hedges

One of the keys to success on multiple-choice tests is paying close attention to every word. This is never truer than with words like almost, most, some, and sometimes. These words are called "hedges" because they indicate that a statement is not totally true or not true in every place and time. An absolute statement will contain no hedges, but in many subjects, the answers are not always straightforward or absolute. There are always exceptions to the rules in these subjects. For this reason, you should favor those multiple-choice questions that contain hedging language. The presence of qualifying words indicates that the author is taking special care with his or her words, which is certainly important when composing the right answer. After all, there are many ways to be wrong, but there is only one way to be right! For this reason, it is wise to avoid answers that are absolute when taking a multiple-choice test. An absolute answer is one that says things are either all one way or all another. They often include words like *every*, *always*, *best*, and *never*. If you are taking a multiple-choice test in a subject that doesn't lend itself to absolute answers, be on your guard if you see any of these words.

12. Long Answers

In many subject areas, the answers are not simple. As already mentioned, the right answer often requires hedges. Another common feature of the answers to a complex or subjective question are qualifying clauses, which are groups of words that subtly modify the meaning of the sentence. If the question or answer choice describes a rule to which there are exceptions or the subject matter is complicated, ambiguous, or confusing, the correct answer will require many words in order to be expressed clearly and accurately. In essence, you should not be deterred by answer choices that seem excessively long. Oftentimes, the author of the text will not be able to write the correct answer without offering some qualifications and modifications. Your job is to read the answer choices thoroughly and completely and to select the one that most accurately and precisely answers the question.

13. Restating to Understand

Sometimes, a question on a multiple-choice test is difficult not because of what it asks but because of how it is written. If this is the case, restate the question or answer choice in different words. This process serves a couple of important purposes. First, it forces you to concentrate on the core of the question. In order to rephrase the question accurately, you have to understand it well. Rephrasing the question will concentrate your mind on the key words and ideas. Second, it will present the information to your mind in a fresh way. This process may trigger your memory and render some useful scrap of information picked up while studying.

14. True Statements

Sometimes an answer choice will be true in itself, but it does not answer the question. This is one of the main reasons why it is essential to read the question carefully and completely before proceeding to the answer choices. Too often, test takers skip ahead to the answer choices and look for true statements. Having found one of these, they are content to select it without reference to the question above. Obviously, this provides an easy way for test makers to play tricks. The savvy test taker will always read the entire question before turning to the answer choices. Then, having settled on a correct answer choice, he or she will refer to the original question and ensure that the selected answer is relevant. The mistake of choosing a correct-but-irrelevant answer choice is especially common on questions related to specific pieces of objective knowledge. A prepared test taker will have a wealth of factual knowledge at his or her disposal, and should not be careless in its application.

15. No Patterns

One of the more dangerous ideas that circulates about multiple-choice tests is that the correct answers tend to fall into patterns. These erroneous ideas range from a belief that B and C are the most common right answers, to the idea that an unprepared test-taker should answer "A-B-A-C-A-D-A-B-A." It cannot be emphasized enough that pattern-seeking of this type is exactly the WRONG way to approach a multiple-choice test. To begin with, it is highly unlikely that the test maker will plot the correct answers according to some predetermined pattern. The questions are scrambled and delivered in a random order. Furthermore, even if the test maker was following a pattern in the assignation of correct answers, there is no reason why the test taker would know which pattern he or she was using. Any attempt to discern a pattern in the answer choices is a waste of time and a distraction from the real work of taking the test. A test taker would be much better served by extra preparation before the test than by reliance on a pattern in the answers.

FREE DVD OFFER

Don't forget that doing well on your exam includes both understanding the test content and understanding how to use what you know to do well on the test. We offer a completely FREE Test Taking Tips DVD that covers world class test taking tips that you can use to be even more successful when you are taking your test.

All that we ask is that you email us your feedback about your study guide. To get your **FREE Test Taking Tips DVD**, email freedvd@studyguideteam.com with "FREE DVD" in the subject line and the following information in the body of the email:

- The title of your study guide.
- Your product rating on a scale of 1-5, with 5 being the highest rating.
- Your feedback about the study guide. What did you think of it?
- Your full name and shipping address to send your free DVD.

Introduction to the PAX

Function of the Test

The National League for Nursing Pre-Admission Examination (NLN PAX) is an entrance exam designed for students seeking acceptance into nursing programs in the United States. Although there were previously two versions of the PAX (the RN and the PN), the NLN has streamlined the exam offerings and combined these versions into the sole PAX exam. To be eligible for the exam, candidates must have obtained a high school diploma or GED. Each nursing program can set their own minimum passing score required for prospective candidates.

There are three main content domains on the NLN PAX: Verbal, Math, and Science. As such, the exam is designed to assess the background knowledge and skills in these academic areas, as well as the general reasoning ability of prospective nursing students.

Test Administration

The NLN PAX is a multiple-choice exam with 160 questions administered via computer. Candidates can register online through the NLN testing services website and test at proctored locations (usually nursing schools) across the country; alternatively, some nursing programs offer registration and dates of administration directly on their websites. Test takers should review the websites or admissions information of the programs for which they seek entry.

Special accommodations are available for students with documented disabilities. Official requests must be made on the NLN testing services website. Candidates with disabilities should contact the nursing school where they will be taking the test to make the necessary arrangements.

Test Format

The NLN PAX has three sections: Verbal, Math, and Science. The questions in the verbal section assesses word knowledge, reading comprehension, and critical thinking. In the mathematics section, questions address basic computations and quantitative reasoning skills, conversions, graphs, algebra, geometry, and word problems. The science section includes questions about general biology, chemistry, physics, human health, and human anatomy and physiology. Each of the three sections lasts 40 minutes. There are 160 questions on the exam. The breakdown is as follows:

Section	Number of Questions	Time Allotted
Verbal	60	40 minutes
Math	40	40 minutes
Science	60	40 minutes
Total	160	2 hours

Note that additional, unscored items may also be added to each section. As these are unscored, they do not affect the percentage of questions answered correctly in the section nor the overall score. Some nursing programs allow the use of calculators, while others do not. Candidates will need to confirm the policy at the school administering their exam.

Scoring

Score reports are available four hours after completing the exam. Test takers can log in to their NLN account and access their results on the Reports tab. There is no set "passing score;" instead, each nursing program sets their own standards. These percentiles are usually published in the information about admissions on their website. If a candidate "fails" one section, the entire test must be retaken. A score (from 1-200) and percentile rank for each of the three sections is reported as well as an overall composite percentile rank.

Verbal

Word Knowledge

Synonyms

Synonyms are words that mean the same or nearly the same if given a list of words in the same language. When presented with several words and asked to choose the synonym, more than one word may be similar to the original. However, one word is generally the strongest match. Synonyms should always share the same part of speech. For instance, *shy* and *timid* are both adjectives and hold similar meanings. The words *shy* and *loner* are similar, but shy is an adjective, while loner is a noun. Another way to test for the best synonym is to reread the question with each possible word and determine which one makes the most sense. Consider the words: adore, sweet, kind, and nice.

Now consider the following sentence: *He will love you forever.*

He will adore you forever.

He will sweet you forever.

He will kind you forever.

He will nice you forever.

In the first sentence, the word *love* is used as a verb. The best synonym from the list that shares the same part of speech is *adore*. Adore is a verb, and when substituted in the sentence, it is the only substitution that makes grammatical and semantic sense.

Synonyms can be found for nouns, adjectives, verbs, adverbs, and prepositions. Here are some examples of synonyms from different parts of speech:

- Nouns: clothes, wardrobe, attire, apparel
- Verbs: run, spring, dash
- Adjectives: fast, quick, rapid, swift
- Adverbs: slowly, nonchalantly, leisurely
- Prepositions: near, proximal, neighboring, close

Here are several more examples of synonyms in the English language:

Word	Synonym	Meaning
smart	intelligent	having or showing a high level of intelligence
exact	specific	clearly identified
almost	nearly	not quite but very close
to annoy	to bother	to irritate
to answer	to reply	to form a written or verbal response
building	edifice	a structure that stands on its own with a roof and four walls
business	commerce	the act of purchasing, negotiating, trading, and selling
defective	faulty	when a device is not working or not working well

Vocabulary

In order to understand synonyms, one must have a good foundation of vocabulary. *Vocabulary* is the words a person uses on a daily basis. Having a good vocabulary is important. It's important in writing and also when you talk to people. Many of the questions on the test may have words that you don't know. Therefore, it's important to learn ways to find out a word's meaning.

It's hard to use vocabulary correctly. Imagine being thrust into a foreign country. If you didn't know right words to use to ask for the things you need, you could run into trouble! Asking for help from people who don't share the same vocabulary is hard. Language helps us understand each other. The more vocabulary words a person knows, the easier they can ask for things they need. This section of the study guide focuses on getting to know vocabulary through basic grammar.

Prefixes and Suffixes

In this section, we will look at the *meaning* of various prefixes and suffixes when added to a root word. A *prefix* is a combination of letters found at the beginning of a word. A *suffix* is a combination of letters found at the end. A *root word* is the word that comes after the prefix, before the suffix, or between them both. Sometimes a root word can stand on its own without either a prefix or a suffix. More simply put:

Prefix + Root Word = Word

Root Word + Suffix = Word

Prefix + Root Word + Suffix = Word

Root Word = Word

Knowing the definitions of common prefixes and suffixes is helpful. It's helpful when you are trying to find out the meaning of a word you don't know. Also, knowing prefixes can help you find out the number of things, the negative of something, or the time and space of an object! Understanding suffixes can help when trying to find out the meaning of an adjective, noun, or verb.

The following charts look at some of the most common prefixes, what they mean, and how they're used to find out a word's meaning:

Number and Quantity Prefixes

Prefix	Definition	Example
bi-	two	bicycle, bilateral
mono-	one, single	monopoly, monotone
poly-	many	polygamy, polygon
semi-	half, partly	semiannual, semicircle
uni-	one	unicycle, universal

Here's an example of a number prefix:

The girl rode on a *bicycle* to school.

Look at the word *bicycle*. The root word (*cycle*)comes from the Greek and means *wheel*. The prefix *bi-* means *two*. The word *bicycle* means two wheels! When you look at any bicycles, they all have two wheels. If you had a unicycle, your bike would only have one wheel, because *uni-* means *one*.

Negative Prefixes

Prefix	Definition	Example
a-	without, lack of	amoral, atypical
in-	not, opposing	inability, inverted
non-	not	nonexistent, nonstop
un-	not, reverse	unable, unspoken

Here's an example of a negative prefix:

The girl was *insensitive* to the boy who broke his leg.

Look at the word *insensitive.* In the chart above, the prefix *in-* means *not* or *opposing*. Replace the prefix with *not*. Now place *not* in front of the word *sensitive.* Now we see that the girl was "not sensitive" to the boy who broke his leg. In simpler terms, she showed that she did not care. These are easy ways to use prefixes and suffixes in order to find out what a word means.

Time and Space Prefixes

Prefix	Definition	Example
a-	in, on, of, up, to	aloof, associate
ab-	from, away, off	abstract, absent
ad-	to, towards	adept, adjacent
ante-	before, previous	antebellum, antenna
anti-	against, opposing	anticipate, antisocial
cata-	down, away, thoroughly	catacomb, catalogue
circum-	around	circumstance, circumvent
com-	with, together, very	combine, compel
contra-	against, opposing	contraband, contrast
de-	from	decrease, descend
dia-	through, across, apart	diagram, dialect
dis-	away, off, down, not	disregard, disrespect
epi-	upon	epidemic, epiphany
ex-	out	example, exit
hypo-	under, beneath	hypoallergenic, hypothermia
inter-	among, between	intermediate, international
intra-	within	intrapersonal, intravenous
ob-	against, opposing	obtain, obscure
per-	through	permanent, persist
peri-	around	periodontal, periphery
post-	after, following	postdate, postoperative
pre-	before, previous	precede, premeditate
pro-	forward, in place of	program, propel
retro-	back, backward	retroactive, retrofit
sub-	under, beneath	submarine, substantial
super-	above, extra	superior, supersede
trans-	across, beyond, over	transform, transmit
ultra-	beyond, excessively	ultraclean, ultralight

Here's an example of a space prefix:

> The teacher's motivational speech helped *propel* her students toward greater academic achievement.

Look at the word *propel.* The prefix *pro-* means *forward. Forward* means something related to time and space. *Propel* means to drive or move in a forward direction. Therefore, knowing the prefix *pro-* helps interpret that the students are moving forward *toward greater academic achievement.*

Miscellaneous Prefixes

Prefix	Definition	Example
belli-	war, warlike	bellied, belligerent
bene-	well, good	benediction, beneficial
equi-	equal	equidistant, equinox
for-	away, off, from	forbidden, forsaken
fore-	previous	forecast, forebode
homo-	same, equal	homogeneous, homonym
hyper-	excessive, over	hyperextend, hyperactive
in-	in, into	insignificant, invasive
magn-	large	magnetic, magnificent
mal-	bad, poorly, not	maladapted, malnourished
mis-	bad, poorly, not	misplace, misguide
mor-	death	mortal, morgue
neo-	new	neoclassical, neonatal
omni-	all, everywhere	omnipotent, omnipresent
ortho-	right, straight	orthodontist, orthopedic
over-	above	overload, overstock,
pan-	all, entire	panacea, pander
para-	beside, beyond	paradigm, parameter
phil-	love, like	philanthropy, philosophic
prim-	first, early	primal, primer
re-	backward, again	reload, regress
sym-	with, together	symmetry, symbolize
vis-	to see	visual, visibility

Here's another prefix example:

> The computer was *primitive*; it still had a floppy disk drive!

The word *primitive* has the prefix *prim-*. The prefix *prim-* indicates being *first* or *early*. *Primitive* refers to the historical development of something. Therefore, the sentence is saying that the computer is an older model, because it still has a floppy disk drive.

The charts that follow review some of the most common suffixes. They also include examples of how the suffixes are used to determine the meaning of a word. Remember, suffixes are added to the *end* of a root word:

Adjective Suffixes

Suffix	Definition	Example
-able (-ible)	capable of being	teachable, accessible
-esque	in the style of, like	humoresque, statuesque
-ful	filled with, marked by	helpful, deceitful
-ic	having, containing	manic, elastic
-ish	suggesting, like	malnourish, tarnish
-less	lacking, without	worthless, fearless
-ous	marked by, given to	generous, previous

Here's an example of an adjective suffix:

The live model looked so *statuesque* in the window display; she didn't even move!

Look at the word *statuesque*. The suffix *-esque* means *in the style of* or *like*. If something is *statuesque*, it's *like a statue*. In this sentence, the model looks like a statue.

Noun Suffixes

Suffix	Definition	Example
-acy	state, condition	literacy, legacy
-ance	act, condition, fact	distance, importance
-ard	one that does	leotard, billiard
-ation	action, state, result	legislation, condemnation
-dom	state, rank, condition	freedom, kingdom
-er (-or)	office, action	commuter, spectator
-ess	feminine	caress, princess
-hood	state, condition	childhood, livelihood
-ion	action, result, state	communion, position
-ism	act, manner, doctrine	capitalism, patriotism
-ist	worker, follower	stylist, activist
-ity (-ty)	state, quality, condition	community, dirty
-ment	result, action	empowerment, segment
-ness	quality, state	fitness, rudeness
-ship	position	censorship, leadership
-sion (-tion)	state, result	tension, transition
-th	act, state, quality	twentieth, wealth
-tude	quality, state, result	attitude, latitude

Look at the following example of a noun suffix:

The *spectator* cheered when his favorite soccer team scored a goal.

Look at the word *spectator*. The suffix *-or* means *action*. In this sentence, the *action* is to *spectate* (watch something). Therefore, a *spectator* is someone involved in watching something.

Verb Suffixes

Suffix	Definition	Example
-ate	having, showing	facilitate, integrate
-en	cause to be, become	frozen, written
-fy	make, cause to have	modify, rectify
-ize	cause to be, treat with	realize, sanitize

Here's an example of a verb suffix:

The preschool had to *sanitize* the toys every Tuesday and Thursday.

In the word *sanitize*, the suffix *-ize* means *cause to be* or *treat with*. By adding the suffix *-ize* to the root word *sanitary*, the meaning of the word becomes active: *cause to be sanitary*.

Context Clues

It's common to find words that aren't familiar in writing. When you don't know a word, there are some "tricks" that can be used to find out its meaning. *Context clues* are words or phrases in a sentence or paragraph that provide hints about a word and what it means. For example, if an unknown word is attached to a noun with other surrounding words as clues, these can help you figure out the word's meaning. Consider the following example:

> After the treatment, Grandma's natural rosy cheeks looked *wan* and ghostlike.

The word we don't know is *wan*. The first clue to its meaning is in the phrase *After the treatment,* which tells us that something happened after a procedure (possibly medical). A second clue is the word *rosy,* which describes Grandma's natural cheek color that changed after the treatment. Finally, the word *ghostlike* infers that Grandma's cheeks now look white. By using the context clues in the sentence, we can figure out that the meaning of the word *wan* means *pale*.

Below are more ways to use context clues to find out the meaning of a word we don't know:

Contrasts
Look for context clues that *contrast* the unknown word. When reading a sentence with a word we don't know, look for an opposite word or idea. Here's an example:

> Since Mary didn't cite her research sources, she lost significant points for *plagiarizing* the content of her report.

In this sentence, *plagiarizing* is the word we don't know. Notice that when Mary *didn't cite her research sources,* it resulted in her losing points for *plagiarizing the content of her report*. These contrasting ideas tell us that Mary did something wrong with the content. This makes sense because the definition of *plagiarizing* is "taking the work of someone else and passing it off as your own."

Contrasts often use words like *but, however, although,* or phrases like *on the other hand.* For example:

> The *gargantuan* television won't fit in my car, but it will cover the entire wall in the den.

The word we don't know is *gargantuan*. Notice that the television is too big to fit in a car, <u>but</u> *it will cover the entire wall in the den*. This tells us that the television is extremely large. The word *gargantuan* means *enormous*.

Synonyms
Another way to find out a word you don't know is to think of synonyms for that word. *Synonyms* are words with the same meaning. To do this, replace synonyms one at a time. Then read the sentence after each synonym to see if the meaning is clear. By replacing a word we don't know with a word we do know, it's easier to uncover its meaning. For example:

> Gary's clothes were *saturated* after he fell into the swimming pool.

In this sentence, we don't know the word *saturated*. To brainstorm synonyms for *saturated,* think about what happens to Gary's clothes after falling into the swimming pool. They'd be *soaked* or *wet*. These both turn out to be good synonyms to try. The actual meaning of *saturated* is "thoroughly soaked."

Antonyms

Sometimes sentences contain words or phrases that oppose each other. Opposite words are known as *antonyms*. An example of an antonym is *hot* and *cold*. For example:

> Although Mark seemed *tranquil,* you could tell he was actually nervous as he paced up and down the hall.

The word we don't know is *tranquil*. The sentence says that Mark was in fact not *tranquil.* He was *actually nervous*. The opposite of the word *nervous* is *calm. Calm* is the meaning of the word *tranquil.*

Explanations or Descriptions

Explanations or descriptions of other things in the sentence can also provide clues to an unfamiliar word. Take the following example:

> Golden Retrievers, Great Danes, and Pugs are the top three *breeds* competing in the dog show.

We don't know the word *breeds*. Look at the sentence for a clue. The subjects (*Golden Retrievers, Great Danes,* and *Pugs*) describe different types of dogs. This description helps uncover the meaning of the word *breeds.* The word *breeds* means "a particular type of animal."

Inferences

Inferences are clues to an unknown word that tell us its meaning. These inferences can be found within the sentence where the word appears. Or, they can be found in a sentence before the word or after the word. Look at the following example:

> The *wretched* old lady was kicked out of the restaurant. She was so mean and nasty to the waiter!

Here, we don't know the word *wretched*. The first sentence says that the *old lady was kicked out of the restaurant*, but it doesn't say why. The sentence after tells us why: *She was so mean and nasty to the waiter!* This infers that the old lady was *kicked out* because she was *so mean and nasty* or, in other words, *wretched*.

When you prepare for a vocabulary test, try reading harder materials to learn new words. If you don't know a word on the test, look for prefixes and suffixes to find out what the word means and get rid of wrong answers. If two answers both seem right, see if there are any differences between them. Then select the word that best fits. Context clues in the sentence or paragraph can also help you find the meaning of a word you don't know. By learning new words, a person can expand their knowledge. They can also improve the quality of their writing.

Reading Comprehension

Events, Plots, Characters, Settings, and Ideas

Putting Events in Order

One of the most crucial skills for conquering the Reading Comprehension questions is the ability to recognize the sequences of events for each passage and place them in the correct order. Every passage has a plot, whether it is from a short story, a manual, a newspaper article or editorial, or a history text. And each plot has a logical order, which is also known as a sequence. Some of the most straightforward sequences can be found in technology directions, science experiments, instructional materials, and recipes. These forms of writing list actions that must occur in a proper sequence in order to get sufficient results. Other forms of writing, however, use style and ideas in ways that completely change the sequence of events. Poetry, for instance, may introduce repetitions that make the events seem cyclical. Postmodern writers are famous for experimenting with different concepts of place and time, creating "cut scenes" that distort straightforward sequences and abruptly transport the audience to different contexts or times. Even everyday newspaper articles, editorials, and historical sources may experiment with different sequential forms for stylistic effect.

Most questions that call for test takers to apply their sequential knowledge use key words such as **sequence**, **sequence of events**, or **sequential order** to cue the test taker in to the task at hand. In social studies or history passages, the test questions might employ key words such as **chronology** or **chronological order** to cue the test taker. In some cases, sequence can be found through comprehension techniques. These literal passages number the sequences, or they use key words such as *firstly*, *secondly*, *finally*, *next*, or *then*. The sequences of these stories can be found by rereading the passage and charting these numbers or key words. In most cases, however, readers have to correctly order events through inferential and evaluative reading techniques; they have to place events in a logical order without explicit cues.

Making Inferences

Predictions

Some texts use suspense and foreshadowing to captivate readers. For example, an intriguing aspect of murder mysteries is that the reader is never sure of the culprit until the author reveals the individual's identity. Authors often build suspense and add depth and meaning to a work by leaving clues to provide hints or predict future events in the story; this is called foreshadowing. While some instances of foreshadowing are subtle, others are quite obvious.

Inferences

Another way to read actively is to identify examples of inference within text. Making an inference requires the reader to read between the lines and look for what is implied rather than what is directly stated. That is, using information that is known from the text, the reader is able to make a logical assumption about information that is *not* directly stated but is probably true.

Authors employ literary devices such as tone, characterization, and theme to engage the audience by showing details of the story instead of merely telling them. For example, if an author said *Bob is selfish*, there's little left to infer. If the author said, *Bob cheated on his test, ignored his mom's calls, and parked illegally*, the reader can infer Bob is selfish. Authors also make implications through character dialogue, thoughts, effects on others, actions, and looks. Like in life, readers must assemble all the clues to form a complete picture.

Read the following passage:

"Hey, do you wanna meet my new puppy?" Jonathan asked.

"Oh, I'm sorry but please don't—" Jacinta began to protest, but before she could finish, Jonathan had already opened the passenger side door of his car and a perfect white ball of fur came bouncing towards Jacinta.

"Isn't he the cutest?" beamed Jonathan.

"Yes—achoo!—he's pretty—aaaachooo!!—adora—aaa—aaaachoo!" Jacinta managed to say in between sneezes. "But if you don't mind, I—I—achoo!—need to go inside."

Which of the following can be inferred from Jacinta's reaction to the puppy?
a. she hates animals
b. she is allergic to dogs
c. she prefers cats to dogs
d. she is angry at Jonathan

An inference requires the reader to consider the information presented and then form their own idea about what is probably true. Based on the details in the passage, what is the best answer to the question? Important details to pay attention to include the tone of Jacinta's dialogue, which is overall polite and apologetic, as well as her reaction itself, which is a long string of sneezes. Answer choices (a) and (d) both express strong emotions ("hates" and "angry") that are not evident in Jacinta's speech or actions. Answer choice (c) mentions cats, but there is nothing in the passage to indicate Jacinta's feelings about cats. Answer choice (b), "she is allergic to dogs," is the most logical choice—based on the fact that she began sneezing as soon as a fluffy dog approached her, it makes sense to guess that Jacinta might be allergic to dogs. So even though Jacinta never directly states, "Sorry, I'm allergic to dogs!" using the clues in the passage, it is still reasonable to guess that this is true.

Making inferences is crucial for readers of literature, because literary texts often avoid presenting complete and direct information to readers about characters' thoughts or feelings, or they present this information in an unclear way, leaving it up to the reader to interpret clues given in the text. In order to make inferences while reading, readers should ask themselves:

- What details are being presented in the text?
- Is there any important information that seems to be missing?
- Based on the information that the author *does* include, what else is probably true?
- Is this inference reasonable based on what is already known?

Conclusions
Active readers should also draw conclusions. When doing so, the reader should ask the following questions: What is this piece about? What does the author believe? Does this piece have merit? Do I believe the author? Would this piece support my argument? The reader should first determine the author's intent. Identify the author's viewpoint and connect relevant evidence to support it. Readers may then move to the most important step: deciding whether to agree and determining whether they are correct. Always read cautiously and critically. Interact with text, and record reactions in the margins. These active reading skills help determine not only what the author thinks, but what the you as the reader thinks.

Analyzing Relationships within Passages
Inferences are useful in gaining a deeper understanding of how people, events, and ideas are connected in a passage. Readers can use the same strategies used with general inferences and analyzing texts— paying attention to details and using them to make reasonable guesses about the text—to read between the lines and get a more complete picture of how (and why) characters are thinking, feeling, and acting.

Read the following passage from O. Henry's story "The Gift of the Magi":

> One dollar and eighty-seven cents. That was all. And sixty cents of it was in pennies. Pennies saved one and two at a time by bulldozing the grocer and the vegetable man and the butcher until one's cheeks burned with the silent imputation of parsimony that such close dealing implied. Three times Della counted it. One dollar and eighty-seven cents. And the next day would be Christmas.
>
> There was clearly nothing to do but flop down on the shabby little couch and howl. So Della did it.

These paragraphs introduce the reader to the character Della. Even though the author doesn't include a direct description of Della, the reader can already form a general impression of her personality and emotions. One detail that should stick out to the reader is repetition: "one dollar and eighty-seven cents." This amount is repeated twice in the first paragraph, along with other descriptions of money: "sixty cents of it was in pennies," "pennies saved one and two at a time." The story's preoccupation with money parallels how Della herself is constantly thinking about her finances—"three times Della counted" her meager savings. Already the reader can guess that Della is having money problems. Next, think about her emotions. The first paragraph describes haggling over groceries "until one's cheeks burned"—another way to describe blushing. People tend to blush when they are embarrassed or ashamed, so readers can infer that Della is ashamed by her financial situation. This inference is also supported by the second paragraph, when she flops down and howls on her "shabby little couch." Clearly, she's in distress. Without saying, "Della has no money and is embarrassed to be poor," O. Henry is able to communicate the same impression to readers through his careful inclusion of details.

A character's **motive** is their reason for acting a certain way. Usually, characters are motivated by something that they want. In the passage above, why is Della upset about not having enough money? There's an important detail at the end of the first paragraph: "the next day would be Christmas." Why is money especially important around Christmas? Christmas is a holiday when people exchange gifts. If Della is struggling with money, she's probably also struggling to buy gifts. So a shrewd reader should be able to guess that Della's motivation is wanting to buy a gift for someone—but she's currently unable to afford it, leading to feelings of shame and frustration.

In order to understand characters in a text, readers should keep the following questions in mind:

- What words does the author use to describe the character? Are these words related to any specific emotions or personality traits (for example, characteristics like rude, friendly, unapproachable, or innocent)?

- What does the character say? Does their dialogue seem to be straightforward, or are they hiding some thoughts or emotions?

- What actions can be observed from this character? How do their actions reflect their feelings?

- What does the character want? What do they do to get it?

Understanding Main Ideas and Details

Determining the Relationship Between Ideas

It is very important to know the difference between the topic and the main idea of the text. Even though these two are similar because they both present the central point of a text, they have distinctive differences. A **topic** is the subject of the text; it can usually be described in a one- to two-word phrase and appears in the simplest form. On the other hand, the **main idea** is more detailed and provides the author's central point of the text. It can be expressed through a complete sentence and is often found in the beginning, middle, or end of a paragraph. In most nonfiction books, the first sentence of the passage usually (but not always) states the main idea.

Review the passage below to explore the topic versus the main idea:

> Cheetahs are one of the fastest mammals on the land, reaching up to 70 miles an hour over short distances. Even though cheetahs can run as fast as 70 miles an hour, they usually only have to run half that speed to catch up with their choice of prey. Cheetahs cannot maintain a fast pace over long periods of time because their bodies will overheat. After a chase, cheetahs need to rest for approximately 30 minutes prior to eating or returning to any other activity.

In the example above, the topic of the passage is "Cheetahs" simply because that is the subject of the text. The main idea of the text is "Cheetahs are one of the fastest mammals on the land but can only maintain a fast pace for shorter distances." While it covers the topic, it is more detailed and refers to the text in its entirety. The text continues to provide additional details called **supporting details**, which will be discussed in the next section.

How Details Develop the Main Idea

Supporting details help readers better develop and understand the main idea. Supporting details answer questions like *who, what, where, when, why,* and *how*. Different types of supporting details include examples, facts and statistics, anecdotes, and sensory details.

Persuasive and informative texts often use supporting details. In persuasive texts, authors attempt to make readers agree with their points of view, and supporting details are often used as "selling points." If authors make a statement, they need to support the statement with evidence in order to adequately persuade readers. Informative texts use supporting details such as examples and facts to inform readers. Review the previous "Cheetahs" passage to find examples of supporting details.

> Cheetahs are one of the fastest mammals on the land, reaching up to 70 miles an hour over short distances. Even though cheetahs can run as fast as 70 miles an hour, they usually only have to run half that speed to catch up with their choice of prey. Cheetahs cannot maintain a fast pace over long periods of time because their bodies will overheat. After a chase, cheetahs need to rest for approximately 30 minutes prior to eating or returning to any other activity.

In the example, supporting details include:

- Cheetahs reach up to 70 miles per hour over short distances.
- They usually only have to run half that speed to catch up with their prey.
- Cheetahs will overheat if they exert a high speed over longer distances.
- Cheetahs need to rest for 30 minutes after a chase.

Look at the diagram below (applying the cheetah example) to help determine the hierarchy of topic, main idea, and supporting details.

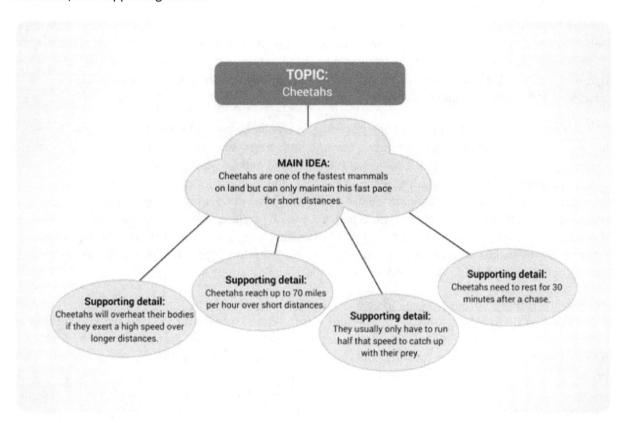

Point of View and Purpose

Author's Point of View and Purpose

When it comes to an author's writing, readers should always identify a **position** or **stance**. No matter how objective a text may seem, readers should assume the author has preconceived beliefs. One can reduce the likelihood of accepting an invalid argument by looking for multiple articles on the topic, including those with varying opinions. If several opinions point in the same direction and are backed by reputable peer-reviewed sources, it's more likely that the author has a valid argument. Positions that run contrary to widely held beliefs and existing data should invite scrutiny. There are exceptions to the rule, so readers should be careful consumers of information.

While themes, symbols, and motifs are buried deep within the text and can sometimes be difficult to infer, an author's **purpose** is usually obvious from the beginning. There are four purposes of writing: to inform, to persuade, to describe, and to entertain. **Informative** writing presents facts in an accessible way. **Persuasive** writing appeals to emotions and logic to inspire the reader to adopt a specific stance. Readers should be wary of this type of writing, as it can mask a lack of objectivity with powerful emotion. **Descriptive** writing is designed to paint a picture in the reader's mind, while texts that **entertain** are often narratives designed to engage and delight the reader.

The various writing styles are usually blended, with one purpose dominating the rest. A persuasive text, for example, might begin with a humorous tale to make readers more receptive to the persuasive message, or a recipe in a cookbook designed to inform might be preceded by an entertaining anecdote that makes the recipes more appealing.

Author's Position and Response to Different Viewpoints

If an author presents a differing opinion or a counterargument in order to refute it, the reader should consider how and why this information is being presented. It is meant to strengthen the original argument and shouldn't be confused with the author's intended conclusion, but it should also be considered in the reader's final evaluation.

Authors can also use bias if they ignore the opposing viewpoint or present their side in an unbalanced way. A strong argument considers the opposition and finds a way to refute it. Critical readers should look for an unfair or one-sided presentation of the argument and be skeptical, as a bias may be present. Even if this bias is unintentional, if it exists in the writing, the reader should be wary of the validity of the argument. Readers should also look for the use of stereotypes, which refer to specific groups. Stereotypes are often negative connotations about a person or place and should always be avoided. When a critical reader finds stereotypes in a piece of writing, they should be critical of the argument, and consider the validity of anything the author presents. Stereotypes reveal a flaw in the writer's thinking and may suggest a lack of knowledge or understanding about the subject.

Inferring the Author's Purpose in the Passage

In nonfiction writing, authors employ argumentative techniques to present their opinion to readers in the most convincing way. First of all, persuasive writing usually includes at least one type of appeal: an appeal to logic (**logos**), emotion (**pathos**), or credibility and trustworthiness (**ethos**). When a writer appeals to logic, they are asking readers to agree with them based on research, evidence, and an established line of reasoning. An author's argument might also appeal to readers' emotions, perhaps by including personal stories and anecdotes (a short narrative of a specific event). A final type of appeal— appeal to authority—asks the reader to agree with the author's argument on the basis of their expertise or credentials. Consider three different approaches to arguing the same opinion:

Logic (Logos)

Below is an example of an appeal to logic. The author uses evidence to disprove the logic of the school's rule (the rule was supposed to reduce discipline problems; the number of problems has not been reduced; therefore, the rule is not working) and he or she calls for its repeal.

> Our school should abolish its current ban on cell phone use on campus. This rule was adopted last year as an attempt to reduce class disruptions and help students focus more on their lessons. However, since the rule was enacted, there has been no change in the number of disciplinary problems in class. Therefore, the rule is ineffective and should be done away with.

Emotion (Pathos)

An author's argument might also appeal to readers' emotions, perhaps by including personal stories and anecdotes. The next example presents an appeal to emotion. By sharing the personal anecdote of one student and speaking about emotional topics like family relationships, the author invokes the reader's empathy in asking them to reconsider the school rule.

> Our school should abolish its current ban on cell phone use on campus. If they aren't able to use their phones during the school day, many students feel isolated from their loved ones. For example, last semester, one student's grandmother had a heart attack in the morning. However, because he couldn't use his cell phone, the student didn't know about his grandmother's condition until the end of the day—when she had already passed away and it was too late to say

goodbye. By preventing students from contacting their friends and family, our school is placing undue stress and anxiety on students.

Credibility (Ethos)
Finally, an appeal to authority includes a statement from a relevant expert. In this case, the author uses a doctor in the field of education to support the argument. All three examples begin from the same opinion—the school's phone ban needs to change—but rely on different argumentative styles to persuade the reader.

> Our school should abolish its current ban on cell phone use on campus. According to Dr. Bartholomew Everett, a leading educational expert, "Research studies show that cell phone usage has no real impact on student attentiveness. Rather, phones provide a valuable technological resource for learning. Schools need to learn how to integrate this new technology into their curriculum." Rather than banning phones altogether, our school should follow the advice of experts and allow students to use phones as part of their learning.

Rhetorical Questions
Another commonly used argumentative technique is asking **rhetorical questions**, questions that do not actually require an answer but that push the reader to consider the topic further.

> I wholly disagree with the proposal to ban restaurants from serving foods with high sugar and sodium contents. Do we really want to live in a world where the government can control what we eat? I prefer to make my own food choices.

Here, the author's rhetorical question prompts readers to put themselves in a hypothetical situation and imagine how they would feel about it.

Tone and Figurative Language

How Words Affect Tone
Tone refers to the writer's attitude toward the subject matter. For example, the tone conveys how the writer feels about the topic he or she is writing about. A lot of nonfiction writing has a neutral tone, which is an important tone for the writer to take. A neutral tone demonstrates that the writer is presenting a topic impartially and letting the information speak for itself.

On the other hand, nonfiction writing can be just as effective and appropriate if the tone isn't neutral. For instance, consider this example:

> Seat belts save more lives than any other automobile safety feature. Many studies show that airbags save lives as well; however, not all cars have airbags. For instance, some older cars don't. Furthermore, air bags aren't entirely reliable. For example, studies show that in 15% of accidents, airbags don't deploy as designed; but, on the other hand, seat belt malfunctions are extremely rare. The number of highway fatalities has plummeted since laws requiring seat belt usage were enacted.

In this passage, the writer mostly chooses to retain a neutral tone when presenting information. If the writer would instead include their own personal experience of losing a friend or family member in a car accident, the tone would change dramatically. The tone would no longer be neutral and would show that the writer has a personal stake in the content, allowing them to interpret the information in a different way. When analyzing tone, consider what the writer is trying to achieve in the text and how they *create* the tone using style.

An author's choice of words—also referred to as **diction**—helps to convey his or her meaning in a particular way. Through diction, an author can convey a particular tone—e.g., a humorous tone, a serious tone—in order to support the thesis in a meaningful way to the reader.

Connotation and Denotation
Connotation is when an author chooses words or phrases that invoke ideas or feelings other than their literal meaning. An example of the use of connotation is the word *cheap*, which suggests something is poor in value or negatively describes a person as reluctant to spend money. When something or someone is described this way, the reader is more inclined to have a particular image or feeling about it or him/her. Thus, connotation can be a very effective language tool in creating emotion and swaying opinion. However, connotations are sometimes hard to pin down because varying emotions can be associated with a word. Generally, though, connotative meanings tend to be fairly consistent within a specific cultural group.

Denotation refers to words or phrases that mean exactly what they say. It is helpful when a writer wants to present hard facts or vocabulary terms with which readers may be unfamiliar. Some examples of denotation are the words *inexpensive* and *frugal*. *Inexpensive* refers to the cost of something, not its value, and *frugal* indicates that a person is conscientiously watching his or her spending. These terms do not elicit the same emotions that *cheap* does.

Authors sometimes choose to use both, but what they choose and when they use it is what critical readers need to differentiate. One method isn't inherently better than the other; however, one may create a better effect, depending upon an author's intent. If, for example, an author's purpose is to inform, to instruct, and to familiarize readers with a difficult subject, his or her use of connotation may be helpful. However, it may also undermine credibility and confuse readers. An author who wants to create a credible, scholarly effect in his or her text would most likely use denotation, which emphasizes literal, factual meaning and examples.

How Figurative Language Affects the Meaning of Words
It's important to be able to recognize and interpret **figurative,** or non-literal, language. Literal statements rely directly on the denotations of words and express exactly what's happening in reality. Figurative language uses non-literal expressions to present information in a creative way. Consider the following sentences:

   a. His pillow was very soft and he fell asleep quickly.

   b. His pillow was a fluffy cloud and he floated away on it to the dream world.

Sentence *A* is literal, employing only the real meanings of each word. Sentence *B* is figurative. It employs a metaphor by stating that his pillow was a cloud. Of course, he isn't actually sleeping on a cloud, but the reader can draw on images of clouds as light, soft, fluffy, and relaxing to get a sense of how the character felt as he fell asleep. Also, in sentence *B*, the pillow becomes a vehicle that transports him to a magical dream world. The character isn't literally floating through the air—he's simply falling asleep! But by utilizing figurative language, the author creates a scene of peace, comfort, and relaxation that conveys stronger emotions and more creative imagery than the purely literal sentence. While there are countless types of figurative language, there are a few common ones that any reader should recognize.

Simile and **metaphor** are comparisons between two things, but their formats differ slightly. A simile says that two things are *similar* and makes a comparison using "like" or "as"—*A is like B*, or *A is as [some characteristic] as B*—whereas a metaphor states that two things are exactly the same—*A is B*. In both cases, simile and metaphor invite the reader to think more deeply about the characteristics of the two subjects and consider where they overlap. An example of metaphor can be found in the above sentence about the sleeper ("His pillow was a fluffy cloud"). For an example of simile, look at the first line of Robert Burns' famous poem:

> My love is like a red, red rose

This is comparison using "like," and the two things being compared are love and a rose. Some characteristics of a rose are that it's fragrant, beautiful, blossoming, colorful, vibrant—by comparing his love to a rose, Burns asks the reader to apply these qualities to his love. In this way, he implies that his love is also fresh, blossoming, and brilliant.

Similes can also compare things that appear dissimilar. Here's a song lyric from Florence and the Machine:

> Happiness hit her like a bullet in the back

"Happiness" has a very positive connotation, but getting "a bullet in the back" seems violent and aggressive, not at all related to happiness. By using an unexpected comparison, the writer forces readers to think more deeply about the comparison and ask themselves how could getting shot be similar to feeling happy. "A bullet in the back" is something that she doesn't see coming; it's sudden and forceful; and presumably, it has a strong impact on her life. So, in this way, the author seems to be saying that unexpected happiness made a sudden and powerful change in her life.

Another common form of figurative language is **personification,** when a non-human object is given human characteristics. William Blake uses personification here:

> . . . the stars threw down their spears,

> And watered heaven with their tears

He imagines the stars as combatants in a heavenly battle, giving them both action (throwing down their spears) and emotion (the sadness and disappointment of their tears). Personification helps to add emotion or develop relationships between characters and non-human objects. In fact, most people use personification in their everyday lives:

> My alarm clock betrayed me! It didn't go off this morning!

> The last piece of chocolate cake was staring at me from the refrigerator.

Next is **hyperbole,** a type of figurative language that uses extreme exaggeration. Sentences like, "I love you to the moon and back," or "I will love you for a million years," are examples of hyperbole. They aren't literally true—unfortunately, people cannot jump to outer space or live for a million years—but they're creative expressions that communicate the depth of feeling of the author.

Another way that writers add deeper meaning to their work is through **allusions.** An allusion is a reference to something from history, literature, or another cultural source. When the text is from a different culture or a time period, readers may not be familiar with every allusion. However, allusions tend to be well-known because the author wants the reader to make a connection between what's happening in the text and what's being referenced.

> I can't believe my best friend told our professor that I was skipping class to finish my final project! What a Judas!

This sentence contains a Biblical allusion to Judas, a friend and follower of Jesus who betrayed Jesus to the Romans. In this case, the allusion to Judas is used to give a deeper impression of betrayal and disloyalty from a trusted friend. Commonly used allusions in Western texts may come from the Bible, Greek or Roman mythology, or well-known literature such as Shakespeare. By familiarizing themselves with these touchstones of history and culture, readers can be more prepared to recognize allusions.

How Figurative Language Influences the Author's Purpose

A **rhetorical strategy**—also referred to as a **rhetorical mode**—is the structural way an author chooses to present his/her argument. Though the terms noted below are similar to the organizational structures noted earlier, these strategies do not imply that the entire text follows the approach. For example, a cause and effect organizational structure is solely that, nothing more. A persuasive text may use cause and effect as a strategy to convey a singular point. Thus, an argument may include several of the strategies as the author strives to convince his or her audience to take action or accept a different point of view. It's important that readers are able to identify an author's thesis and position on the topic in order to be able to identify the careful construction through which the author speaks to the reader.

The following are some of the more common rhetorical strategies:

- **Cause and effect**—establishing a logical correlation or causation between two ideas

- **Classification/division**—the grouping of similar items together or division of something into parts

- **Comparison/contrast**—the distinguishing of similarities/differences to expand on an idea

- **Definition**—used to clarify abstract ideas, unfamiliar concepts, or to distinguish one idea from another

- **Description**—use of vivid imagery, active verbs, and clear adjectives to explain ideas

- **Exemplification**—the use of examples to explain an idea

- **Narration**—anecdotes or personal experience to present or expand on a concept

- **Problem/Solution**—presentation of a problem or problems, followed by proposed solution(s)

How Rhetorical Language Conveys Meaning, Emotion, or Persuades Readers

A **rhetorical device** is the phrasing and presentation of an idea that reinforces and emphasizes a point in an argument. A rhetorical device is often quite memorable. One of the more famous uses of a rhetorical device is in John F. Kennedy's 1961 inaugural address: "Ask not what your country can do for you, ask what you can do for your country." The contrast of ideas presented in the phrasing is an example of the rhetorical device of antimetabole. Some other common examples are provided in the following chart, but test takers should be aware that this is not a complete list.

Observe this chart:

Device	Definition	Example
Allusion	A reference to a famous person, event, or significant literary text as a form of significant comparison	"We are apt to shut our eyes against a painful truth, and listen to the song of that siren till she transforms us into beasts." Patrick Henry
Anaphora	The repetition of the same words at the beginning of successive words, phrases, or clauses, designed to emphasize an idea	"We shall not flag or fail. We shall go on to the end. We shall fight in France, we shall fight on the seas and oceans, we shall fight with growing confidence ... we shall fight in the fields and in the streets, we shall fight in the hills. We shall never surrender." Winston Churchill
Understatement	A statement meant to portray a situation as less important than it actually is to create an ironic effect	"The war in the Pacific has not necessarily developed in Japan's favor." Emperor Hirohito, surrendering Japan in World War II
Parallelism	A syntactical similarity in a structure or series of structures used for impact of an idea, making it memorable	"A penny saved is a penny earned." Ben Franklin
Rhetorical question	A question posed that is not answered by the writer though there is a desired response, most often designed to emphasize a point	"Can anyone look at our reduced standing in the world today and say, 'Let's have four more years of this?'" Ronald Reagan

Organizing Ideas

How a Section Fits into a Passage and Helps Develop the Ideas
Being able to determine what is most important while reading is critical to synthesis. It is the difference between being able to tell what is necessary to full comprehension and that which is interesting but not necessary.

When determining the importance of an author's ideas, consider the following:

- Ask how critical an author's particular idea, assertion, or concept is to the overall message.

- Ask "is this an interesting fact or is this information essential to understanding the author's main idea?"

- Make a simple chart. On one side, list all of the important, essential points an author makes and on the other, list all of the interesting yet non-critical ideas.

- Highlight, circle, or underline any dates or data in non-fiction passages. Pay attention to headings, captions, and any graphs or diagrams.

- When reading a fictional passage, delineate important information such as theme, character, setting, conflict (what the problem is), and resolution (how the problem is fixed). Most often, these are the most important aspects contained in fictional text.

- If a non-fiction passage is instructional in nature, take physical note of any steps in the order of their importance as presented by the author. Look for words such as *first*, *next*, *then*, and *last*.

Determining the importance of an author's ideas is critical to synthesis in that it requires the test taker to parse out any unnecessary information and demonstrate they have the ability to make sound determination on what is important to the author, and what is merely a supporting or less critical detail.

<u>Analyzing How a Text is Organized</u>
Depending on what the author is attempting to accomplish, certain formats or text structures work better than others. For example, a sequence structure might work for narration but not when identifying similarities and differences between dissimilar concepts. Similarly, a comparison-contrast structure is not useful for narration. It's the author's job to put the right information in the correct format.

Readers should be familiar with the five main literary structures:

Sequence Structure
Sequence structure (sometimes referred to as the order structure) is when the order of events proceeds in a predictable order. In many cases, this means the text goes through the plot elements: exposition, rising action, climax, falling action, and resolution. Readers are introduced to characters, setting, and conflict in the **exposition**. In the **rising action**, there's an increase in tension and suspense. The **climax** is the height of tension and the point of no return. **Tension** decreases during the falling action. In the **resolution**, any conflicts presented in the exposition are resolved, and the story concludes. An informative text that is structured sequentially will often go in order from one step to the next.

Problem-Solution
In the **problem-solution structure**, authors identify a potential problem and suggest a solution. This form of writing is usually divided into two paragraphs and can be found in informational texts. For example, cell phone, cable, and satellite providers use this structure in manuals to help customers troubleshoot or identify problems with services or products.

Comparison-Contrast
When authors want to discuss similarities and differences between separate concepts, they arrange thoughts in a **comparison-contrast paragraph structure**. **Venn diagrams** are an effective graphic organizer for comparison-contrast structures because they feature two overlapping circles that can be used to organize similarities and differences. A comparison-contrast essay organizes one paragraph based on similarities and another based on differences. A comparison-contrast essay can also be arranged with the similarities and differences of individual traits addressed within individual paragraphs. Words such as *however*, *but*, and *nevertheless* help signal a contrast in ideas.

Descriptive

Descriptive writing is designed to appeal to your senses. Much like an artist who constructs a painting, good descriptive writing builds an image in the reader's mind by appealing to the five senses: *sight, hearing, taste, touch,* and *smell.* However, overly descriptive writing can become tedious; likewise, sparse descriptions can make settings and characters seem flat. Good authors strike a balance by applying descriptions only to facts that are integral to the passage.

Cause and Effect

Passages that use the **cause and effect structure** are simply asking *why* by demonstrating some type of connection between ideas. Words such as *if, since, because, then,* or *consequently* indicate a relationship. By switching the order of a complex sentence, the writer can rearrange the emphasis on different clauses. Saying *If Sheryl is late, we'll miss the dance* is different from saying *We'll miss the dance if Sheryl is late.* One emphasizes Sheryl's tardiness while the other emphasizes missing the dance. Paragraphs can also be arranged in a cause and effect format. Since the format—before and after—is sequential, it is useful when authors wish to discuss the impact of choices. Researchers often apply this paragraph structure to the scientific method.

Understanding the Meaning and Purpose of Transition Words

The writer should act as a guide, showing the reader how all the sentences fit together. Consider this example:

> Seat belts save more lives than any other automobile safety feature. Many studies show that airbags save lives as well. Not all cars have airbags. Many older cars don't. Air bags aren't entirely reliable. Studies show that in 15% of accidents, airbags don't deploy as designed. Seat belt malfunctions are extremely rare.

There's nothing wrong with any of these sentences individually, but together they're disjointed and difficult to follow. The best way for the writer to communicate information is through the use of transition words. Here are examples of transition words and phrases that tie sentences together, enabling a more natural flow:

- To show causality: *as a result, therefore,* and *consequently*
- To compare and contrast: *however, but,* and *on the other hand*
- To introduce examples: *for instance, namely,* and *including*
- To show order of importance: *foremost, primarily, secondly,* and *lastly*

Note: This is not a complete list of transitions. There are many more that can be used; however, most fit into these or similar categories. The point is that the words should clearly show the relationship between sentences, supporting information, and the main idea.

Here is an update to the previous example using transition words. These changes make it easier to read and bring clarity to the writer's points:

> Seat belts save more lives than any other automobile safety feature. Many studies show that airbags save lives as well; however, not all cars have airbags. For instance, some older cars don't. Furthermore, air bags aren't entirely reliable. For example, studies show that in 15% of accidents, airbags don't deploy as designed; but, on the other hand, seat belt malfunctions are extremely rare.

Also, be prepared to analyze whether the writer is using the best transition word or phrase for the situation. Take this sentence for example: "As a result, seat belt malfunctions are extremely rare." This sentence doesn't make sense in the context above because the writer is trying to show the contrast between seat belts and airbags, not the causality.

How the Passage Organization Supports the Author's Ideas

Even if the writer includes plenty of information to support their point, the writing is only coherent when the information is in a logical order. **Logical sequencing** is really just common sense, but it's an important writing technique. First, the writer should introduce the main idea, whether for a paragraph, a section, or the entire piece. Then they should present evidence to support the main idea by using transitional language. This shows the reader how the information relates to the main idea and the sentences around it. The writer should then take time to interpret the information, making sure necessary connections are obvious to the reader. Finally, the writer can summarize the information in a closing section.

Note: Though most writing follows this pattern, it isn't a set rule. Sometimes writers change the order for effect. For example, the writer can begin with a surprising piece of supporting information to grab the reader's attention, and then transition to the main idea. Thus, if a passage doesn't follow the logical order, don't immediately assume it's wrong. However, most writing usually settles into a logical sequence after a nontraditional beginning.

Introductions and Conclusions

Examining the writer's strategies for introductions and conclusions puts the reader in the right mindset to interpret the rest of the text. Look for methods the writer might use for **introductions** such as:

- Stating the main point immediately, followed by outlining how the rest of the piece supports this claim.

- Establishing important, smaller pieces of the main idea first, and then grouping these points into a case for the main idea.

- Opening with a quotation, anecdote, question, seeming paradox, or other piece of interesting information, and then using it to lead to the main point.

- Whatever method the writer chooses, the introduction should make their intention clear, establish their voice as a credible one, and encourage a person to continue reading.

Conclusions tend to follow a similar pattern. In them, the writer restates their main idea a final time, often after summarizing the smaller pieces of that idea. If the introduction uses a quote or anecdote to grab the reader's attention, the conclusion often makes reference to it again. Whatever way the writer chooses to arrange the conclusion, the final restatement of the main idea should be clear and simple for the reader to interpret. Finally, conclusions shouldn't introduce any new information.

Comparing Different Ways of Presenting Ideas

Evaluating Two Different Texts

Every passage has its own unique scope, purpose, and emphasis, or what it covers, why it is written, and what its specific focus is centered upon. Additionally, each passage is written with a particular audience in mind, and each passage affects its audience differently. The scope, purpose, and emphasis of each passage can be found by comparing the parts of the piece with the whole framework of the piece. Word choices, grammatical choices, and syntactical choices can help the reader figure out the scope, purpose, and emphasis. These choices are embedded in the words and sentences of the passage (the parts). They help show the intentions and goals of the author (the "whole"). For example, if an author uses strong language like *enrage*, *ignite*, *infuriate*, and *antagonize*, then they may be cueing the reader in to their own rage, or they may be trying to incite anger in others. Likewise, if an author continually uses short, simple sentences, he or she might be trying to incite excitement or nervousness. These different choices and styles affect the overall message, or purpose. Sometimes the subject matter or audience is discussed explicitly, but often, test takers have to break a passage down, also known as decoding the passage. In this way, test takers can find the passage's target audience and intentions. Meanwhile, the impact of the article can be personal or historical, depending upon the passage—it can either speak to the test taker personally or capture a historical era.

When two passages are analyzed in juxtaposition—or side-by-side—it can help the audience have a clearer picture of the scope, purpose, emphasis, audience, and impact. Evaluating and comparing passages side-by-side helps shed light on similarities and differences that are helpful for test takers. The key is to figure out both the parts and the "wholes" of each passage. Compare the word choices, grammatical choices, and syntactical choices of each passage, and then compare the big picture of each passage. As a result, test takers will have a stronger basis for understanding the intricate details and broader frameworks of all passages they encounter.

Evaluating Two Different Passages

Every passage offered has its own view, tone, style, organization, purpose, or impact. It is extremely important to compare the parts to the "wholes" of each passage. Additionally, these parts and "wholes" are better understood through **intertextual analysis** (for example, comparing the texts as if they were side by side). The viewpoint of the text can be found through a close analysis of the author's biases, or personal opinions or perceptions. All biases are embedded in the word choices, grammatical choices, and syntactical choices of each passage. For example, if an author continually uses negative words like *dislike*, *hate*, *despise*, *detrimental*, or *loathe*, they are trying to illustrate their own hatred of something or convey a character's hatred of something. These negative terms inevitably affect the view and tone of a passage. Comparing terminologies and biases can help a test taker better understand the similarities and differences of two or more passages. Similarly, the purposes of each can be better highlighted with a closer examination of word choices, grammatical choices, and syntactical choices.

Organization, on the other hand, is more easily understood by studying the passage on its own. Organizational differences on the page are likely to jump out at the test taker. A poetry passage, for instance, is traditionally organized differently than a prose passage. Test takers can see the differences in structures: one uses paragraphs, while the other uses stanzas. If organizational differences cannot be deduced through visual analysis, test takers should try to take a closer look at the sequence of events or the content of each paragraph. Organization, nevertheless, is not something that is separate from view, tone, purpose, style, and impact. It can skew or connect a viewpoint, shift or solidify tone, reinforce or undermine purpose, express or conceal a particular style, or establish or disestablish the impact of passage. Organization is the backbone of every form of written expression—it unifies all the parts and sets the parameters for the wholes. Thus, organization should be analyzed strategically when comparing passages.

Critical Thinking

The Relationship Between Evidence and Main Ideas and Details

Summarizing Information from a Passage

Summarizing is an effective way to draw a conclusion from a passage. A summary is a shortened version of the original text, written by the reader in his/her own words. Focusing on the main points of the original text and including only the relevant details can help readers reach a conclusion. It's important to retain the original meaning of the passage.

Like summarizing, **paraphrasing** can also help a reader fully understand different parts of a text. Paraphrasing calls for the reader to take a small part of the passage and list or describe its main points. Paraphrasing is more than rewording the original passage, though. It should be written in the reader's own words, while still retaining the meaning of the original source. This will indicate an understanding of the original source, yet still help the reader expand on his/her interpretation.

Readers should pay attention to the **sequence**, or the order in which details are laid out in the text, as this can be important to understanding its meaning as a whole. Writers will often use transitional words to help the reader understand the order of events and to stay on track. Words like *next, then, after*, and *finally* show that the order of events is important to the author. In some cases, the author omits these transitional words, and the sequence is implied. Authors may even purposely present the information out of order to make an impact or have an effect on the reader. An example might be when a narrative writer uses **flashback** to reveal information.

Relationship Between the Main Idea and Details of a Passage

In order to understand any text, readers first must determine the **topic**, or what the text is about. In non-fiction writing, the topic can generally be expressed in a few words. For example, a passage might be about college education, moving to a new neighborhood, or dog breeds. Slightly more specific information is found in the **main idea**, or what the writer wants readers to know about the topic. An article might be about the history of popular dog breeds; another article might tell how certain dog breeds are unfairly stereotyped. In both cases, the topic is the same—dog breeds—but the main ideas are quite different. Each writer has a distinct purpose for writing and a different set of details for what they want us to know about dog breeds. When a writer expresses their main idea in one sentence, this is known as a **thesis statement**. If a writer uses a thesis statement, it can generally be found at the beginning of the passage. Finally, the most specific information in a text is in the **supporting details**. An article about dog breed stereotyping might discuss a case study of pit bulls and provide statistics about how many dog attacks are caused by pit bulls versus other breeds.

Main Idea of a Passage

Topics and main ideas are critical parts of writing. The **topic** is the subject matter of the piece. An example of a topic would be *the use of cell phones in a classroom*.

The **main idea** is what the writer wants to say about that topic. A writer may make the point that the use of cell phones in a classroom is a serious problem that must be addressed in order for students to learn better. Therefore, the topic is cell phone usage in a classroom, and the main idea is that it's *a serious problem needing to be addressed*. The topic can be expressed in a word or two, but the main idea should be a complete thought.

An author will likely identify the topic immediately within the title or the first sentence of the passage. The main idea is usually presented in the introduction. In a single passage, the main idea may be identified in the first or last sentence, but it will most likely be directly stated and easily recognized by the reader. Because it is not always stated immediately in a passage, it's important that readers carefully read the entire passage to identify the main idea.

The main idea should not be confused with the thesis statement. A **thesis statement** is a clear statement of the writer's specific stance and can often be found in the introduction of a nonfiction piece. The thesis is a specific sentence (or two) that offers the direction and focus of the discussion.

In order to illustrate the main idea, a writer will use **supporting details**, which provide evidence or examples to help make a point. Supporting details are typically found in nonfiction pieces that seek to inform or persuade the reader.

Determining Which Details Support a Main Idea
An important skill is the ability to determine which details in a passage support the main idea. In the example of cell phone usage in the classroom, where the author's main idea is to show the seriousness of this problem and the need to "unplug", supporting details would be critical for effectively making that point. Supporting details used here might include statistics on a decline in student focus and studies showing the impact of digital technology usage on students' attention spans. The author could also include testimonies from teachers surveyed on the topic.

It's important that readers evaluate the author's supporting details to be sure that they are credible, provide evidence of the author's point, and directly support the main idea. Although shocking statistics grab readers' attention, their use may provide ineffective information in the piece. Details like this are crucial to understanding the passage and evaluating how well the author presents his or her argument and evidence.

Though there are several types of conflicts and several potential themes within them, the following are the most common:

- Individual against the self—relevant to themes of self-awareness, internal struggles, pride, coming of age, facing reality, fate, free will, vanity, loss of innocence, loneliness, isolation, fulfillment, failure, and disillusionment

- Individual against nature— relevant to themes of knowledge vs. ignorance, nature as beauty, quest for discovery, self-preservation, chaos and order, circle of life, death, and destruction of beauty

- Individual against society— relevant to themes of power, beauty, good, evil, war, class struggle, totalitarianism, role of men/women, wealth, corruption, change vs. tradition, capitalism, destruction, heroism, injustice, and racism

- Individual against another individual— relevant to themes of hope, loss of love or hope, sacrifice, power, revenge, betrayal, and honor

For example, in Hawthorne's *The Scarlet Letter*, one possible narrative conflict could be the individual against the self, with a relevant theme of internal struggles. This theme is alluded to through characterization—Dimmesdale's moral struggle with his love for Hester and Hester's internal struggles with the truth and her daughter, Pearl. It's also alluded to through plot—Dimmesdale's suicide and Hester helping the very townspeople who initially condemned her.

Sometimes, a text can convey a **message** or **universal lesson**—a truth or insight that the reader infers from the text, based on analysis of the literary and/or poetic elements. This message is often presented as a statement. For example, a potential message in Shakespeare's *Hamlet* could be "Revenge is what ultimately drives the human soul." This message can be immediately determined through plot and characterization in numerous ways, but it can also be determined through the setting of Norway, which is bordering on war.

How Authors Develop Theme
Authors employ a variety of techniques to present a theme. They may compare or contrast characters, events, places, ideas, or historical or invented settings to speak thematically. They may use analogies, metaphors, similes, allusions, or other literary devices to convey the theme. An author's use of diction, syntax, and tone can also help convey the theme. Authors will often develop themes through the development of characters, use of the setting, repetition of ideas, use of symbols, and through contrasting value systems. Authors of both fiction and nonfiction genres will use a variety of these techniques to develop one or more themes.

Regardless of the literary genre, there are commonalities in how authors, playwrights, and poets develop themes or central ideas.

Authors often do research, the results of which contributes to theme. In prose fiction and drama, this research may include real historical information about the setting the author has chosen or include elements that make fictional characters, settings, and plots seem realistic to the reader. In nonfiction, research is critical since the information contained within this literature must be accurate and, moreover, accurately represented.

In fiction, authors present a narrative conflict that will contribute to the overall theme. In fiction, this conflict may involve the storyline itself and some trouble within characters that needs resolution. In nonfiction, this conflict may be an explanation or commentary on factual people and events.

Authors will sometimes use character motivation to convey theme, such as in the example from *Hamlet* regarding revenge. In fiction, the characters an author creates will think, speak, and act in ways that effectively convey the theme to readers. In nonfiction, the characters are factual, as in a biography, but authors pay particular attention to presenting those motivations to make them clear to readers.

Authors also use literary devices as a means of conveying theme. For example, the use of moon symbolism in Shelley's *Frankenstein* is significant, as its phases can be compared to the phases that the Creature undergoes as he struggles with his identity.

The selected point of view can also contribute to a work's theme. The use of first-person point of view in a fiction or non-fiction work engages the reader's response differently than third person point of view. The central idea or theme from a first-person narrative may differ from a third-person limited text.

In literary nonfiction, authors usually identify the purpose of their writing, which differs from fiction, where the general purpose is to entertain. The purpose of nonfiction is usually to inform, persuade, or entertain the audience. The stated purpose of a non-fiction text will drive how the central message or theme, if applicable, is presented.

Authors identify an audience for their writing, which is critical in shaping the theme of the work. For example, the audience for J.K. Rowling's *Harry Potter* series would be different than the audience for a biography of George Washington. The audience an author chooses to address is closely tied to the purpose of the work. The choice of an audience also drives the choice of language and level of diction an author uses. Ultimately, the intended audience determines the level to which that subject matter is presented and the complexity of the theme.

Drawing Conclusions, Making Inferences, and Evaluating Evidence

Making Generalizations Based on Evidence

One way to make generalizations is to look for main topics. When doing so, pay particular attention to any titles, headlines, or opening statements made by the author. Topic sentences or repetitive ideas can be clues in gleaning inferred ideas. For example, if a passage contains the phrase *DNA testing, while some consider it infallible, is an inherently flawed technique,* the test taker can infer the rest of the passage will contain information that points to DNA testing's infallibility.

The test taker may be asked to make a generalization based on prior knowledge but may also be asked to make predictions based on new ideas. For example, the test taker may have no prior knowledge of DNA other than its genetic property to replicate. However, if the reader is given passages on the flaws of DNA testing with enough factual evidence, the test taker may arrive at the inferred conclusion or generalization that the author does not support the infallibility of DNA testing in all identification cases.

When making generalizations, it is important to remember that the critical thinking process involved must be fluid and open to change. While a reader may infer an idea from a main topic, general statement, or other clues, they must be open to receiving new information within a particular passage. New ideas presented by an author may require the test taker to alter a generalization. Similarly, when asked questions that require making an inference, it's important to read the entire test passage and all of the answer options. Often, a test taker will need to refine a generalization based on new ideas that may be presented within the text itself.

Using Main Ideas to Draw Conclusions

Determining conclusions requires being an active reader, as a reader must make a prediction and analyze facts to identify a conclusion. There are a few ways to determine a logical conclusion, but careful reading is the most important. It's helpful to read a passage a few times, noting details that seem important to the text. A reader should also identify key words in a passage to determine the logical conclusion or determination that flows from the information presented.

Textual evidence within the details helps readers draw a conclusion about a passage. **Textual evidence** refers to information—facts and examples that support the main point. Textual evidence will likely come from outside sources and can be in the form of quoted or paraphrased material. In order to draw a conclusion from evidence, it's important to examine the credibility and validity of that evidence as well as how (and if) it relates to the main idea.

If an author presents a differing opinion or a **counterargument** in order to refute it, the reader should consider how and why this information is being presented. It is meant to strengthen the original argument and shouldn't be confused with the author's intended conclusion, but it should also be considered in the reader's final evaluation.

Sometimes, authors explicitly state the conclusion they want readers to understand. Alternatively, a conclusion may not be directly stated. In that case, readers must rely on the implications to form a logical conclusion:

> On the way to the bus stop, Michael realized his homework wasn't in his backpack. He ran back to the house to get it and made it back to the bus just in time.

In this example, though it's never explicitly stated, it can be inferred that Michael is a student on his way to school in the morning. When forming a conclusion from implied information, it's important to read the text carefully to find several pieces of evidence in the text to support the conclusion.

Describing the Steps of an Argument

Strong arguments tend to follow a fairly defined format. In the introduction, background information regarding the problem is shared, the implications of the issue, and the author's thesis or claims. Supporting evidence is then presented in the body paragraphs, along with the counterargument, which then gets refuted with specific evidence. Lastly, in the conclusion, the author summarizes the points and claims again.

Evidence Used to Support a Claim or Conclusion

Premises are the why, and **conclusions** are the what. Stated differently, premises are the evidence or facts supporting why the conclusion is logical and valid. Reading Comprehension questions do not require evaluation of the factual accuracy of the arguments; instead, the questions evaluate the test taker's ability to assess an argument's logical strength. For example, John eats all red food. Apples are red. Therefore, John eats apples. This argument is logically sound, despite having no factual basis in reality. Below is an example of a practice argument.

> Julie is an American track athlete. She's the star of the number one collegiate team in the country. Her times are consistently at the top of national rankings. Julie is extremely likely to represent the United States at the upcoming Olympics.

In this example, the conclusion, or the *what*, is that she will likely be on the American Olympic team. The author supports this conclusion with two premises. First, Julie is the star of an elite track team. Second, she runs some of the best times of the country. This is the *why* behind the conclusion. The following builds off this basic argument:

> Julie is an American track athlete. She's the star of the number one collegiate team in the country. Her times are consistently at the top of national rankings. Julie is extremely likely to represent the United States at the upcoming Olympics. Julie will continue to develop after the Olympic trials. She will be a frontrunner for the gold. Julie is likely to become a world-famous track star.

These additions to the argument make the conclusion different. Now, the conclusion is that Julie is likely to become a world-famous track star. The previous conclusion, Julie will likely be on the Olympic team, functions as a **sub-conclusion** in this argument. Like conclusions, premises must adequately support sub-conclusions. However, sub-conclusions function like premises, since sub-conclusions also support the overall conclusion.

Determining Whether Evidence is Relevant and Sufficient

A **hasty generalization** involves an argument relying on insufficient statistical data or inaccurately generalizing. One common generalization occurs when a group of individuals under observation have some quality or attribute that is asserted to be universal or true for a much larger number of people than actually documented. Here's an example of a hasty generalization:

> A man smokes a lot of cigarettes, but so did his grandfather. The grandfather smoked nearly two packs per day since his World War II service until he died at ninety years of age. Continuing to smoke cigarettes will clearly not impact the grandson's long-term health.

This argument is a hasty generalization because it assumes that one person's addiction and lack of consequences will naturally be reflected in a different individual. There is no reasonable justification for such extrapolation. It is common knowledge that any smoking is detrimental to everyone's health. The fact that the man's grandfather smoked two packs per day and lived a long life has no logical connection with the grandson engaging in similar behavior. The hasty generalization doesn't take into account other reasons behind the grandfather's longevity. Nor does the author offer evidence that might support the idea that the man would share a similar lifetime if he smokes. It might be different if the author stated that the man's family shares some genetic trait rendering them immune to the effects of tar and chemicals on the lungs. If this were in the argument, we would assume it as truth, like everything else in the Reading Through Language Arts section, and find the generalization to be valid rather than hasty. Of course, this is not the case in our example.

Determining Whether a Statement Is or Is Not Supported

The basic tenant of reading comprehension is the ability to read and understand text. One way to understand text is to look for information that supports the author's main idea, topic, or position statement. This information may be factual or it may be based on the author's opinion. This section will focus on the test taker's ability to identify factual information, as opposed to opinionated bias. The test will ask test takers to read passages containing factual information, and then logically relate those passages by drawing conclusions based on evidence.

In order to identify factual information within one or more text passages, begin by looking for statements of fact. Factual statements can be either true or false. Identifying factual statements as opposed to opinion statements is important in demonstrating full command of evidence in reading. For example, the statement *The temperature outside was unbearably hot* may seem like a fact; however, it's not. While anyone can point to a temperature gauge as factual evidence, the statement itself reflects only an opinion. Some people may find the temperature unbearably hot. Others may find it comfortably warm. Thus, the sentence, *The temperature outside was unbearably hot,* reflects the opinion of the author who found it unbearable. If the text passage followed up the sentence with atmospheric conditions indicating heat indices above 140 degrees Fahrenheit, then the reader knows there is factual information that supports the author's assertion of *unbearably hot*.

In looking for information that can be proven or disproven, it's helpful to scan for dates, numbers, timelines, equations, statistics, and other similar data within any given text passage. These types of indicators will point to proven particulars. For example, the statement, *The temperature outside was unbearably hot on that summer day, July 10, 1913,* most likely indicates factual information, even if the reader is unaware that this is the hottest day on record in the United States. Be careful when reading biased words from an author. Biased words indicate opinion, as opposed to fact.

See the list of biased words below and keep in mind that it's not an inclusive list:

- Good/bad
- Great/greatest
- Better/best/worst
- Amazing
- Terrible/bad/awful
- Beautiful/handsome/ugly
- More/most
- Exciting/dull/boring
- Favorite
- Very
- Probably/should/seem/possibly

Remember, most of what is written is actually opinion or carefully worded information that seems like fact when it isn't. To say, *duplicating DNA results is not cost-effective* sounds like it could be a scientific fact, but it isn't. Factual information can be verified through independent sources.

The simplest type of test question may provide a text passage, then ask the test taker to distinguish the correct factual supporting statement that best answers the corresponding question on the test. However, be aware that most questions may ask the test taker to read more than one text passage and identify which answer best supports an author's topic. While the ability to identify factual information is critical, these types of questions require the test taker to identify chunks of details, and then relate them to one another.

Assessing Whether an Argument is Valid

Although different from conditions and If/Then Statements, **reasonableness** is another important foundational concept. Evaluating an argument for reasonableness and validity entails evaluating the evidence presented by the author to justify their conclusions. Everything contained in the argument should be considered, but remember to ignore outside biases, judgments, and knowledge. For the purposes of this test, the test taker is a one-person jury at a criminal trial using a standard of reasonableness under the circumstances presented by the argument.

These arguments are encountered on a daily basis through social media, entertainment, and cable news. An example is:

> Although many believe it to be a natural occurrence, some believe that the red tide that occurs in Florida each year may actually be a result of human sewage and agricultural runoff. However, it is arguable that both natural and human factors contribute to this annual phenomenon. On one hand, the red tide has been occurring every year since the time of explorers like Cabeza de Vaca in the 1500's. On the other hand, the red tide seems to be getting worse each year, and scientists from the Florida Fish & Wildlife Conservation say the bacteria found inside the tide feed off of nutrients found in fertilizer runoff.

The author's conclusion is that both natural phenomena and human activity contribute to the red tide that happens annually in Florida. The author backs this information up by historical data to prove the natural occurrence of the red tide, and then again with scientific data to back up the human contribution to the red tide. Both of these statements are examples of the premises in the argument.

Evaluating the strength of the logical connection between the premises and conclusion is how reasonableness is determined. Another example is:

> The local railroad is a disaster. Tickets are exorbitantly priced, bathrooms leak, and the floor is sticky.

The author is clearly unhappy with the railroad service. They cite three examples of why they believe the railroad to be a disaster. An argument more familiar to everyday life is:

> Alexandra said the movie she just saw was amazing. We should go see it tonight.

Although not immediately apparent, this is an argument. The author is making the argument that they should go see the movie. This conclusion is based on the premise that Alexandra said the movie was amazing. There's an inferred note that Alexandra is knowledgeable on the subject, and she's credible enough to prompt her friends to go see the movie. This seems like a reasonable argument. A less reasonable argument is:

> Alexandra is a film student, and she's written the perfect romantic comedy script. We should put our life savings toward its production as an investment in our future.

The author's conclusion is that they should invest their life savings into the production of a movie, and it is justified by referencing Alexandra's credibility and current work. However, the premises are entirely too weak to support the conclusion. Alexandra is only a film *student*, and the script is seemingly her first work. This is not enough evidence to justify investing one's life savings in the film's success.

Assumptions in an Argument

Think of assumptions as unwritten premises. Although they never explicitly appear in the argument, the author is relying on it to defend the argument, just like a premise. Assumptions are the most important part of an argument that will never appear in an argument.

An argument in the abstract is: The author concludes Z based on W and X premises. But the W and X premises actually depend on the unmentioned assumption of Y. Therefore, what the author is really saying is that, X, W, and Y make Z correct, but Y is assumed.

People assume all of the time. Assumptions and inferences allow the human mind to process the constant flow of information. Many assumptions underlie even the most basic arguments. However, in the world of Legal Reasoning arguments, assumptions must be avoided. An argument must be fully presented to be valid; relying on an assumption is considered weak. The test requires that test takers identify these underlying assumptions. One example is:

> Peyton Manning is the most over-rated quarterback of all time. He lost more big games than anyone else. Plus, he allegedly assaulted his female trainer in college. Peyton clearly shouldn't make the Hall of Fame.

The author certainly relies on a lot of assumptions. A few assumptions are:

- Peyton Manning plays quarterback.

- He is considered to be a great quarterback by at least some people.

- He played in many big games.

- Allegations and past settlements without any admission of guilt from over a decade ago can be relied upon as evidence against Hall of Fame acceptance.

- The Hall of Fame voqters factor in off-the-field incidents, even if true.

- The best players should make the Hall of Fame.

- Losing big games negates, at least in part, the achievement of making it to those big games

- Peyton Manning is retired, and people will vote on whether he makes the Hall of Fame at some point in the future.

The author is relying on all of these assumptions. Some are clearly more important to his argument than others. In fact, disproving a necessary assumption can destroy a premise and possibly an entire conclusion. For example, what if the Hall of Fame did not factor in any of the off-the-field incidents? Then the alleged assault no longer factors into the argument. Even worse, what if making the big games actually was more important than losing those games in the eyes of the Hall of Fame voters? Then the whole conclusion falls apart. The conclusion is no longer justified if that premise is disproven.

Assumption questions test this exact point by asking the test taker to identify which assumption the argument relies upon. If the author is making numerous assumptions, then the most important *one* assumption must be chosen.

If the author truly relies on an assumption, then the argument will completely fall apart if the assumption isn't true. **Negating** a necessary assumption will *always* make the argument fall apart. This is a universal rule of logic and should be the first thing done in testing answer choices.

Here are some ways that underlying assumptions will appear as questions:

- Which of the following is a hidden assumption that the author makes to advance his argument?
- Which assumption, if true, would support the argument's conclusion (make it more logical)?
- The strength of the argument depends on which of the following?
- Upon which of the following assumptions does the author rely?
- Which assumption does the argument presuppose?

An example is:

> Frank Underwood is a terrible president. The man is a typical spend, spend, spend liberal. His employment program would exponentially increase the annual deficit and pile on the national debt. Not to mention, Underwood is also on the verge of starting a war with Russia.

Upon which of the following assumptions does the author's argument most rely?
a. Frank Underwood is a terrible president.
b. The United States cannot afford Frank Underwood's policy plans without spending more than the country raises in revenue.
c. No spend, spend, spend liberal has ever succeeded as president.
d. Starting a war with Russia is beneficial to the United States.

Use the negation rule to find the correct answer in the choices below.

Choice *A* is not an assumption—it is the author's conclusion. This type of restatement will never be the correct answer, but test it anyway. After negating the choice, what remains is: *Frank Underwood is a fantastic president.* Does this make the argument fall apart? No, it just becomes the new conclusion. The argument is certainly worse since it does not seem reasonable for someone to praise a president for being a spend, spend, spend liberal or raising the national debt; however, the argument still makes *logical* sense. Eliminate this choice.

Choice *B* is certainly an assumption. It underlies the premises that the country cannot afford Underwood's economic plans. When reversed to: *The United States can afford Frank Underwood's policy plans without spending more than the country raises in revenue,* this destroys the argument. If the United States can afford his plans, then the annual deficit and national debt won't increase; therefore, Underwood being a terrible president would only be based on the final premise. The argument is much weaker without the two sentences involving the financials. Keep it as a benchmark while working through the remaining choices.

Choice *C* is irrelevant. The author is not necessarily claiming that all loose-pocket liberals make for bad presidents. His argument specifically pertains to Underwood. Negate it— *Some spend, spend, spend liberals have succeeded as president.* This does not destroy the argument. Some other candidate could have succeeded as president. However, the author is pointing out that those policies would be disastrous considering the rising budget and debt. The author is not making an appeal to historical precedent. Although not a terrible choice, it is certainly weaker than Choice *B*. Eliminate this choice.

Choice *D* is definitely not an assumption made by the author. The author is assuming that a war with Russia is disastrous. Negate it anyway—*Starting a war with Russia is not beneficial for the United States.* This does not destroy the argument; it makes it stronger. Eliminate this choice.

<u>Analyzing Two Arguments and Evaluating the Types of Evidence Used to Support Each Claim</u>
Arguments use evidence and reasoning to support a position or prove a point. Claims are typically controversial and may be faced with some degree of contention. Thus, authors support claims with evidence. Two arguments might present different types of evidence that readers will need to evaluate for merit, worthiness, accuracy, relevance, and impact. Evidence can take on many forms such as numbers (statistics, measurements, numerical data, etc.), expert opinions or quotes, testimonies, anecdotal evidence or stories from individuals, and textual evidence, such as that obtained from documents like diaries, newspapers, and laws.

Verbal Questions

Word Knowledge

Select the word that most correctly completes the sentence.

1. When the baseball game was over, the first thing Jackson did was run towards the dugout to grab his water bottle to relieve his arid throat. Arid means:
    a. humid
    b. scorched
    c. parched
    d. dusty

2. Driving across the United States, the two friends became inseparable each time they arrived in a new state. They shared many good memories on that trip they would remember for the rest of their lives. Inseparable means:
    a. closer
    b. distant
    c. suffering
    d. irritable

3. After Kira wrote her first book, she pledged to her fans the sequel would be just as exciting as the first. Pledged to means:
    a. denied
    b. promised
    c. invigorated
    d. germinated

4. When I heard the wolf howl from my tent, my hands started trembling and my heart stopped . . . hopefully I would make it through this night alive! Trembling means:
    a. dancing
    b. glowing
    c. shaking
    d. throbbing

5. Unlike Leo, who always played basketball in the park after school, Gabriel would consistently go to the library and study after school. Consistently means:
    a. infrequently
    b. occasionally
    c. hardly
    d. usually

6. As soon as the shot rang out, the runners dashed toward the finish line. Dashed means:
    a. sprinted
    b. skipped
    c. rejoiced
    d. herded

7. Resolved to get an *A* on her paper, LaShonda began writing it two weeks before it was due. Resolved means:
    a. resumed
    b. content
    c. enthusiastic
    d. determined

8. After Colby's mom picked him up from school, they went to the bank to install a check. Install means:
    a. celebrate
    b. neutralize
    c. eliminate
    d. deposit

9. The sale at the grocery store motivated my dad to buy four avocados instead of two. Motivated means:
    a. intimidated
    b. inspired
    c. dismayed
    d. berated

10. My mom recently started drinking fruit and vegetable smoothies in order to enhance the quality of her health. Enhance means:
    a. increase
    b. decrease
    c. curtail
    d. request

11. In the middle of our vacation, we had a sojourn in a remote cabin in the woods. Believe it or not, we got snowed in and had to stay for two weeks! Sojourn means:
    a. soiree
    b. presentation
    c. layover
    d. cohort

12. Cooking dinner was her favorite activity until she triggered the fire alarm by burning the casserole in the oven. Triggered means:
    a. activated
    b. offended
    c. unplugged
    d. disbanded

13. Much to her consternation, she had to go to the dentist's office to get a tooth pulled, so she did some breathing exercises before she walked in. Consternation means:
    a. refresh
    b. creative
    c. rapture
    d. dread

14. The yellow feathers and purple markings told us that this bird was native to the southeast part of the United States. Native means:
   a. entertaining
   b. indigenous
   c. impudent
   d. monotonous

15. When we caught the eels, their bodies wriggled out of our hands and back into the water. Wriggled means:
   a. exploded
   b. deteriorated
   c. thundered
   d. slithered

16. Even though at the restaurant my mom requested the eggplant with no cheese, she received a huge serving of parmesan on top. Serving means:
   a. portion
   b. directed
   c. mourning
   d. endorsement

Reading Comprehension

Questions 17–22 are based upon the following passage:

My gentleness and good behaviour had gained so far on the emperor and his court, and indeed upon the army and people in general, that I began to conceive hopes of getting my liberty in a short time. I took all possible methods to cultivate this favourable disposition. The natives came, by degrees, to be less apprehensive of any danger from me. I would sometimes lie down, and let five or six of them dance on my hand; and at last the boys and girls would venture to come and play at hide-and-seek in my hair. I had now made a good progress in understanding and speaking the language. The emperor had a mind one day to entertain me with several of the country shows, wherein they exceed all nations I have known, both for dexterity and magnificence. I was diverted with none so much as that of the rope-dancers, performed upon a slender white thread, extended about two feet, and twelve inches from the ground. Upon which I shall desire liberty, with the reader's patience, to enlarge a little.

This diversion is only practised by those persons who are candidates for great employments, and high favour at court. They are trained in this art from their youth, and are not always of noble birth, or liberal education. When a great office is vacant, either by death or disgrace (which often happens,) five or six of those candidates petition the emperor to entertain his majesty and the court with a dance on the rope; and whoever jumps the highest, without falling, succeeds in the office. Very often the chief ministers themselves are commanded to show their skill, and to convince the emperor that they have not lost their faculty. Flimnap, the treasurer, is allowed to cut a caper on the straight rope, at least an inch higher than any other lord in the whole empire. I have seen him do the summerset several times together, upon a trencher fixed on a rope which is no thicker than a common packthread in England. My friend

Reldresal, principal secretary for private affairs, is, in my opinion, if I am not partial, the second after the treasurer; the rest of the great officers are much upon a par.

from Jonathan Swift's *Gulliver's Travels into Several Remote Nations of the World*

17. Which of the following statements best summarize the central purpose of this text?
    a. Gulliver details his fondness for the archaic yet interesting practices of his captors.
    b. Gulliver conjectures about the intentions of the aristocratic sector of society.
    c. Gulliver becomes acquainted with the people and practices of his new surroundings.
    d. Gulliver's differences cause him to become penitent around new acquaintances.

18. What is the word *principal* referring to in the following text?
    My friend Reldresal, principal secretary for private affairs, is, in my opinion, if I am not partial, the second after the treasurer; the rest of the great officers are much upon a par.

    a. Primary or chief
    b. An acolyte
    c. An individual who provides nurturing
    d. One in a subordinate position

19. What can the reader infer from this passage?
    I would sometimes lie down, and let five or six of them dance on my hand; and at last the boys and girls would venture to come and play at hide-and-seek in my hair.

    a. The children tortured Gulliver.
    b. Gulliver traveled because he wanted to meet new people.
    c. Gulliver is considerably larger than the children who are playing around him.
    d. Gulliver has a genuine love and enthusiasm for people of all sizes.

20. What is the significance of the word *mind* in the following passage?
    The emperor had a mind one day to entertain me with several of the country shows, wherein they exceed all nations I have known, both for dexterity and magnificence.

    a. The ability to think
    b. A collective vote
    c. A definitive decision
    d. A mythological question

21. Which of the following assertions does not support the fact that games are a commonplace event in this culture?
    a. My gentlest and good behavior . . . short time.
    b. They are trained in this art from their youth . . . liberal education.
    c. Very often the chief ministers themselves are commanded to show their skill . . . not lost their faculty.
    d. Flimnap, the treasurer, is allowed to cut a caper on the straight rope . . . higher than any other lord in the whole empire.

22. How do the roles of Flimnap and Reldresal serve as evidence of the community's emphasis in regards to the correlation between physical strength and leadership abilities?
  a. Only children used Gulliver's hands as a playground.
  b. The two men who exhibited superior abilities held prominent positions in the community.
  c. Only common townspeople, not leaders, walk the straight rope.
  d. No one could jump higher than Gulliver.

Questions 23–28 are based upon the following passage:

Three years ago, I think there were not many bird-lovers in the United States, who believed it possible to prevent the total extinction of both egrets from our fauna. All the known rookeries accessible to plume-hunters had been totally destroyed. Two years ago, the secret discovery of several small, hidden colonies prompted William Dutcher, President of the National Association of Audubon Societies, and Mr. T. Gilbert Pearson, Secretary, to attempt the protection of those colonies. With a fund contributed for the purpose, wardens were hired and duly commissioned. As previously stated, one of those wardens was shot dead in cold blood by a plume hunter. The task of guarding swamp rookeries from the attacks of money-hungry desperadoes to whom the accursed plumes were worth their weight in gold, is a very chancy proceeding. There is now one warden in Florida who says that "before they get my rookery they will first have to get me."

Thus far the protective work of the Audubon Association has been successful. Now there are twenty colonies, which contain all told, about 5,000 egrets and about 120,000 herons and ibises which are guarded by the Audubon wardens. One of the most important is on Bird Island, a mile out in Orange Lake, central Florida, and it is ably defended by Oscar E. Baynard. To-day, the plume hunters who do not dare to raid the guarded rookeries are trying to study out the lines of flight of the birds, to and from their feeding-grounds, and shoot them in transit. Their motto is—"Anything to beat the law, and get the plumes." It is there that the state of Florida should take part in the war.

The success of this campaign is attested by the fact that last year a number of egrets were seen in eastern Massachusetts—for the first time in many years. And so to-day the question is, can the wardens continue to hold the plume-hunters at bay?

from *Our Vanishing Wildlife*, by William T. Hornaday

23. The author's use of first person pronoun in the following text does NOT have which of the following effects?

Three years ago, I think there were not many bird-lovers in the United States, who believed it possible to prevent the total extinction of both egrets from our fauna.

  a. The phrase *I think* acts as a sort of hedging, where the author's tone is less direct and/or absolute.
  b. It allows the reader to more easily connect with the author.
  c. It encourages the reader to empathize with the egrets.
  d. It distances the reader from the text by overemphasizing the story.

24. What purpose does the quote serve at the end of the first paragraph?
    a. The quote shows proof of a hunter threatening one of the wardens.
    b. The quote lightens the mood by illustrating the colloquial language of the region.
    c. The quote provides an example of a warden protecting one of the colonies.
    d. The quote provides much needed comic relief in the form of a joke.

25. What is the meaning of the word *rookeries* in the following text?
    To-day, the plume hunters who do not dare to raid the guarded rookeries are trying to study out the lines of flight of the birds, to and from their feeding-grounds, and shoot them in transit.

    a. Houses in a slum area
    b. A place where hunters gather to trade tools
    c. A place where wardens go to trade stories
    d. A colony of breeding birds

26. What is on Bird Island?
    a. Hunters selling plumes
    b. An important bird colony
    c. Bird Island Battle between the hunters and the wardens
    d. An important egret with unique plumes

27. What is the main purpose of the passage?
    a. To persuade the audience to act in preservation of the bird colonies
    b. To show the effect hunting egrets has had on the environment
    c. To argue that the preservation of bird colonies has had a negative impact on the environment.
    d. To demonstrate the success of the protective work of the Audubon Association

28. Why are hunters trying to study the lines of flight of the birds?
    a. To study ornithology, one must know the lines of flight that birds take.
    b. To help wardens preserve the lives of the birds
    c. To have a better opportunity to hunt the birds
    d. To builds their homes under the lines of flight because they believe it brings good luck

Questions 29–34 are based upon the following passage:

Insects as a whole are preeminently creatures of the land and the air. This is shown not only by the possession of wings by a vast majority of the class, but by the mode of breathing to which reference has already been made, a system of branching air-tubes carrying atmospheric air with its combustion-supporting oxygen to all the insect's tissues. The air gains access to these tubes through a number of paired air-holes or spiracles, arranged segmentally in series.

It is of great interest to find that, nevertheless, a number of insects spend much of their time under water. This is true of not a few in the perfect winged state, as for example aquatic beetles and water-bugs ('boatmen' and 'scorpions') which have some way of protecting their spiracles when submerged, and, possessing usually the power of flight, can pass on occasion from pond or stream to upper air. But it is advisable in connection with our present subject to dwell especially on some insects that remain continually under water till they are ready to undergo their final moult and attain the winged state, which they pass entirely in the air. The preparatory instars of such insects are aquatic;

the adult instar is aerial. All may-flies, dragon-flies, and caddis-flies, many beetles and two-winged flies, and a few moths thus divide their life-story between the water and the air. For the present we confine attention to the Stone-flies, the May-flies, and the Dragon-flies, three well-known orders of insects respectively called by systematists the Plecoptera, the Ephemeroptera and the Odonata.

In the case of many insects that have aquatic larvae, the latter are provided with some arrangement for enabling them to reach atmospheric air through the surface-film of the water. But the larva of a stone-fly, a dragon-fly, or a may-fly is adapted more completely than these for aquatic life; it can, by means of gills of some kind, breathe the air dissolved in water.

from *The Life-Story of Insects*, by Geo H. Carpenter

29. Which statement best details the central idea in this passage?
    a. It introduces certain insects that transition from water to air.
    b. It delves into entomology, especially where gills are concerned.
    c. It defines what constitutes as insects' breathing.
    d. It invites readers to have a hand in the preservation of insects.

30. Which definition most closely relates to the usage of the word *moult* in the passage?
    a. An adventure of sorts, especially underwater
    b. Mating act between two insects
    c. The act of shedding part or all of the outer shell
    d. Death of an organism that ends in a revival of life

31. What is the purpose of the first paragraph in relation to the second paragraph?
    a. The first paragraph serves as a cause and the second paragraph serves as an effect.
    b. The first paragraph serves as a contrast to the second.
    c. The first paragraph is a description for the argument in the second paragraph.
    d. The first and second paragraphs are merely presented in a sequence.

32. What does the following sentence most nearly mean?
    The preparatory instars of such insects are aquatic; the adult instar is aerial.

    a. The volume of water is necessary to prep the insect for transition rather than the volume of the air.
    b. The abdomen of the insect is designed like a star in the water as well as the air.
    c. The stage of preparation in between molting is acted out in the water, while the last stage is in the air.
    d. These insects breathe first in the water through gills yet continue to use the same organs to breathe in the air.

33. Which of the statements reflect information that one could reasonably infer based on the author's tone?
    a. The author's tone is persuasive and attempts to call the audience to action.
    b. The author's tone is passionate due to excitement over the subject and personal narrative.
    c. The author's tone is informative and exhibits interest in the subject of the study.
    d. The author's tone is somber, depicting some anger at the state of insect larvae.

34. Which statement best describes stoneflies, mayflies, and dragonflies?
    a. They are creatures of the land and the air.
    b. They have a way of protecting their spiracles when submerged.
    c. Their larvae can breathe the air dissolved in water through gills of some kind.
    d. The preparatory instars of these insects are aerial.

Questions 35–41 are based on the following passage.

In the quest to understand existence, modern philosophers must question if humans can fully comprehend the world. Classical western approaches to philosophy tend to hold that one can understand something, be it an event or object, by standing outside of the phenomena and observing it. It is then by unbiased observation that one can grasp the details of the world. This seems to hold true for many things. Scientists conduct experiments and record their findings, and thus many natural phenomena become comprehendible. However, several of these observations were possible because humans used tools in order to make these discoveries.

This may seem like an extraneous matter. After all, people invented things like microscopes and telescopes in order to enhance their capacity to view cells or the movement of stars. While humans are still capable of seeing things, the question remains if human beings have the capacity to fully observe and see the world in order to understand it. It would not be an impossible stretch to argue that what humans see through a microscope is not the exact thing itself, but a human interpretation of it.

This would seem to be the case in the "Business of the Holes" experiment conducted by Richard Feynman. To study the way electrons behave, Feynman set up a barrier with two holes and a plate. The plate was there to indicate how many times the electrons would pass through the hole(s). Rather than casually observe the electrons acting under normal circumstances, Feynman discovered that electrons behave in two totally different ways depending on whether or not they are observed. The electrons that were observed had passed through either one of the holes or were caught on the plate as particles. However, electrons that weren't observed acted as waves instead of particles and passed through both holes. This indicated that electrons have a dual nature. Electrons seen by the human eye act like particles, while unseen electrons act like waves of energy.

This dual nature of the electrons presents a conundrum. While humans now have a better understanding of electrons, the fact remains that people cannot entirely perceive how electrons behave without the use of instruments. We can only observe one of the mentioned behaviors, which only provides a partial understanding of the entire function of electrons. Therefore, we're forced to ask ourselves whether the world we observe is objective or if it is subjectively perceived by humans. Or, an alternative question: can man understand the world only through machines that will allow them to observe natural phenomena?

Both questions humble man's capacity to grasp the world. However, those ideas don't take into account that many phenomena have been proven by human beings without the use of machines, such as the discovery of gravity. Like all philosophical questions, whether man's reason and observation alone can understand the universe can be approached from many angles.

35. What is the author's motivation for writing the passage?
    a. Bring to light an alternative view on human perception by examining the role of technology in human understanding.
    b. Educate the reader on the latest astroparticle physics discovery and offer terms that may be unfamiliar to the reader.
    c. Argue that humans are totally blind to the realities of the world by presenting an experiment that proves that electrons are not what they seem on the surface.
    d. Reflect on opposing views of human understanding.

36. Which of the following most closely resembles the way in which paragraph four is structured?
    a. It offers one solution, questions the solution, and then ends with an alternative solution.
    b. It presents an inquiry, explains the detail of that inquiry, and then offers a solution.
    c. It presents a problem, explains the details of that problem, and then ends with more inquiry.
    d. It gives a definition, offers an explanation, and then ends with an inquiry.

37. For the classical approach to understanding to hold true, which of the following must be required?
    a. A telescope.
    b. The person observing must prove their theory beyond a doubt.
    c. Multiple witnesses present.
    d. The person observing must be unbiased.

38. Which best describes how the electrons in the experiment behaved like waves?
    a. The electrons moved up and down like actual waves.
    b. The electrons passed through both holes and then onto the plate.
    c. The electrons converted to photons upon touching the plate.
    d. Electrons were seen passing through one hole or the other.

39. The author mentions "gravity" in the last paragraph in order to do what?
    a. In order to show that different natural phenomena test man's ability to grasp the world.
    b. To prove that since man has not measured it with the use of tools or machines, humans cannot know the true nature of gravity.
    c. To demonstrate an example of natural phenomena humans discovered and understand without the use of tools or machines.
    d. To show an alternative solution to the nature of electrons that humans have not thought of yet.

40. Which situation best parallels the revelation of the dual nature of electrons discovered in Feynman's experiment?
    a. A man is born color-blind and grows up observing everything in lighter or darker shades. With the invention of special goggles he puts on, he discovers that there are other colors in addition to different shades.
    b. The coelacanth was thought to be extinct, but a live specimen was just recently discovered. There are now two living species of coelacanth known to man, and both are believed to be endangered.
    c. In the Middle Ages, blacksmiths added carbon to iron, thus inventing steel. The consequences of this important discovery would have its biggest effects during the industrial revolution.
    d. In order to better examine and treat broken bones, the x-ray machine was invented and put to use in hospitals and medical centers.

41. Which statement about technology would the author likely disagree with?
    a. Technology can help expand the field of human vision.
    b. Technology renders human observation irrelevant.
    c. Developing tools used in observation and research indicates growing understanding of our world in itself.
    d. Studying certain phenomena necessitates the use of tools and machines.

Questions 42–47 are based upon the following passage:

Fellow citizens—Pardon me, and allow me to ask, why am I called upon to speak here today? What have I, or those I represent, to do with your national independence? Are the great principles of political freedom and of natural justice embodied in that Declaration of Independence, Independence extended to us? And am I therefore called upon to bring our humble offering to the national altar, and to confess the benefits, and express devout gratitude for the blessings, resulting from your independence to us?

Would to God, both for your sakes and ours, ours that an affirmative answer could be truthfully returned to these questions! Then would my task be light, and my burden easy and delightful. For who is there so cold that a nation's sympathy could not warm him? Who so obdurate and dead to the claims of gratitude that would not thankfully acknowledge such priceless benefits? Who so stolid and selfish, that would not give his voice to swell the hallelujahs of a nation's jubilee, when the chains of servitude had been torn from his limbs? I am not that man. In a case like that, the dumb may eloquently speak, and the lame man leap as an hart.

But, such is not the state of the case. I say it with a sad sense of the disparity between us. I am not included within the pale of this glorious anniversary. Oh pity! Your high independence only reveals the immeasurable distance between us. The blessings in which you this day rejoice, I do not enjoy in common. The rich inheritance of justice, liberty, prosperity, and independence, bequeathed by your fathers, is shared by *you*, not by *me*. This Fourth of July is *yours,* not *mine*. You may rejoice, *I* must mourn. To drag a man in fetters into the grand illuminated temple of liberty, and call upon him to join you in joyous anthems, were inhuman mockery and sacrilegious irony. Do you mean, citizens, to mock me, by asking me to speak today? If so there is a parallel to your conduct. And let me warn you that it is dangerous to copy the example of a nation whose crimes, towering up to heaven, were thrown down by the breath of the Almighty, burying that nation and irrecoverable ruin! I can today take up the plaintive lament of a peeled and woe-smitten people.

By the rivers of Babylon, there we sat down. Yea! We wept when we remembered Zion. We hanged our harps upon the willows in the midst thereof. For there, they that carried us away captive, required of us a song; and they who wasted us required of us mirth, saying, "Sing us one of the songs of Zion." How can we sing the Lord's song in a strange land? If I forget thee, O Jerusalem, let my right hand forget her cunning. If I do not remember thee, let my tongue cleave to the roof of my mouth.

From "What to the Slave is the Fourth of July?" by Frederick Douglass, Rochester, New York July 5, 1852

42. What is the tone of the first paragraph of this passage?
    a. Exasperated
    b. Inclusive
    c. Contemplative
    d. Nonchalant

43. Which word CANNOT be used synonymously with the term *obdurate* as it is conveyed in the text below?

      Who so obdurate and dead to the claims of gratitude, that would not thankfully acknowledge such priceless benefits?

    a. Steadfast
    b. Stubborn
    c. Contented
    d. Unwavering

44. What is the central purpose of this text?
    a. To demonstrate the author's extensive knowledge of the Bible
    b. To address the feelings of exclusion expressed by African Americans after the establishment of the Fourth of July holiday
    c. To convince wealthy landowners to adopt new holiday rituals
    d. To explain why minorities often relished the notion of segregation in government institutions

45. Which statement serves as evidence of the question above?
    a. By the rivers of Babylon . . . down.
    b. Fellow citizens . . . today.
    c. I can . . . woe-smitten people.
    d. The rich inheritance of justice . . . *not by me.*

46. The statement below features an example of which of the following literary devices?

      Oh pity! Your high independence only reveals the immeasurable distance between us.

    a. Assonance
    b. Parallelism
    c. Amplification
    d. Hyperbole

47. The speaker's use of biblical references, such as "rivers of Babylon" and the "songs of Zion," helps the reader to do all of the following EXCEPT:
    a. Identify with the speaker through the use of common text.
    b. Convince the audience that injustices have been committed by referencing another group of people who have been previously affected by slavery.
    c. Display the equivocation of the speaker and those that he represents.
    d. Appeal to the listener's sense of humanity.

The next question is based on the following passage.

A famous children's author recently published a historical fiction novel under a pseudonym; however, it did not sell as many copies as her children's books. In her earlier years, she had majored in history and earned a graduate degree in Antebellum American History, which is the time frame of her new novel. Critics praised this newest work far more than the children's series that made her famous. In fact, her new novel was nominated for the prestigious Albert J. Beveridge Award, but still isn't selling like her children's books, which fly off the shelves because of her name alone.

48. Which one of the following statements might be accurately inferred based on the above passage?
    a. The famous children's author produced an inferior book under her pseudonym.
    b. The famous children's author is the foremost expert on Antebellum America.
    c. The famous children's author did not receive the bump in publicity for her historical novel that it would have received if it were written under her given name.
    d. People generally prefer to read children's series than historical fiction.

Questions 49–54 are based on the following passage:

Dana Gioia argues in his article that poetry is dying, now little more than a limited art form confined to academic and college settings. Of course, poetry remains healthy in the academic setting, but the idea of poetry being limited to this academic subculture is a stretch. New technology and social networking alone have contributed to poets and other writers' work being shared across the world. YouTube has emerged to be a major asset to poets, allowing live performances to be streamed to billions of users. Even now, poetry continues to grow and voice topics that are relevant to the culture of our time. Poetry is not in the spotlight as it may have been in earlier times, but it's still a relevant art form that continues to expand in scope and appeal.

Furthermore, Gioia's argument does not account for live performances of poetry. Not everyone has taken a poetry class or enrolled in university—but most everyone is online. The Internet is a perfect launching point to get all creative work out there. An example of this was the performance of Buddy Wakefield's *Hurling Crowbirds at Mockingbars*. Wakefield is a well-known poet who has published several collections of contemporary poetry. One of my favorite works by Wakefield is *Crowbirds*, specifically his performance at New York University in 2009. Although his reading was a campus event, views of his performance online number in the thousands. His poetry attracted people outside of the university setting.

Naturally, the poem's popularity can be attributed both to Wakefield's performance and the quality of his writing. *Crowbirds* touches on themes of core human concepts such as faith, personal loss, and growth. These are not ideas that only poets or students of literature understand, but all human beings: "You acted like I was hurling crowbirds at mockingbars / and abandoned me for not making sense. / Evidently, I don't experience things as rationally as you do" (Wakefield 15-17). Wakefield weaves together a complex description of the perplexed and hurt emotions of the speaker undergoing a separation from a romantic interest. The line "You acted like I was hurling crowbirds at mockingbars" conjures up an image of someone confused, seemingly out of their mind . . . or in the case of the speaker, passionately trying to grasp at a relationship that is fading. The speaker is looking back and finding the words that described how he wasn't making sense. This poem is particularly human and gripping in its message, but the entire effect of the poem is enhanced through the physical performance.

At its core, poetry is about addressing issues/ideas in the world. Part of this is also addressing the perspectives that are exiguously considered. Although the platform may look different, poetry continues to have a steady audience due to the emotional connection the poet shares with the audience.

49. Which one of the following best explains how the passage is organized?
a. The author begins with a long definition of the main topic, and then proceeds to prove how that definition has changed over the course of modernity.
b. The author presents a puzzling phenomenon and uses the rest of the passage to showcase personal experiences in order to explain it.
c. The author contrasts two different viewpoints, then builds a case showing preference for one over the other.
d. The passage is an analysis of another theory in which the author has no stake in.

50. The author of the passage would likely agree most with which of the following?
a. Buddy Wakefield is a genius and is considered at the forefront of modern poetry.
b. Poetry is not irrelevant; it is an art form that adapts to the changing time while containing its core elements.
c. Spoken word is the zenith of poetic forms and the premier style of poetry in this decade.
d. Poetry is on the verge of vanishing from our cultural consciousness.

51. Which one of the following words, if substituted for the word *exiguously* in the last paragraph, would LEAST change the meaning of the sentence?
a. Indolently
b. Inaudibly
c. Interminably
d. Infrequently

52. Which of the following is most closely analogous to the author's opinion of Buddy Wakefield's performance in relation to modern poetry?
a. Someone's refusal to accept that the Higgs Boson will validate the Standard Model.
b. An individual's belief that soccer will lose popularity within the next fifty years.
c. A professor's opinion that poetry contains the language of the heart, while fiction contains the language of the mind.
d. A student's insistence that psychoanalysis is a subset of modern psychology.

53. What is the primary purpose of the passage?
a. To educate readers on the development of poetry and describe the historical implications of poetry in media.
b. To disprove Dana Gioia's stance that poetry is becoming irrelevant and is only appreciated in academia.
c. To inform readers of the brilliance of Buddy Wakefield and to introduce them to other poets that have influence in contemporary poetry.
d. To prove that Gioia's article does have some truth to it and to shed light on its relevance to modern poetry.

54. What is the author's main reason for including the quote in the passage?
    a. The quote opens up opportunity to disprove Gioia's views.
    b. To demonstrate that people are still writing poetry even if the medium has changed in current times.
    c. To prove that poets still have an audience to write for even if the audience looks different than it did centuries ago.
    d. The quote illustrates the complex themes poets continue to address, which still draws listeners and appreciation.

Questions 55–59 are based on the following passage:

The Middle Ages were a time of great superstition and theological debate. Many beliefs were developed and practiced, while some died out or were listed as heresy. Boethianism is a Medieval theological philosophy that attributes sin to gratification and righteousness with virtue and God's providence. Boethianism holds that sin, greed, and corruption are means to attain temporary pleasure, but that they inherently harm the person's soul as well as other human beings.

In *The Canterbury Tales,* we observe more instances of bad actions punished than goodness being rewarded. This would appear to be some reflection of Boethianism. In the "Pardoner's Tale," all three thieves wind up dead, which is a result of their desire for wealth. Each wrong doer pays with their life, and they are unable to enjoy the wealth they worked to steal. Within his tales, Chaucer gives reprieve to people undergoing struggle, but also interweaves stories of contemptible individuals being cosmically punished for their wickedness. The thieves idolize physical wealth, which leads to their downfall. This same theme and ideological principle of Boethianism is repeated in the "Friar's Tale," whose summoner character attempts to gain further wealth by partnering with a demon. The summoner's refusal to repent for his avarice and corruption leads to the demon dragging his soul to Hell. Again, we see the theme of the individual who puts faith and morality aside in favor for a physical prize. The result, of course, is that the summoner loses everything.

The examples of the righteous being rewarded tend to appear in a spiritual context within the *Canterbury Tales*. However, there are a few instances where we see goodness resulting in physical reward. In the Prioress' Tale, we see corporal punishment for barbarism *and* a reward for goodness. The Jews are punished for their murder of the child, giving a sense of law and order (though racist) to the plot. While the boy does die, he is granted a lasting reward by being able to sing even after his death, a miracle that marks that the murdered youth led a pure life. Here, the miracle represents eternal favor with God.

Again, we see the theological philosophy of Boethianism in Chaucer's *The Canterbury Tales* through acts of sin and righteousness and the consequences that follow. When pleasures of the world are sought instead of God's favor, we see characters being punished in tragic ways. However, the absence of worldly lust has its own set of consequences for the characters seeking to obtain God's favor.

55. What would be a potential reward for living a good life, as described in Boethianism?
    a. A long life sustained by the good deeds one has done over a lifetime
    b. Wealth and fertility for oneself and the extension of one's family line
    c. Vengeance for those who have been persecuted by others who have a capacity for committing wrongdoing
    d. God's divine favor for one's righteousness

56. What might be the main reason why the author chose to discuss Boethianism through examining The Canterbury Tales?
    a. *The Canterbury Tales* is a well-known text.
    b. *The Canterbury Tales* is the only known fictional text that contains use of Boethianism.
    c. *The Canterbury Tales* presents a manuscript written in the medieval period that can help illustrate Boethianism through stories and show how people of the time might have responded to the idea.
    d. Within each individual tale in *The Canterbury Tales*, the reader can read about different levels of Boethianism and how each level leads to greater enlightenment.

57. What "ideological principle" is the author referring to in the middle of the second paragraph when talking about the "Friar's Tale"?
    a. The principle that the act of ravaging another's possessions is the same as ravaging one's soul.
    b. The principle that thieves who idolize physical wealth will be punished in an earthly sense as well as eternally.
    c. The principle that fraternization with a demon will result in one losing everything, including his or her life.
    d. The principle that a desire for material goods leads to moral malfeasance punishable by a higher being.

58. Which of the following words, if substituted for the word *avarice* in paragraph two, would LEAST change the meaning of the sentence?
    a. Perniciousness
    b. Pithiness
    c. Parsimoniousness
    d. Precariousness

59. Based on the passage, what view does Boethianism take on desire?
    a. Desire does not exist in the context of Boethianism
    b. Desire is a virtue and should be welcomed
    c. Having desire is evidence of demonic possession
    d. Desire for pleasure can lead toward sin

60. The following exchange occurred after the Baseball Coach's team suffered a heartbreaking loss in the final inning.

Reporter: The team clearly did not rise to the challenge. I'm sure that getting zero hits in twenty at-bats with runners in scoring position hurt the team's chances at winning the game. What are your thoughts on this devastating loss?

Baseball Coach: Hitting with runners in scoring position was not the reason we lost this game. We made numerous errors in the field, and our pitchers gave out too many free passes. Also, we did not even need a hit with runners in scoring position. Many of those at-bats could have driven in the run by simply making contact. Our team did not deserve to win the game.

Which of the following best describes the main point of dispute between the reporter and baseball coach?
    a. Whether the loss was heartbreaking.
    b. Whether getting zero hits in twenty at-bats with runners in scoring position caused the loss.
    c. Numerous errors in the field and pitchers giving too many free passes caused the loss.
    d. Whether the team deserved to win the game.

61. Conservative Politician: Social welfare programs are destroying our country. These programs are not only adding to the annual deficit, which increases the national debt, but they also discourage hard work. Our country must continue producing leaders who bootstrap their way to the top. None of our country's citizens truly *need* assistance from the government; rather, the assistance just makes things easier.

Liberal Politician: Our great country is founded on the principle of hope. The country is built on the backs of immigrants who came here with nothing, except for the hope of a better life. Our country is too wealthy not to provide basic necessities for the less fortunate. Recent immigrants, single mothers, historically disenfranchised, disabled persons, and the elderly all require an ample safety net.

What is the main point of dispute between the politicians?
    a. Spending on social welfare programs increases the national debt.
    b. Certain classes of people rely on social welfare programs to meet their basic needs.
    c. Certain classes of people would be irreparably harmed if the country failed to provide a social welfare program.
    d. All of the country's leaders have bootstrapped their way to the top.

Questions 62–67 are based upon the following passage:

> My Good Friends,—When I first imparted to the committee of the projected Institute my particular wish that on one of the evenings of my readings here the main body of my audience should be composed of working men and their families, I was animated by two desires; first, by the wish to have the great pleasure of meeting you face to face at this Christmas time, and accompany you myself through one of my little Christmas books; and second, by the wish to have an opportunity of stating publicly in your presence, and in the presence of the committee, my earnest hope that the Institute will, from the beginning, recognise one great principle—strong in reason and justice—which I believe to be essential to the very life of such an Institution. It is, that the working man shall, from the first unto the last, have a share in the management of an Institution which is designed for his benefit, and which calls itself by his name.

I have no fear here of being misunderstood—of being supposed to mean too much in this. If there ever was a time when any one class could of itself do much for its own good, and for the welfare of society—which I greatly doubt—that time is unquestionably past. It is in the fusion of different classes, without confusion; in the bringing together of employers and employed; in the creating of a better common understanding among those whose interests are identical, who depend upon each other, who are vitally essential to each other, and who never can be in unnatural antagonism without deplorable results, that one of the chief principles of a Mechanics' Institution should consist. In this world, a great deal of the bitterness among us arises from an imperfect understanding of one another. Erect in Birmingham a great Educational Institution, properly educational; educational of the feelings as well as of the reason; to which all orders of Birmingham men contribute; in which all orders of Birmingham men meet; wherein all orders of Birmingham men are faithfully represented—and you will erect a Temple of Concord here which will be a model edifice to the whole of England.

Contemplating as I do the existence of the Artisans' Committee, which not long ago considered the establishment of the Institute so sensibly, and supported it so heartily, I earnestly entreat the gentlemen—earnest I know in the good work, and who are now among us—by all means to avoid the great shortcoming of similar institutions; and in asking the working man for his confidence, to set him the great example and give him theirs in return. You will judge for yourselves if I promise too much for the working man, when I say that he will stand by such an enterprise with the utmost of his patience, his perseverance, sense, and support; that I am sure he will need no charitable aid or condescending patronage; but will readily and cheerfully pay for the advantages which it confers; that he will prepare himself in individual cases where he feels that the adverse circumstances around him have rendered it necessary; in a word, that he will feel his responsibility like an honest man, and will most honestly and manfully discharge it. I now proceed to the pleasant task to which I assure you I have looked forward for a long time.

from Charles Dickens' speech in Birmingham in England on December 30, 1853 on behalf of the Birmingham and Midland Institute.

62. Which word is most closely synonymous with the word *patronage* as it appears in the following statement?

...that I am sure he will need no charitable aid or condescending patronage

a. Auspices
b. Aberration
c. Acerbic
d. Adulation

63. Which term is most closely aligned with the definition of the term *working man* as it is defined in the following passage?

> You will judge for yourselves if I promise too much for the working man, when I say that he will stand by such an enterprise with the utmost of his patience, his perseverance, sense, and support...

    a. Plebian
    b. Viscount
    c. Entrepreneur
    d. Bourgeois

64. Which of the following statements most closely correlates with the definition of the term *working man* as it is defined in Question 41?
    a. A working man is not someone who works for institutions or corporations, but someone who is well-versed in the workings of the soul.
    b. A working man is someone who is probably not involved in social activities because the physical demand for work is too high.
    c. A working man is someone who works for wages among the middle class.
    d. The working man has historically taken to the field, to the factory, and now to the screen.

65. Based upon the contextual evidence provided in the passage above, what is the meaning of the term *enterprise* in the third paragraph?
    a. Company
    b. Courage
    c. Game
    d. Cause

66. The speaker addresses his audience as *My Good Friends.* What kind of credibility does this salutation give to the speaker?
    a. The speaker is an employer addressing his employees, so the salutation is a way for the boss to bridge the gap between himself and his employees.
    b. The speaker's salutation is one from an entertainer to his audience, and uses the friendly language to connect to his audience before a serious speech.
    c. The salutation is used ironically to give a somber tone to the serious speech that follows.
    d. The speech is one from a politician to the public, so the salutation is used to grab the audience's attention.

67. According to the passage, what is the speaker's second desire for his time in front of the audience?
    a. To read a Christmas story
    b. For the working man to have a say in his institution, which is designed for his benefit.
    c. To have an opportunity to stand in their presence
    d. For the life of the institution to be essential to the audience as a whole

"MANKIND being originally equals in the order of creation, the equality could only be destroyed by some subsequent circumstance; the distinctions of rich, and poor, may in a great measure be accounted for, and that without having recourse to the harsh ill sounding names of oppression and avarice. Oppression is often the consequence, but seldom or never the means of riches; and though avarice will preserve a man from being necessitously poor, it generally makes him too timorous to be wealthy.

But there is another and greater distinction for which no truly natural or religious reason can be assigned, and that is, the distinction of men into KINGS and SUBJECTS. Male and female are the distinctions of nature, good and bad the distinctions of heaven; but how a race of men came into the world so exalted above the rest, and distinguished like some new species, is worth enquiring into, and whether they are the means of happiness or of misery to mankind.

In the early ages of the world, according to the scripture chronology, there were no kings; the consequence of which was there were no wars; it is the pride of kings which throw mankind into confusion Holland without a king hath enjoyed more peace for this last century than any of the monarchical governments in Europe. Antiquity favors the same remark; for the quiet and rural lives of the first patriarchs hath a happy something in them, which vanishes away when we come to the history of Jewish royalty.

Government by kings was first introduced into the world by the Heathens, from whom the children of Israel copied the custom. It was the most prosperous invention the Devil ever set on foot for the promotion of idolatry. The Heathens paid divine honors to their deceased kings, and the Christian world hath improved on the plan by doing the same to their living ones. How impious is the title of sacred majesty applied to a worm, who in the midst of his splendor is crumbling into dust!

As the exalting one man so greatly above the rest cannot be justified on the equal rights of nature, so neither can it be defended on the authority of scripture; for the will of the Almighty, as declared by Gideon and the prophet Samuel, expressly disapproves of government by kings. All anti-monarchical parts of scripture have been very smoothly glossed over in monarchical governments, but they undoubtedly merit the attention of countries, which have their governments yet to form. "Render unto Caesar the things which are Caesar's" is the scripture doctrine of courts, yet it is no support of monarchical government, for the Jews at that time were without a king, and in a state of vassalage to the Romans.

Near three thousand years passed away from the Mosaic account of the creation, till the Jews under a national delusion requested a king. Till then their form of government (except in extraordinary cases, where the Almighty interposed) was a kind of republic administered by a judge and the elders of the tribes. Kings they had none, and it was held sinful to acknowledge any being under that title but the Lord of Hosts. And when a man seriously reflects on the idolatrous homage which is paid to the persons of Kings, he need not wonder, that the Almighty ever jealous of his honor, should disapprove of a form of government which so impiously invades the prerogative of heaven.

from Thomas Paine, "Common Sense"

68. According to passage, what role does avarice, or greed, play in poverty?
   a. It can make a man very wealthy
   b. It is the consequence of wealth
   c. Avarice can prevent a man from being poor, but too fearful to be very wealthy
   d. Avarice is what drives a person to be very wealthy

69. Of these distinctions, which does the author believe to be beyond natural or religious reason?
   a. Good and bad
   b. Male and female
   c. Human and animal
   d. King and subjects

70. According to the passage, what are the Heathens responsible for?
   a. Government by kings
   b. Quiet and rural lives of patriarchs
   c. Paying divine honors to their living kings
   d. Equal rights of nature

71. Which of the following best states Paine's rationale for the denouncement of monarchy?
   a. It is against the laws of nature
   b. It is against the equal rights of nature and is denounced in scripture
   c. Despite scripture, a monarchal government is unlawful
   d. Neither the law nor scripture denounce monarchy

72. Based on the passage, what is the best definition of the word *idolatrous*?
   a. Worshipping heroes
   b. Being deceitful
   c. Sinfulness
   d. Engaging in illegal activities

73. What is the essential meaning of lines 41-44?

   And when a man seriously reflects on the idolatrous homage which is paid to the persons of Kings, he need not wonder, that the Almighty ever jealous of his honor, should disapprove of a form of government which so impiously invades the prerogative of heaven.

   a. God would disapprove of the irreverence of a monarchical government.
   b. With careful reflection, men should realize that heaven is not promised.
   c. God will punish those that follow a monarchical government.
   d. Belief in a monarchical government cannot coexist with belief in God.

Questions 74–79 are based on the following passage:

   When I got on the coach the driver had not taken his seat, and I saw him talking with the landlady. They were evidently talking of me, for every now and then they looked at me, and some of the people who were sitting on the bench outside the door came and listened, and then looked at me, most of them pityingly. I could hear a lot of words often repeated, queer words, for there were many nationalities in the crowd; so I quietly got my polyglot dictionary from my bag and looked them out. I must say they weren't cheering to me, for amongst them were "Ordog"—Satan, "pokol"—hell, "stregoica"—witch, "vrolok" and "vlkoslak"—both of which mean the same thing, one being Slovak and the other Servian for something that is either were-wolf or vampire.

When we started, the crowd round the inn door, which had by this time swelled to a considerable size, all made the sign of the cross and pointed two fingers towards me. With some difficulty I got a fellow-passenger to tell me what they meant; he wouldn't answer at first, but on learning that I was English, he explained that it was a charm or guard against the evil eye. This was not very pleasant for me, just starting for an unknown place to meet an unknown man; but everyone seemed so kind-hearted, and so sorrowful, and so sympathetic that I couldn't but be touched. I shall never forget the last glimpse which I had of the inn-yard and its crowd of picturesque figures, all crossing themselves, as they stood round the wide archway, with its background of rich foliage of oleander and orange trees in green tubs clustered in the centre of the yard. Then our driver cracked his big whip over his four small horses, which ran abreast, and we set off on our journey.

I soon lost sight and recollection of ghostly fears in the beauty of the scene as we drove along, although had I known the language, or rather languages, which my fellow-passengers were speaking, I might not have been able to throw them off so easily. Before us lay a green sloping land full of forests and woods, with here and there steep hills, crowned with clumps of trees or with farmhouses, the blank gable end to the road. There was everywhere a bewildering mass of fruit blossom—apple, plum, pear, cherry; and as we drove by I could see the green grass under the trees spangled with the fallen petals. In and out amongst these green hills of what they call here the "Mittel Land" ran the road, losing itself as it swept round the grassy curve, or was shut out by the straggling ends of pine woods, which here and there ran down the hillsides like tongues of flame. The road was rugged, but still we seemed to fly over it with a feverish haste. I couldn't understand then what the haste meant, but the driver was evidently bent on losing no time in reaching Borgo Prund.

74. What type of narrator is found in this passage?
   a. First person
   b. Second person
   c. Third-person limited
   d. Third-person omniscient

75. Which of the following is true of the traveler?
   a. He wishes the driver would go faster.
   b. He's returning to the country of his birth.
   c. He has some familiarity with the local customs.
   d. He doesn't understand all of the languages being used.

76. How does the traveler's mood change between the second and third paragraphs?
   a. From relaxed to rushed
   b. From fearful to charmed
   c. From confused to enlightened
   d. From comfortable to exhausted

77. Who is the traveler going to meet?
    a. A kind landlady
    b. A distant relative
    c. A friendly villager
    d. A complete stranger

78. Based on the details in this passage, what can readers probably expect to happen in the story?
    a. The traveler will become a farmer.
    b. The traveler will arrive late at his destination.
    c. The traveler will soon encounter danger or evil.
    d. The traveler will have a pleasant journey and make many new friends.

79. Which sentence from the passage provides a clue for question 39?
    a. "I must say they weren't cheering to me, for amongst them were "Ordog"—Satan, "pokol"—hell, "stregoica"—witch, "vrolok" and "vlkoslak"—both of which mean the same thing, one being Slovak and the other Servian for something that is either were-wolf or vampire."
    b. "When I got on the coach the driver had not taken his seat, and I saw him talking with the landlady."
    c. "Then our driver cracked his big whip over his four small horses, which ran abreast, and we set off on our journey."
    d. "There was everywhere a bewildering mass of fruit blossom—apple, plum, pear, cherry; and as we drove by I could see the green grass under the trees spangled with the fallen petals."

Questions 80–85 are based on the following passage:

I heartily accept the motto, "that government is best which governs least," and I should like to see it acted up to more rapidly and systematically. Carried out, it finally amounts to this, which also I believe—"that government is best which governs not at all," and when men are prepared for it, that will be the kind of government which they will have. Government is at best but an expedient; but most governments are usually, and all governments are sometimes, inexpedient. The objections which have been brought against a standing army, and they are many and weighty, and deserve to prevail, may also at last be brought against a standing government. The standing army is only an arm of the standing government. The government itself, which is only the mode which the people have chosen to execute their will, is equally liable to be abused and perverted before the people can act through it. Witness the present Mexican war, the work of comparatively a few individuals using the standing government as their tool; for, in the outset, the people would not have consented to this measure.

This American government—what is it but a tradition, though a recent one, endeavoring to transmit itself unimpaired to posterity, but each instant losing some of its integrity? It has not the vitality and force of a single living man; for a single man can bend it to his will. It is a sort of wooden gun to the people themselves. But it is not the less necessary for this; for the people must have some complicated machinery or other, and hear its din, to satisfy that idea of government which they have. Governments show thus how successfully men can be imposed on, even impose on themselves, for their own advantage. It is excellent, we must all allow. Yet this government never of itself furthered any enterprise, but by the alacrity with which it got out of its way. It does not keep the country free. It does not settle the West. It does not educate. The character inherent in the American people has done all that has been accomplished; and it would have done somewhat more, if the government had not sometimes got in its way. For government is an expedient by which men would fain succeed in letting one another alone; and, as has been said, when it is most expedient, the governed are most let alone by it. Trade and commerce, if they were not made of india-rubber, would never manage to bounce over the obstacles which legislators are continually putting in their way; and, if one were to judge these men wholly by the effects of their actions and not partly by their intentions, they would deserve to be classed and punished with those mischievous persons who put obstructions on the railroads.

But, to speak practically and as a citizen, unlike those who call themselves no-government men, I ask for, not at once no government, but at once a better government. Let every man make known what kind of government would command his respect, and that will be one step toward obtaining it.

The following passage is an excerpt from Civil Disobedience, by Henry David Thoreau

80. Which phrase best encapsulates Thoreau's use of the term *expedient* in the first paragraph?
    a. A dead end
    b. A state of order
    c. A means to an end
    d. Rushed construction

81. Which best describes Thoreau's view on the Mexican War?
    a. Government is inherently corrupt because it must wage war.
    b. Government can easily be manipulated by a few individuals for their own agenda.
    c. Government is a tool for the people, but it can also act against their interest.
    d. The Mexican War was a necessary action, but not all the people believed this.

82. What is Thoreau's purpose for writing?
    a. His goal is to illustrate how government can function if ideals are maintained.
    b. He wants to prove that true democracy is the best government, but it can be corrupted easily.
    c. Thoreau reflects on the stages of government abuses.
    d. He is seeking to prove that government is easily corruptible and inherently restrictive of individual freedoms that can simultaneously affect the whole state.

83. Which example best supports Thoreau's argument?
    a. A vote carries in the Senate to create a new road tax.
    b. The president vetoes the new FARM bill.
    c. Prohibition is passed to outlaw alcohol.
    d. Trade is opened between the United States and Iceland.

84. Which best summarizes this section from the following passage?

"This American government—what is it but a tradition, though a recent one, endeavoring to transmit itself unimpaired to posterity, but each instant losing some of its integrity? It has not the vitality and force of a single living man; for a single man can bend it to his will. It is a sort of wooden gun to the people themselves."

    a. The government may be instituted to ensure the protections of freedoms, but this is weakened by the fact that it is easily manipulated by individuals.
    b. Unlike an individual, government is uncaring.
    c. Unlike an individual, government has no will, making it more prone to be used as a weapon against the people.
    d. American government is modeled after other traditions but actually has greater potential to be used to control people.

85. According to Thoreau, what's the main reason why government eventually fails to achieve progress?
    a. There are too many rules.
    b. Legislation eventually becomes a hindrance to the lives and work of everyday people.
    c. Trade and wealth eventually become the driving factor of those in government.
    d. Government doesn't separate religion and state.

Answer Explanations

Word Knowledge

1. C: Jackson wanted to relieve his *parched* throat. *Parched* is the correct answer because it means *thirsty*, or *arid*. Choice *A*, humid, means moist, and usually refers to the weather. Choice *B*, scorched, means blackened or baked, and doesn't fit in this context. Choice *D* is incorrect; although *dusty* can cause dryness, it is not the same as the word *thirsty* or *arid*.

2. A: The two friends became inseparable, or *closer*. For this question, it's important to look at the context of the sentence. The second sentence says the friends shared good memories on the trip, which would not make the friends distant or irritable, Choices *B* and *D*. Choice *C*, suffering, carries a negative connotation, and *closer* or *inseparable* are positive words. Therefore, Choice *A* is correct.

3. B: She pledged to, or *promised* her fans the sequel would be just as exciting as the first. Choice *A*, denied, is the opposite of the word *promised* and does not fit with the word *excited*. Choice *C*, invigorated, means energized, and might fit the tone of the sentence with the word *excited*. However, *promised* is the better word to use here. Choice *D*, germinated, means to grow.

4. C: My hands started shaking and my heart stopped. *Shaking* is most closely related to the word *trembling*. Choice *A*, dancing, is not a synonym of shaking. Choice *B*, glowing, is incorrect; hands usually do not glow when one is afraid of something. Choice *D*, throbbing, is closer than *A* or *B*, but Choice *C*, shaking, is closer to the answer than *throbbing*.

5. D: Gabriel would consistently, or *usually* go to the library and study after school. Consistently and usually mean similar things. *Infrequently*, *occasionally*, and *hardly* are the opposite of *consistently* so they do not fit here.

6. A: The runners sprinted, or *dashed* toward the finish line. Choice *B* is incorrect; runners who begin a race usually don't skip toward the finish line. Choice *C* is incorrect, as *rejoice* means to celebrate, not dash or run. Choice *D*, herded, means to gather around something; usually *herded* is used for animals and not for runners.

7. D: *Resolved* means driven or determined, Choice *D*. Choice *A*, resumed, means to start again. Choice *B*, content, means to be satisfied with something. Choice *C*, enthusiastic, means hopeful.

8. D: They went to the bank to install, or *deposit* a check. When people go to the bank with a check, they usually don't celebrate it, Choice *A*, but do something more practical with it, like deposit it. Choice *B*, neutralize, means to counteract something, and is incorrect in this sentence. Choice *C*, eliminate, means to get rid of something, and is also incorrect here.

9. B: The sale at the grocery store inspired, or *motivated* my dad to buy four avocados instead of two. The rest of the words (intimidated, dismayed, and berated) have negative connotations and therefore do not fit within the context of the sentence.

10. A: In order to increase, or *enhance* the quality of her health. Enhance or increase means to make better. Becoming healthier is a direct effect of consuming fruits and vegetables, so Choice *A* is the best answer choice here. Becoming healthier might lead to Choices *B*, *C*, and *D*, but these are not synonyms of *enhance*.

11. C: Sojourn means a brief stop, *layover*, or break. Choice *A*, soiree, means party. Choice *B*, presentation, means something displayed or proposed. Choice *D*, cohort, means partner in activity.

12. A: Until she activated, or *triggered* the fire alarm by burning the casserole in the oven. Triggered means to activate something or initiate something. Choice *B*, offended, is the wrong choice here. You can offend a person because they have emotions, but you cannot offend a fire alarm. Choice *C*, unplugged, is also incorrect. Choice *D*, disbanded, is the opposite of *activated* and is incorrect in this context.

13. D: Consternation means dread or dismay. Choice *A*, refresh, is not an adjective used to describe a dentist's office, especially when the patient is about to take care of a cavity. Choices *B*, creative, is not a synonym of consternation. Choice *C*, rapture, means ecstatic or happy, and is the opposite sentiment of what we are looking for.

14. B: Told us that the bird was indigenous, or *native* to the southeast part of the United States. Indigenous means native or belonging to a certain area, so Choice *B* is the best answer here. Choice *A*, entertaining, means amusing. Choice *C*, impudent, means bold or shameless. Choice *D*, monotonous, means remaining the same or dull.

15. D: Their bodies wriggled, or *slithered* out of our hands and back into the water. Choices *A* and *C*, exploded and thundered, are too extreme for the context. Deteriorated, Choice *B*, means to crumble or disintegrate, which is not a synonym of wriggled. Choice *D* is the best answer for this sentence.

16. A: Serving means *portion*, Choice *A*. Directed, Choice *B*, means to supervise or conduct, and does not make sense in the context of the sentence. Choice *C*, mourning, means to grieve over, and is also incorrect. Choice *D*, endorsement, means to approve or support something.

Reading Comprehension

17. C: Gulliver becomes acquainted with the people and practices of his new surroundings. Choice *C* is the correct answer because it most extensively summarizes the entire passage. While Choices *A* and *B* are reasonable possibilities, they reference portions of Gulliver's experiences, not the whole. Choice *D* is incorrect because Gulliver doesn't express repentance or sorrow in this particular passage.

18. A: Principal refers to *chief* or *primary* within the context of this text. Choice *A* is the answer that most closely aligns with this answer. Choices *B* and *D* make reference to a helper or followers while Choice *C* doesn't meet the description of Gulliver from the passage.

19. C: One can reasonably infer that Gulliver is considerably larger than the children who were playing around him because multiple children could fit into his hand. Choice *B* is incorrect because there is no indication of stress in Gulliver's tone. Choices *A* and *D* aren't the best answer because though Gulliver seems fond of his new acquaintances, he didn't travel there with the intentions of meeting new people or to express a definite love for them in this particular portion of the text.

20. C: The emperor made a *definitive decision* to expose Gulliver to their native customs. In this instance, the word *mind* was not related to a vote, question, or cognitive ability.

21. A: Choice *A* is correct. This assertion does *not* support the fact that games are a commonplace event in this culture because it mentions conduct, not games. Choices *B*, *C*, and *D* are incorrect because these do support the fact that games were a commonplace event.

22. B: Choice *B* is the only option that mentions the correlation between physical ability and leadership positions. Choices *A* and *D* are unrelated to physical strength and leadership abilities. Choice *C* does not make a deduction that would lead to the correct answer—it only comments upon the abilities of common townspeople.

23. D: The use of "I" could have all of the effects for the reader; it could serve to have a "hedging" effect, allow the reader to connect with the author in a more personal way, and cause the reader to empathize more with the egrets. However, it doesn't distance the reader from the text, thus eliminating Choice *D*.

24. C: The quote provides an example of a warden protecting one of the colonies. Choice *A* is incorrect because the speaker of the quote is a warden, not a hunter. Choice B is incorrect because the quote does not lighten the mood but shows the danger of the situation between the wardens and the hunters. Choice *D* is incorrect because there is no humor found in the quote.

25. D: A *rookery* is a colony of breeding birds. Although *rookery* could mean Choice *A*, houses in a slum area, it does not make sense in this context. Choices *B* and *C* are both incorrect, as this is not a place for hunters to trade tools or for wardens to trade stories.

26. B: An important bird colony. The previous sentence is describing "twenty colonies" of birds, so what follows should be a bird colony. Choice *A* may be true, but we have no evidence of this in the text. Choice *C* does touch on the tension between the hunters and wardens, but there is no official "Bird Island Battle" mentioned in the text. Choice *D* does not exist in the text.

27. D: To demonstrate the success of the protective work of the Audubon Association. The text mentions several different times how and why the association has been successful and gives examples to back this fact. Choice *A* is incorrect because although the article, in some instances, calls certain people to act, it is not the purpose of the entire passage. There is no way to tell if Choices *B* and *C* are correct, as they are not mentioned in the text.

28. C: To have a better opportunity to hunt the birds. Choice *A* might be true in a general sense, but it is not relevant to the context of the text. Choice *B* is incorrect because the hunters are not studying lines of flight to help wardens, but to hunt birds. Choice *D* is incorrect because nothing in the text mentions that hunters are trying to build homes underneath lines of flight of birds for good luck.

29. A: It introduces certain insects that transition from water to air. Choice *B* is incorrect because although the passage talks about gills, it is not the central idea of the passage. Choices *C* and *D* are incorrect because the passage does not "define" or "invite," but only serves as an introduction to stoneflies, dragonflies, and mayflies and their transition from water to air.

30. C: The act of shedding part or all of the outer shell. Choices *A*, *B*, and *D* are incorrect.

31. B: The first paragraph serves as a contrast to the second. Notice how the first paragraph goes into detail describing how insects are able to breathe air. The second paragraph acts as a contrast to the first by stating "[i]t is of great interest to find that, nevertheless, a number of insects spend much of their time under water." Watch for transition words such as "nevertheless" to help find what type of passage you're dealing with.

32: C: The stage of preparation in between molting is acted out in the water, while the last stage is in the air. Choices *A, B,* and *D* are all incorrect. *Instars* is the phase between two periods of molting, and the text explains when these transitions occur.

33. C: The author's tone is informative and exhibits interest in the subject of the study. Overall, the author presents us with information on the subject. One moment where personal interest is depicted is when the author states, "It is of great interest to find that, nevertheless, a number of insects spend much of their time under water."

34. C: Their larva can breathe the air dissolved in water through gills of some kind. This is stated in the last paragraph. Choice *A* is incorrect because the text mentions this in a general way at the beginning of the passage concerning "insects as a whole." Choice *B* is incorrect because this is stated of beetles and water-bugs, and not the insects in question. Choice *D* is incorrect because this is the opposite of what the text says of instars.

35. A: Bring to light an alternative view on human perception by examining the role of technology in human understanding. This is a challenging question because the author's purpose is somewhat open-ended. The author concludes by stating that the questions regarding human perception and observation can be approached from many angles. Thus, they do not seem to be attempting to prove one thing or another. Choice B is incorrect because we cannot know for certain whether the electron experiment is the latest discovery in astroparticle physics because no date is given. Choice *C* is a broad generalization that does not reflect accurately on the writer's views. While the author does appear to reflect on opposing views of human understanding (Choice *D*), the best answer is Choice *A*.

36. C: It presents a problem, explains the details of that problem, and then ends with more inquiry. The beginning of this paragraph literally "presents a conundrum," explains the problem of partial understanding, and then ends with more questions, or inquiry. There is no solution offered in this paragraph, making Choices *A* and *B* incorrect. Choice *D* is incorrect because the paragraph does not begin with a definition.

37. D: Looking back in the text, the author describes that classical philosophy holds that understanding can be reached by careful observation. This will not work if they are overly invested or biased in their pursuit. Choices *A* and *C* are in no way related and are completely unnecessary. A specific theory is not necessary to understanding, according to classical philosophy mentioned by the author. Again, the key to understanding is observing the phenomena outside of it, without biased or predisposition. Thus, Choice *B* is wrong.

38. B: The electrons passed through both holes and then onto the plate. Choices *A* and *C* are wrong because such movement is not mentioned at all in the text. In the passage the author says that electrons that were physically observed appeared to pass through one hole or another. Remember, the electrons that were observed doing this were described as acting like particles. Therefore, Choice D is wrong. Recall that the plate actually recorded electrons passing through both holes simultaneously and hitting the plate This behavior, the electron activity that wasn't seen by humans, was characteristic of waves. Thus, Choice *B* is the right answer.

39. C: To demonstrate an example of natural phenomena humans discovered and understand without the use of tools or machines. Choice *A* mirrors the language in the beginning of the paragraph but is incorrect in its intent. Choice *B* is incorrect; the paragraph mentions nothing of "not knowing the true nature of gravity." Choice *D* is incorrect as well. There is no mention of an "alternative solution" in this paragraph.

40. A: The important thing to keep in mind is that we must choose a scenario that best parallels, or is most similar to, the discovery of the experiment mentioned in the passage. The important aspects of the experiment can be summed up like so: humans directly observed one behavior of electrons and then through analyzing a tool (the plate that recorded electron hits), discovered that there was another electron behavior that could not be physically seen by human eyes. This best parallels the scenario in Choice A. Like Feynman, the colorblind person is able to observe one aspect of the world but through the special goggles (a tool) he is able to see a natural phenomenon that he could not physically see on his own. While Choice D is compelling, the x-ray helps humans see the broken bone, not necessarily revealing that the bone is broken in the first place. The other choices do not parallel the scenario in question. Therefore, Choice A is the best choice.

41. B: The author would not agree that technology renders human observation irrelevant. Choice A is incorrect because much of the passage discusses how technology helps humans observe what cannot be seen with the naked eye, therefore the author would agree with this statement. This line of reasoning is also why the author would agree with Choice D, making it incorrect as well. As indicated in the second paragraph, the author seems to think that humans create inventions and tools with the goal of studying phenomena more precisely. This indicates increased understanding as people recognize limitations and develop items to help bypass the limitations and learn. Therefore, Choice C is incorrect as well. Again, the author doesn't attempt to disprove or dismiss classical philosophy.

42. A: The tone is exasperated. While contemplative is an option because of the inquisitive nature of the text, Choice A is correct because the speaker is annoyed by the thought of being included when he felt that the fellow members of his race were being excluded. The speaker is not nonchalant, nor accepting of the circumstances which he describes.

43. C: Choice C, *contented*, is the only word that has different meaning. Furthermore, the speaker expresses objection and disdain throughout the entire text.

44. B: To address the feelings of exclusion expressed by African Americans after the establishment of the Fourth of July holiday. While the speaker makes biblical references, it is not the main focus of the passage, thus eliminating Choice A as an answer. The passage also makes no mention of wealthy landowners and doesn't speak of any positive response to the historical events, so Choices C and D are not correct.

45. D: Choice D is the correct answer because it clearly makes reference to justice being denied.

46. D: Hyperbole. Choices A and B are unrelated. Assonance is the repetition of sounds and commonly occurs in poetry. Parallelism refers to two statements that correlate in some manner. Choice C is incorrect because amplification normally refers to clarification of meaning by broadening the sentence structure, while hyperbole refers to a phrase or statement that is being exaggerated.

47. C: Display the equivocation of the speaker and those that he represents. Choice C is correct because the speaker is clear about his intention and stance throughout the text. Choice A could be true, but the words "common text" is arguable. Choice B is also partially true, as another group of people affected by slavery are being referenced. However, the speaker is not trying to convince the audience that injustices have been committed, as it is already understood there have been injustices committed. Choice D is also close to the correct answer, but it is not the *best* answer choice possible.

48. C: We are looking for an inference—a conclusion that is reached on the basis of evidence and reasoning—from the passage that will likely explain why the famous children's author did not achieve her usual success with the new genre (despite the book's acclaim). Choice *A* is wrong because the statement is false according to the passage. Choice *B* is wrong because, although the passage says the author has a graduate degree on the subject, it would be an unrealistic leap to infer that she is the foremost expert on Antebellum America. Choice *D* is wrong because there is nothing in the passage to lead us to infer that people generally prefer a children's series to historical fiction. In contrast, Choice *C* can be logically inferred since the passage speaks of the great success of the children's series and the declaration that the fame of the author's name causes the children's books to "fly off the shelves." Thus, she did not receive any bump from her name since she published the historical novel under a pseudonym, and Choice *C* is correct.

49. C: The author contrasts two different viewpoints, then builds a case showing preference for one over the other. Choice *A* is incorrect because the introduction does not contain an impartial definition, but rather, an opinion. Choice *B* is incorrect. There is no puzzling phenomenon given, as the author doesn't mention any peculiar cause or effect that is in question regarding poetry. Choice *D* does contain another's viewpoint at the beginning of the passage; however, to say that the author has no stake in this argument is incorrect; the author uses personal experiences to build their case.

50. B: Choice *B* accurately describes the author's argument in the text: that poetry is not irrelevant. While the author does praise, and even value, Buddy Wakefield as a poet, the author never heralds him as a genius. Eliminate Choice *A*, as it is an exaggeration. Not only is Choice *C* an exaggerated statement, but the author never mentions spoken word poetry in the text. Choice *D* is wrong because this statement contradicts the writer's argument.

51. D: *Exiguously* means not occurring often, or occurring rarely, so Choice *D* would LEAST change the meaning of the sentence. Choice *A*, *indolently*, means unhurriedly, or slow, and does not fit the context of the sentence. Choice *B*, *inaudibly*, means quietly or silently. Choice *C*, *interminably*, means endlessly, or all the time, and is the opposite of the word *exiguously*.

52. D: A student's insistence that psychoanalysis is a subset of modern psychology is the most analogous option. The author of the passage tries to insist that performance poetry is a subset of modern poetry, and therefore, tries to prove that modern poetry is not "dying," but thriving on social media for the masses. Choice *A* is incorrect, as the author is not refusing any kind of validation. Choice *B* is incorrect; the author's insistence is that poetry will *not* lose popularity. Choice *C* mimics the topic but compares two different genres, while the author does no comparison in this passage.

53. B: The author's purpose is to disprove Gioia's article claiming that poetry is a dying art form that only survives in academic settings. In order to prove his argument, the author educates the reader about new developments in poetry (Choice *A*) and describes the brilliance of a specific modern poet (Choice *C*), but these serve as examples of a growing poetry trend that counters Gioia's argument. Choice *D* is incorrect because it contradicts the author's argument.

54. D: This question is difficult because the choices offer real reasons as to why the author includes the quote. However, the question specifically asks for the *main reason* for including the quote. The quote from a recently written poem shows that people are indeed writing, publishing, and performing poetry (Choice *B*). The quote also shows that people are still listening to poetry (Choice *C*). These things are true, and by their nature, serve to disprove Gioia's views (Choice *A*), which is the author's goal. However, Choice *D* is the most direct reason for including the quote, because the article analyzes the quote for its "complex themes" that "draws listeners and appreciation" right after it's given.

55. D: The author explains that Boethianism is a Medieval theological philosophy that attributes sin to temporary pleasure and righteousness with virtue and God's providence. Besides Choice D, the choices listed are all physical things. While these could still be divine rewards, Boethianism holds that the true reward for being virtuous is in God's favor. It is also stressed in the article that physical pleasures cannot be taken into the afterlife. Therefore, the best choice is D, God's favor.

56. C: *The Canterbury Tales* presents a manuscript written in the medieval period that can help illustrate Boethianism through stories and show how people of the time might have responded to the idea. Choices A and B are generalized statements, and we have no evidence to support Choice B. Choice D is very compelling, but it looks at Boethianism in a way that the author does not. The author does not mention "different levels of Boethianism" when discussing the tales, only that the concept appears differently in different tales. Boethianism also doesn't focus on enlightenment.

57. D: The author is referring to the principle that a desire for material goods leads to moral malfeasance punishable by a higher being. Choice A is incorrect; while the text does mention thieves ravaging others' possessions, it is only meant as an example and not as the principle itself. Choice B is incorrect for the same reason as A. Choice C is mentioned in the text and is part of the example that proves the principle, and also not the principle itself.

58. C: The word *avarice* most nearly means *parsimoniousness*, or an unwillingness to spend money. Choice A means *evil* or *mischief* and does not relate to the context of the sentence. Choice B is also incorrect, because *pithiness* means *shortness* or *conciseness*. Choice D is close because *precariousness* means dangerous or instability, which goes well with the context. However, we are told of the summoner's specific characteristic of greed, which makes Choice C the best answer.

59. D: Desire for pleasure can lead toward sin. Boethianism acknowledges desire as something that leads out of holiness, so Choice A is incorrect. Choice B is incorrect because in the passage, Boethianism is depicted as being wary of desire and anything that binds people to the physical world. Choice C can be eliminated because the author never says that desire indicates demonic.

60. B: Choice A uses similar language, but it is not the main point of disagreement. The reporter calls the loss devastating, and there's no reason to believe that the coach would disagree with this assessment. Eliminate this choice.

Choice B is strong since both passages mention the at-bats with runners in scoring position. The reporter asserts that the team lost due to the team failing to get such a hit. In contrast, the coach identifies several other reasons for the loss, including fielding and pitching errors. Additionally, the coach disagrees that the team even needed a hit in those situations.

Choice C is mentioned by the coach, but not by the reporter. It is unclear whether the reporter would agree with this assessment. Eliminate this choice.

Choice D is mentioned by the coach but not by the reporter. It is not stated whether the reporter believes that the team deserved to win. Eliminate this choice.

Therefore, Choice B is the correct answer.

61. C: Choice *A* is incorrect. The Conservative Politician definitely believes that spending on social welfare programs increases the national debt. However, the Liberal Politician does not address the cost of those programs. Choice *B* is a strong answer choice. The Liberal Politician explicitly agrees that certain classes of people rely on social welfare programs. The Conservative Politician actually agrees that people rely on the programs, but thinks this reliance is detrimental. This answer choice is slightly off base. Eliminate this choice. Choice *C* improves on Choice *B*. The Liberal Politician definitely believes that certain classes of people would be irreparably harmed. In contrast, the Conservative Politician asserts that the programs are actually harmful since people become dependent on the programs. The Conservative Politician concludes that people don't need the assistance and would be better off if left to fend for themselves. This is definitely the main point of disagreement. Choice *D* is not the main point of dispute. Neither of the politicians discusses whether *all* of the nation's leaders have bootstrapped their way to the top. Eliminate this choice.

62. A: The word *patronage* most nearly means *auspices*, which means *protection* or *support*. Choice *B*, *aberration*, means *deformity* and does not make sense within the context of the sentence. Choice *C*, *acerbic*, means *bitter* and also does not make sense in the sentence. Choice *D*, *adulation*, is a positive word meaning *praise*, and thus does not fit with the word *condescending* in the sentence.

63. D: *Working man* is most closely aligned with Choice *D*, *bourgeois*. In the context of the speech, the word *bourgeois* means *working* or *middle class*. Choice *A*, *plebian*, does suggest *common people*; however, this is a term that is specific to ancient Rome. Choice *B*, *viscount*, is a European title used to describe a specific degree of nobility. Choice *C*, *entrepreneur*, is a person who operates their own business.

64. C: In the context of the speech, the term *working man* most closely correlates with Choice *C*, *working man is someone who works for wages among the middle class.* Choice *A* is not mentioned in the passage and is off-topic. Choice *B* may be true in some cases, but it does not reflect the sentiment described for the term *working man* in the passage. Choice *D* may also be arguably true. However, it is not given as a definition but as *acts* of the working man, and the topics of *field, factory,* and *screen* are not mentioned in the passage.

65. D: *Enterprise* most closely means *cause*. Choices *A, B,* and *C* are all related to the term *enterprise*. However, Dickens speaks of a *cause* here, not a company, courage, or a game. *He will stand by such an enterprise* is a call to stand by a cause to enable the working man to have a certain autonomy over his own economic standing. The very first paragraph ends with the statement that the working man *shall . . . have a share in the management of an institution which is designed for his benefit.*

66. B: The speaker's salutation is one from an entertainer to his audience and uses the friendly language to connect to his audience before a serious speech. Recall in the first paragraph that the speaker is there to "accompany [the audience] . . . through one of my little Christmas books," making him an author there to entertain the crowd with his own writing. The speech preceding the reading is the passage itself, and, as the tone indicates, a serious speech addressing the "working man." Although the passage speaks of employers and employees, the speaker himself is not an employer of the audience, so Choice *A* is incorrect. Choice *C* is also incorrect, as the salutation is not used ironically, but sincerely, as the speech addresses the well-being of the crowd. Choice *D* is incorrect because the speech is not given by a politician, but by a writer.

67: B: Choice *A* is incorrect because that is the speaker's *first* desire, not his second. Choices *C* and *D* are tricky because the language of both of these is mentioned after the word *second*. However, the speaker doesn't get to the second wish until the next sentence. Choices *C* and *D* are merely prepositions preparing for the statement of the main clause, Choice *B,* for the working man to have a say in his institution which is designed for his benefit.

68. C: In lines 6 and 7, it is stated that avarice can prevent a man from being necessitously poor, but too timorous, or fearful, to achieve real wealth. According to the passage, avarice does tend to make a person very wealthy. The passage states that oppression, not avarice, is the consequence of wealth. The passage does not state that avarice drives a person's desire to be wealthy.

69. D: Paine believes that the distinction that is beyond a natural or religious reason is between king and subjects. He states that the distinction between good and bad is made in heaven. The distinction between male and female is natural. He does not mention anything about the distinction between humans and animals.

70. A: The passage states that the Heathens were the first to introduce government by kings into the world. The quiet lives of patriarchs came before the Heathens introduced this type of government. It was Christians, not Heathens, who paid divine honors to living kings. Heathens honored deceased kings. Equal rights of nature are mentioned in the paragraph, but not in relation to the Heathens.

71. B: Paine asserts that a monarchy is against the equal rights of nature and cites several parts of scripture that also denounce it. He doesn't say it is against the laws of nature. Because he uses scripture to further his argument, it is not despite scripture that he denounces the monarchy. Paine addresses the law by saying the courts also do not support a monarchical government.

72. A: To be *idolatrous* is to worship idols or heroes, in this case, kings. It is not defined as being deceitful. While idolatry is considered a sin, it is an example of a sin, not a synonym for it. Idolatry may have been considered illegal in some cultures, but it is not a definition for the term.

73. A: The essential meaning of the passage is that the Almighty, God, would disapprove of this type of government. While heaven is mentioned, it is done so to suggest that the monarchical government is irreverent, not that heaven isn't promised. God's disapproval is mentioned, not his punishment. The passage refers to the Jewish monarchy, which required both belief in God and kings.

74. A: First person. This is a straightforward question that requires readers to know that a first-person narrator speaks from an "I" point of view.

75. D: He doesn't understand all of the languages being used. This can be inferred from the fact that the traveler must refer to his dictionary to understand those around him. Choice *A* isn't a good choice because the traveler seems to wonder why the driver needs to drive so fast. Choice *B* isn't mentioned in the passage and doesn't seem like a good answer choice because he seems wholly unfamiliar with his surroundings. This is why Choice C can also be eliminated.

76. B: From fearful to charmed. This can be found in the first sentence of the third paragraph, which states, "I soon lost sight and recollection of ghostly fears in the beauty of the scene as we drove along." Also, readers should get a sense of foreboding from the first two paragraphs, where superstitious villagers seem frightened on the traveler's behalf. However, the final paragraph changes to delighted descriptions of the landscape's natural beauty. Choices *A* and *D* can be eliminated because the traveler is anxious, not relaxed or comfortable at the beginning of the passage. Choice *C* can also be eliminated because the traveler doesn't gain any particular insights in the last paragraph, and in fact continues to lament that he cannot understand the speech of those around him.

77. D: A complete stranger. The answer to this reading comprehension question can be found in the second paragraph, when the traveler is "just starting for an unknown place to meet an unknown man"— in other words, a complete stranger.

78. C: The traveler will soon encounter danger or evil. Answering this prediction question requires readers to understand foreshadowing, or hints that the author gives about what will happen next. There are numerous hints scattered throughout this passage: the villager's sorrow and sympathy for the traveler and their superstitious actions; the spooky words that the traveler overhears; the driver's unexplained haste. All of these point to a danger that awaits the protagonist.

79. A: "I must say they weren't cheering to me, for amongst them were "Ordog"—Satan, "pokol"—hell, "stregoica"—witch, "vrolok" and "vlkoslak"—both of which mean the same thing, one being Slovak and the other Servian for something that is either were-wolf or vampire." As mentioned in question 39, this sentence is an example of how the author hints at evil to come for the traveler. The other answer choices aren't related to the passage's grim foreshadowing.

80. C: This is a tricky question, but it can be solved through careful context analysis and vocabulary knowledge. One can infer that the use of "expedient," while not necessarily very positive, isn't inherently bad in this context either. Note how in the next line, he says, "but most governments are usually, and all governments are sometimes, inexpedient." This use of "inexpedient" indicates that a government becomes a hindrance rather than a solution; it slows progress rather than helps facilitate progress. Thus, Choice *A* and Choice *D* can be ruled out because these are more of the result of government, not the intention or initial design. Choice *B* makes no logical sense. Therefore, Choice *C* is the best description of *expedient*. Essentially, Thoreau is saying that government is constructed as a way of developing order and people's rights, but the rigidness of government soon inhibits justice and human rights.

81. B: While Choice *D* is the only answer that mentions the Mexican War directly, Thoreau clearly thinks the war is unnecessary because the people generally didn't consent to the war. Choices *A*, *B*, and *C* are all correct to a degree, but the answer asks for the best description. Therefore, Choice *B* is the most accurate representation of Thoreau's views. Essentially, Thoreau brings to light the fact that the few people in power can twist government and policy for their own needs.

82. D: Choice *C* and Choice *B* are completely incorrect. Thoreau is not defending government in any way. His views are set against government. As mentioned in the text, he appreciates little government but favors having no government structure at all. The text is reflective by nature, but what makes Choice *D* a more appropriate answer is the presence of evidence in the text. Thoreau cites current events and uses them to illustrate the point he's trying to make.

83. C: One of Thoreau's biggest criticisms of government is its capacity to impose on the people's freedoms and liberties, enacting rules that the people don't want and removing power from the individual. None of the scenarios directly impose specific regulations or restrictions on the people, except Prohibition. Prohibition removed the choice to consume alcohol in favor of abstinence, which was favored by the religious conservatives of the time. Thus, Thoreau would point out that this is a clear violation of free choice and an example of government meddling.

84. A: Choice *B* is totally irrelevant. Choice *C* is also incorrect; Thoreau never personifies government. Also, this doesn't coincide with his wooden gun analogy. Choice *D* is compelling because of its language but doesn't define the statement. Choice *A* is the most accurate summary of the main point of Thoreau's statement.

85. B: Thoreau specifically cites that legislators "are continually putting in their way." This reflects his suspicion and concern of government intervention. Recall that Thoreau continually mentions that government, while meant as a way to establish freedom, is easily used to suppress freedom, piling on regulations and rules that inhibit progress. Choice *B* is the answer that most directly states how Thoreau sees government getting in the way of freedom.

Math

Numbers and Operations

Base-10 Numerals, Number Names, and Expanded Form

Numbers used in everyday life are constituted in a *base-10 system*. Each digit in a number, depending on its location, represents some multiple of 10, or quotient of 10 when dealing with decimals. Each digit to the left of the decimal point represents a higher multiple of 10. Each digit to the right of the decimal point represents a quotient of a higher multiple of 10 for the divisor. For example, consider the number 7,631.42. The digit one represents simply the number one. The digit 3 represents 3×10. The digit 6 represents:

$$6 \times 10 \times 10 \text{ (or } 6 \times 100)$$

The digit 7 represents $7 \times 10 \times 10 \times 10$ (or 7×1000). The digit 4 represents $4 \div 10$. The digit 2 represents $(2 \div 10) \div 10$, or $2 \div (10 \times 10)$ or $2 \div 100$.

A number is written in *expanded form* by expressing it as the sum of the value of each of its digits. The expanded form in the example above, which is written with the highest value first down to the lowest value, is expressed as:

$$7,000 + 600 + 30 + 1 + .4 + .02$$

When verbally expressing a number, the integer part of the number (the numbers to the left of the decimal point) resembles the expanded form without the addition between values. In the above example, the numbers read "seven thousand six hundred thirty-one." When verbally expressing the decimal portion of a number, the number is read as a whole number, followed by the place value of the furthest digit (non-zero) to the right. In the above example, 0.42 is read "forty-two hundredths." Reading the number 7,631.42 in its entirety is expressed as "seven thousand six hundred thirty-one and forty-two hundredths." The word *and* is used between the integer and decimal parts of the number.

Composing and Decomposing Multi-Digit Numbers

Composing and decomposing numbers aids in conceptualizing what each digit of a multi-digit number represents. The standard, or typical, form in which numbers are written consists of a series of digits representing a given value based on their place value. Consider the number 592.7. This number is composed of 5 hundreds, 9 tens, 2 ones, and 7 tenths.

Composing a number requires adding the given numbers for each place value and writing the numbers in standard form. For example, composing 4 thousands, 5 hundreds, 2 tens, and 8 ones consists of adding as follows: $4,000 + 500 + 20 + 8$, to produce 4,528 (standard form).

Decomposing a number requires taking a number written in standard form and breaking it apart into the sum of each place value. For example, the number 83.17 is decomposed by breaking it into the sum of 4 values (for each of the 4 digits): 8 tens, 3 ones, 1 tenth, and 7 hundredths. The decomposed or "expanded" form of 83.17 is:

$$80 + 3 + .1 + .07$$

Place Value of a Given Digit

The number system that is used consists of only ten different digits or characters. However, this system is used to represent an infinite number of values. The *place value system* makes this infinite number of values possible. The position in which a digit is written corresponds to a given value. Starting from the decimal point (which is implied, if not physically present), each subsequent place value to the left represents a value greater than the one before it. Conversely, starting from the decimal point, each subsequent place value to the right represents a value less than the one before it.

The names for the place values to the left of the decimal point are as follows:

...	Billions	Hundred-Millions	Ten-Millions	Millions	Hundred-Thousands	Ten-Thousands	Thousands	Hundreds	Tens	Ones

*Note that this table can be extended infinitely further to the left.

The names for the place values to the right of the decimal point are as follows:

Decimal Point (.)	Tenths	Hundredths	Thousandths	Ten-Thousandths	...

*Note that this table can be extended infinitely further to the right.

When given a multi-digit number, the value of each digit depends on its place value. Consider the number 682,174.953. Referring to the chart above, it can be determined that the digit 8 is in the ten-thousands place. It is in the fifth place to the left of the decimal point. Its value is 8 ten-thousands or 80,000. The digit 5 is two places to the right of the decimal point. Therefore, the digit 5 is in the hundredths place. Its value is 5 hundredths or $\frac{5}{100}$ (equivalent to .05).

Base-10 System

<u>Value of Digits</u>
In accordance with the *base-10 system*, the value of a digit increases by a factor of ten each place it moves to the left. For example, consider the number 7. Moving the digit one place to the left (70), increases its value by a factor of 10 ($7 \times 10 = 70$). Moving the digit two places to the left (700) increases its value by a factor of 10 twice ($7 \times 10 \times 10 = 700$). Moving the digit three places to the left (7,000) increases its value by a factor of 10 three times ($7 \times 10 \times 10 \times 10 = 7,000$), and so on.

Conversely, the value of a digit decreases by a factor of ten each place it moves to the right. (Note that multiplying by $\frac{1}{10}$ is equivalent to dividing by 10). For example, consider the number 40. Moving the digit one place to the right (4) decreases its value by a factor of 10 ($40 \div 10 = 4$). Moving the digit two places to the right (0.4), decreases its value by a factor of 10 twice ($40 \div 10 \div 10 = 0.4$) or ($40 \times \frac{1}{10} \times \frac{1}{10} = 0.4$). Moving the digit three places to the right (0.04) decreases its value by a factor of 10 three times ($40 \div 10 \div 10 \div 10 = 0.04$) or ($40 \times \frac{1}{10} \times \frac{1}{10} \times \frac{1}{10} = 0.04$), and so on.

<u>Exponents to Denote Powers of 10</u>
The value of a given digit of a number in the base-10 system can be expressed utilizing powers of 10. A power of 10 refers to 10 raised to a given exponent such as 10^0, 10^1, 10^2, 10^3, etc. For the number 10^3, 10 is the base and 3 is the exponent. A base raised by an exponent represents how many times the base is multiplied by itself. Therefore, $10^1 = 10$, $10^2 = 10 \times 10 = 100$, $10^3 = 10 \times 10 \times 10 = 1,000$, $10^4 = 10 \times 10 \times 10 \times 10 = 10,000$, etc. Any base with a zero exponent equals one.

Powers of 10 are utilized to decompose a multi-digit number without writing all the zeroes. Consider the number 872,349. This number is decomposed to:

$$800,000 + 70,000 + 2,000 + 300 + 40 + 9$$

When utilizing powers of 10, the number 872,349 is decomposed to:

$$(8 \times 10^5) + (7 \times 10^4) + (2 \times 10^3) + (3 \times 10^2) + (4 \times 10^1) + (9 \times 10^0)$$

The power of 10 by which the digit is multiplied corresponds to the number of zeroes following the digit when expressing its value in standard form. For example, 7×10^4 is equivalent to 70,000 or 7 followed by four zeros.

Rounding Multi-Digit Numbers

Rounding numbers changes the given number to a simpler and less accurate number than the exact given number. Rounding allows for easier calculations which estimate the results of using the exact given number. The accuracy of the estimate and ease of use depends on the place value to which the number is rounded. Rounding numbers consists of:

- Determining what place value the number is being rounded to
- Examining the digit to the right of the desired place value to decide whether to round up or keep the digit
- Replacing all digits to the right of the desired place value with zeros

To round 746,311 to the nearest ten thousands, the digit in the ten thousands place should be located first. In this case, this digit is 4 (746,311). Then, the digit to its right is examined. If this digit is 5 or greater, the number will be rounded up by increasing the digit in the desired place by one. If the digit to the right of the place value being rounded is 4 or less, the number will be kept the same. For the given example, the digit being examined is a 6, which means that the number will be rounded up by increasing the digit to the left by one. Therefore, the digit 4 is changed to a 5. Finally, to write the rounded number, any digits to the left of the place value being rounded remain the same and any to its right are replaced with zeros. For the given example, rounding 746,311 to the nearest ten thousand will produce 750,000. To round 746,311 to the nearest hundred, the digit to the right of the three in the hundreds place is examined to determine whether to round up or keep the same number. In this case, that digit is a one, so the number will be kept the same and any digits to its right will be replaced with zeros. The resulting rounded number is 746,300.

Rounding place values to the right of the decimal follows the same procedure, but digits being replaced by zeros can simply be dropped. To round 3.752891 to the nearest thousandth, the desired place value is located (3.752891) and the digit to the right is examined. In this case, the digit 8 indicates that the number will be rounded up, and the 2 in the thousandths place will increase to a 3. Rounding up and replacing the digits to the right of the thousandths place produces 3.753000 which is equivalent to 3.753. Therefore, the zeros are not necessary and the rounded number should be written as 3.753.

When rounding up, if the digit to be increased is a 9, the digit to its left is increased by 1 and the digit in the desired place value is changed to a zero. For example, the number 1,598 rounded to the nearest ten is 1,600. Another example shows the number 43.72961 rounded to the nearest thousandth is 43.730 or 43.73.

Solving Multistep Mathematical and Real-World Problems

<u>Problem Situations for Operations</u>
Addition and subtraction are *inverse operations*. Adding a number and then subtracting the same number will cancel each other out, resulting in the original number, and vice versa. For example, $8 + 7 - 7 = 8$ and $137 - 100 + 100 = 137$. Similarly, multiplication and division are inverse operations. Therefore, multiplying by a number and then dividing by the same number results in the original number, and vice versa. For example, $8 \times 2 \div 2 = 8$ and $12 \div 4 \times 4 = 12$. Inverse operations are used to work backwards to solve problems. In the case that 7 and a number add to 18, the inverse operation of subtraction is used to find the unknown value ($18 - 7 = 11$). If a school's entire 4th grade was divided evenly into 3 classes each with 22 students, the inverse operation of multiplication is used to determine the total students in the grade ($22 \times 3 = 66$). Additional scenarios involving inverse operations are included in the tables below.

There are a variety of real-world situations in which one or more of the operators is used to solve a problem. The tables below display the most common scenarios.

<u>Addition & Subtraction</u>

	Unknown Result	**Unknown Change**	**Unknown Start**
Adding to	5 students were in class. 4 more students arrived. How many students are in class? $5 + 4 = ?$	8 students were in class. More students arrived late. There are now 18 students in class. How many students arrived late? $8 + ? = 18$ Solved by inverse operations $18 - 8 = ?$	Some students were in class early. 11 more students arrived. There are now 17 students in class. How many students were in class early? $? + 11 = 17$ Solved by inverse operations $17 - 11 = ?$
Taking from	15 students were in class. 5 students left class. How many students are in class now? $15 - 5 = ?$	12 students were in class. Some students left class. There are now 8 students in class. How many students left class? $12 - ? = 8$ Solved by inverse operations $8 + ? = 12 \rightarrow 12 - 8 = ?$	Some students were in class. 3 students left class. Then there were 13 students in class. How many students were in class before? $? - 3 = 13$ Solved by inverse operations $13 + 3 = ?$

	Unknown Total	**Unknown Addends (Both)**	**Unknown Addends (One)**
Putting together/ taking apart	The homework assignment is 10 addition problems and 8 subtraction problems. How many problems are in the homework assignment? $10 + 8 = ?$	Bobby has $9. How much can Bobby spend on candy and how much can Bobby spend on toys? $9 = ? + ?$	Bobby has 12 pairs of pants. 5 pairs of pants are shorts, and the rest are long. How many pairs of long pants does he have? $12 = 5 + ?$ Solved by inverse operations $12 - 5 = ?$

	Unknown Difference	Unknown Larger Value	Unknown Smaller Value
Comparing	Bobby has 5 toys. Tommy has 8 toys. How many more toys does Tommy have than Bobby? $5+?=8$ Solved by inverse operations $8-5=?$ Bobby has $6. Tommy has $10. How many fewer dollars does Bobby have than Tommy? $10-6=?$	Tommy has 2 more toys than Bobby. Bobby has 4 toys. How many toys does Tommy have? $2+4=?$ Bobby has 3 fewer dollars than Tommy. Bobby has $8. How many dollars does Tommy have? $?-3=8$ Solved by inverse operations $8+3=?$	Tommy has 6 more toys than Bobby. Tommy has 10 toys. How many toys does Bobby have? $?+6=10$ Solved by inverse operations $10-6=?$ Bobby has $5 less than Tommy. Tommy has $9. How many dollars does Bobby have? $9-5=?$

Multiplication and Division

	Unknown Product	Unknown Group Size	Unknown Number of Groups
Equal groups	There are 5 students, and each student has 4 pieces of candy. How many pieces of candy are there in all? $5\times4=?$	14 pieces of candy are shared equally by 7 students. How many pieces of candy does each student have? $7\times?=14$ Solved by inverse operations $14\div7=?$	If 18 pieces of candy are to be given out 3 to each student, how many students will get candy? $?\times3=18$ Solved by inverse operations $18\div3=?$
	Unknown Product	**Unknown Factor**	**Unknown Factor**
Arrays	There are 5 rows of students with 3 students in each row. How many students are there? $5\times3=?$	If 16 students are arranged into 4 equal rows, how many students will be in each row? $4\times?=16$ Solved by inverse operations $16\div4=?$	If 24 students are arranged into an array with 6 columns, how many rows are there? $?\times6=24$ Solved by inverse operations $24\div6=?$
	Larger Unknown	**Smaller Unknown**	**Multiplier Unknown**
Comparing	A small popcorn costs $1.50. A large popcorn costs 3 times as much as a small popcorn. How much does a large popcorn cost? $1.50\times3=?$	A large soda costs $6 and that is 2 times as much as a small soda. How much does a small soda cost? $2\times?=6$ Solved by inverse operations $6\div2=?$	A large pretzel costs $3 and a small pretzel costs $2. How many times as much does the large pretzel cost as the small pretzel? $?\times2=3$ Solved by inverse operations $3\div2=?$

Remainders in Division Problems

If a given total cannot be divided evenly into a given number of groups, the amount left over is the *remainder*. Consider the following scenario: 32 textbooks must be packed into boxes for storage. Each box holds 6 textbooks. How many boxes are needed? To determine the answer, 32 is divided by 6, resulting in 5 with a remainder of 2. A remainder may be interpreted three ways:

- Add 1 to the quotient
  How many boxes will be needed? Six boxes will be needed because five will not be enough.

- Use only the quotient
  How many boxes will be full? Five boxes will be full.

- Use only the remainder
  If you only have 5 boxes, how many books will not fit? Two books will not fit.

Strategies and Algorithms to Perform Operations on Rational Numbers

A *rational number* is any number that can be written in the form of a ratio or fraction. Integers can be written as fractions with a denominator of 1:

$$5 = \frac{5}{1}$$

$$-342 = \frac{-342}{1}$$

Decimals that terminate and/or repeat can also be written as fractions:

$$47 = \frac{47}{100}$$

$$.\overline{33} = \frac{1}{3}$$

For more on converting decimals to fractions, see the section *Converting Between Fractions, Decimals, and Percent*.

When adding or subtracting fractions, the numbers must have the same denominators. In these cases, numerators are added or subtracted and denominators are kept the same. For example, $\frac{2}{7} + \frac{3}{7} = \frac{5}{7}$ and $\frac{4}{5} - \frac{3}{5} = \frac{1}{5}$. If the fractions to be added or subtracted do not have the same denominator, a common denominator must be found. This is accomplished by changing one or both fractions to a different but equivalent fraction. Consider the example $\frac{1}{6} + \frac{4}{9}$. First, a common denominator must be found. One method is to find the least common multiple (LCM) of the denominators 6 and 9. This is the lowest number that both 6 and 9 will divide into evenly. In this case the LCM is 18. Both fractions should be changed to equivalent fractions with a denominator of 18. To obtain the numerator of the new fraction, the old numerator is multiplied by the same number by which the old denominator is multiplied. For the fraction $\frac{1}{6}$, 6 multiplied by 3 will produce a denominator of 18.

Therefore, the numerator is multiplied by 3 to produce the new numerator:

$$\left(\frac{1 \times 3}{6 \times 3} = \frac{3}{18}\right)$$

For the fraction $\frac{4}{9}$, multiplying both the numerator and denominator by 2 produces $\frac{8}{18}$. Since the two new fractions have common denominators, they can be added:

$$\left(\frac{3}{18} + \frac{8}{18} = \frac{11}{18}\right)$$

When multiplying or dividing rational numbers, these numbers may be converted to fractions and multiplied or divided accordingly. When multiplying fractions, all numerators are multiplied by each other and all denominators are multiplied by each other. For example:

$$\frac{1}{3} \times \frac{6}{5}$$

$$\frac{1 \times 6}{3 \times 5}$$

$$\frac{6}{15}$$

and

$$\frac{-1}{2} \times \frac{3}{1} \times \frac{11}{100}$$

$$\frac{-1 \times 3 \times 11}{2 \times 1 \times 100}$$

$$\frac{-33}{200}$$

When dividing fractions, the problem is converted by multiplying by the reciprocal of the divisor. This is done by changing division to multiplication and "flipping" the second fraction, or divisor. For example:

$$\frac{1}{2} \div \frac{3}{5} \rightarrow \frac{1}{2} \times \frac{5}{3}$$

and

$$\frac{5}{1} \div \frac{1}{3} \rightarrow \frac{5}{1} \times \frac{3}{1}$$

To complete the problem, the rules for multiplying fractions should be followed.

Note that when adding, subtracting, multiplying, and dividing mixed numbers (ex. $4\frac{1}{2}$), it is easiest to convert these to improper fractions (larger numerator than denominator). To do so, the denominator is kept the same. To obtain the numerator, the whole number is multiplied by the denominator and added to the numerator. For example, $4\frac{1}{2} = \frac{9}{2}$ and $7\frac{2}{3} = \frac{23}{3}$. Also, note that answers involving fractions should be converted to the simplest form.

Rational Numbers and Their Operations

Irregular Products and Quotients

The following shows examples where multiplication does not result in a product greater than both factors, and where division does not result in a quotient smaller than the dividend.

If multiplying numbers where one or more has a value less than one, the product will not be greater than both factors. For example, $6 \times \frac{1}{2} = 3$ and $0.75 \times 0.2 = .15$. When dividing by a number less than one, the resulting quotient will be greater than the dividend. For example, $8 \div \frac{1}{2} = 16$, because division turns into a multiplication problem:

$$8 \div \frac{1}{2}$$

$$8 \times \frac{2}{1}$$

Another example is $0.5 \div 0.2$, which results in 2.5. The problem can be stated by asking how many times 0.2 will go into 0.5. The number being divided is larger than the number that goes into it, so the result will be a number larger than both factors.

Composing and Decomposing Fractions

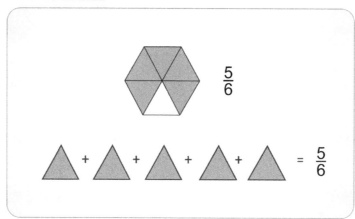

Fractions can be broken apart into sums of fractions with the same denominator. For example, the fraction $\frac{5}{6}$ can be *decomposed* into sums of fractions with all denominators equal to 6 and the numerators adding to 5.

The fraction $\frac{5}{6}$ is decomposed as:

$$\frac{3}{6} + \frac{2}{6}$$

$$\frac{2}{6} + \frac{2}{6} + \frac{1}{6}$$

$$\frac{3}{6} + \frac{1}{6} + \frac{1}{6}$$

$$\frac{1}{6} + \frac{1}{6} + \frac{1}{6} + \frac{2}{6}$$

$$\frac{1}{6} + \frac{1}{6} + \frac{1}{6} + \frac{1}{6} + \frac{1}{6}$$

A unit fraction is a fraction in which the numerator is 1. If decomposing a fraction into unit fractions, the sum will consist of a unit fraction added the number of times equal to the numerator. For example:

$$\frac{3}{4} = \frac{1}{4} + \frac{1}{4} + \frac{1}{4} \text{ (unit fractions } \frac{1}{4} \text{ added 3 times)}$$

Composing fractions is simply the opposite of decomposing. It is the process of adding fractions with the same denominators to produce a single fraction. For example:

$$\frac{3}{7} + \frac{2}{7} = \frac{5}{7}$$

and

$$\frac{1}{5} + \frac{1}{5} + \frac{1}{5} = \frac{3}{5}$$

Decrease in Value of a Unit Fraction

A *unit fraction* is one in which the numerator is 1 ($\frac{1}{2}, \frac{1}{3}, \frac{1}{8}, \frac{1}{20}$, etc.). The denominator indicates the number of *equal pieces* that the whole is divided into. The greater the number of pieces, the smaller each piece will be. Therefore, the greater the denominator of a unit fraction, the smaller it is in value. Unit fractions can also be compared by converting them to decimals. For example, $\frac{1}{2}$ = 0.5, $\frac{1}{3}$ = 0.$\bar{3}$, $\frac{1}{8}$ = 0.125, $\frac{1}{20}$ = 0.05, etc.

Use of the Same Whole when Comparing Fractions

Fractions all represent parts of the same whole. Fractions may have different denominators, but they represent parts of the same one whole, like a pizza. For example, the fractions $\frac{5}{7}$ and $\frac{2}{3}$ can be difficult to compare because they have different denominators. The first fraction may represent a whole divided into seven parts, where five parts are used. The second fraction represents the same whole divided into three parts, where two are used. It may be helpful to convert one or more of the fractions so that they have common denominators for converting to equivalent fractions by finding the LCM of the denominator. Comparing is much easier if fractions are converted to the equivalent fractions of $\frac{15}{21}$ and $\frac{14}{21}$. These fractions show a whole divided into 21 parts, where the numerators can be compared because the denominators are the same.

Order of Operations

When reviewing calculations consisting of more than one operation, the order in which the operations are performed affects the resulting answer. Consider $5 \times 2 + 7$. Performing multiplication then addition results in an answer of 17 ($5 \times 2 = 10$; $10 + 7 = 17$). However, if the problem is written $5 \times (2 + 7)$, the order of operations dictates that the operation inside the parenthesis must be performed first. The resulting answer is 45 ($2 + 7 = 9$, then $5 \times 9 = 45$).

The *order* in which operations should be performed is remembered using the acronym PEMDAS. **PEMDAS** stands for parenthesis, exponents, multiplication/division, and addition/subtraction. Multiplication and division are performed in the same step, working from left to right with whichever comes first. Addition and subtraction are performed in the same step, working from left to right with whichever comes first.

Consider the following example: $8 \div 4 + 8(7 - 7)$. Performing the operation inside the parenthesis produces $8 \div 4 + 8(0)$ or $8 \div 4 + 8 \times 0$. There are no exponents, so multiplication and division are performed next from left to right resulting in: $2 + 8 \times 0$, then $2 + 0$. Finally, addition and subtraction are performed to obtain an answer of 2. Now consider the following example: $6 \times 3 + 3^2 - 6$. Parentheses are not applicable. Exponents are evaluated first, $6 \times 3 + 9 - 6$. Then multiplication/division forms $18 + 9 - 6$. At last, addition/subtraction leads to the final answer of 21.

Properties of Operations

Properties of operations exist that make calculations easier and solve problems for missing values. The following table summarizes commonly used properties of real numbers.

Property	Addition	Multiplication
Commutative	$a + b = b + a$	$a \times b = b \times a$
Associative	$(a + b) + c = a + (b + c)$	$(a \times b) \times c = a \times (bc)$
Identity	$a + 0 = a; 0 + a = a$	$a \times 1 = a; 1 \times a = a$
Inverse	$a + (-a) = 0$	$a \times \frac{1}{a} = 1; a \neq 0$
Distributive	$a(b + c) = ab + ac$	

The commutative property of addition states that the order in which numbers are added does not change the sum. Similarly, the commutative property of multiplication states that the order in which numbers are multiplied does not change the product. The associative property of addition and multiplication state that the grouping of numbers being added or multiplied does not change the sum or product, respectively. The commutative and associative properties are useful for performing calculations. For example, $(47 + 25) + 3$ is equivalent to $(47 + 3) + 25$, which is easier to calculate.

The identity property of addition states that adding zero to any number does not change its value. The identity property of multiplication states that multiplying a number by one does not change its value. The inverse property of addition states that the sum of a number and its opposite equals zero. Opposites are numbers that are the same with different signs (ex. 5 and -5; $-\frac{1}{2}$ and $\frac{1}{2}$). The inverse property of multiplication states that the product of a number (other than zero) and its reciprocal equals one. Reciprocal numbers have numerators and denominators that are inverted (ex. $\frac{2}{5}$ and $\frac{5}{2}$). Inverse properties are useful for canceling quantities to find missing values (see algebra content). For example, $a + 7 = 12$ is solved by adding the inverse of 7(-7) to both sides in order to isolate a.

The distributive property states that multiplying a sum (or difference) by a number produces the same result as multiplying each value in the sum (or difference) by the number and adding (or subtracting) the products. Consider the following scenario: You are buying three tickets for a baseball game. Each ticket costs $18. You are also charged a fee of $2 per ticket for purchasing the tickets online. The cost is calculated: $3 \times 18 + 3 \times 2$. Using the distributive property, the cost can also be calculated $3(18 + 2)$.

Representing Rational Numbers and Their Operations

Concrete Models
Concrete objects are used to develop a tangible understanding of operations of rational numbers. Tools such as tiles, blocks, beads, and hundred charts are used to model problems. For example, a hundred chart (10×10) and beads can be used to model multiplication. If multiplying 5 by 4, beads are placed across 5 rows and down 4 columns producing a product of 20. Similarly, tiles can be used to model division by splitting the total into equal groups. If dividing 12 by 4, 12 tiles are placed one at a time into 4 groups. The result is 4 groups of 3. This is also an effective method for visualizing the concept of remainders.

Representations of objects can be used to expand on the concrete models of operations. Pictures, dots, and tallies can help model these concepts. Utilizing concrete models and representations creates a foundation upon which to build an abstract understanding of the operations.

Rational Numbers on a Number Line
A *number line* typically consists of integers (...3,2,1,0,-1,-2,-3...), and is used to visually represent the value of a rational number. Each rational number has a distinct position on the line determined by comparing its value with the displayed values on the line. For example, if plotting -1.5 on the number line below, it is necessary to recognize that the value of -1.5 is .5 less than -1 and .5 greater than -2. Therefore, -1.5 is plotted halfway between -1 and -2.

Number lines can also be useful for visualizing sums and differences of rational numbers. Adding a value indicates moving to the right (values increase to the right), and subtracting a value indicates moving to the left (numbers decrease to the left). For example, $5 - 7$ is displayed by starting at 5 and moving to the left 7 spaces, if the number line is in increments of 1. This will result in an answer of -2.

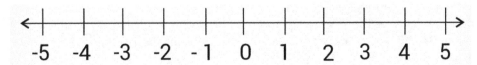

Multiplication and Division Problems

Multiplication and division are *inverse* operations that can be represented by using rectangular arrays, area models, and equations. Rectangular arrays include an arrangement of rows and columns that correspond to the factors and display product totals.

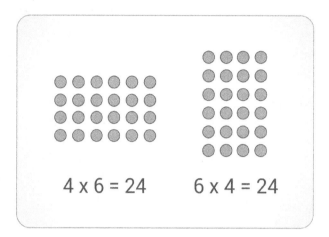

$$4 \times 6 = 24 \qquad 6 \times 4 = 24$$

Another method of multiplication can be done with the use of an *area model*. An area model is a rectangle that is divided into rows and columns that match up to the number of place values within each number. For example, $29 \times 65 = 25 + 4$ and $65 = 60 + 5$. The products of those 4 numbers are found within the rectangle and then summed up to get the answer. The entire process is: $(60 \times 25) + (5 \times 25) + (60 \times 4) + (5 \times 4) = 1,500 + 240 + 125 + 20 = 1,885$. Here is the actual area model:

	25	**4**
60	60x25 1,500	60x4 240
5	5x25 125	5x4 20

$$
\begin{array}{r}
1,500 \\
240 \\
125 \\
+\quad 20 \\
\hline
1,885
\end{array}
$$

Multiplying decimals involves the same procedure as multiplying whole numbers, but including the decimal places in the end result. The problem involves multiplying the two numbers together, ignoring the decimal places, and then inserting the total number of decimal places in the original numbers into the result. For example, given the problem 87.5×0.45, the answer is found by multiplying 875×45 to obtain $39,375$ and then inputting a decimal point three places to the left because there are three total decimal places in the original problem. Therefore, the answer is 39.375.

Dividing a number by a single digit or two digits can be turned into repeated subtraction problems. An area model can be used throughout the problem that represents multiples of the divisor. For example, the answer to 8580 ÷ 55 can be found by subtracting 55 from 8580 one at a time and counting the total number of subtractions necessary.

However, a simpler process involves using larger multiples of 55. First, $100 \times 55 = 5,500$ is subtracted from 8,580, and 3,080 is leftover. Next, $50 \times 55 = 2,750$ is subtracted from 3,080 to obtain 380. $5 \times 55 = 275$ is subtracted from 330 to obtain 55, and finally, $1 \times 55 = 55$ is subtracted from 55 to obtain zero. Therefore, there is no remainder, and the answer is $100 + 50 + 5 + 1 = 156$. Here is a picture of the area model and the repeated subtraction process:

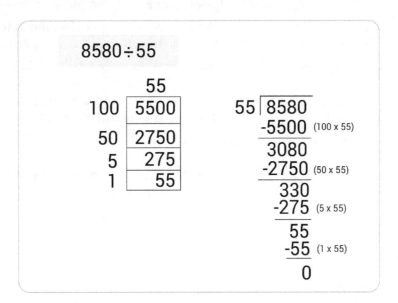

Checking the answer to a division problem involves multiplying the answer—the quotient—times the divisor to see if the dividend is obtained. If there is a remainder, the same process is computed, but the remainder is added on at the end to try to match the dividend. In the previous example, $156 \times 55 = 8580$ would be the checking procedure. Dividing decimals involves the same repeated subtraction process. The only difference would be that the subtractions would involve numbers that include values in the decimal places. Lining up decimal places is crucial in this type of problem.

Comparing, Classifying, and Ordering Rational Numbers

Rational numbers are any number that can be written as a fraction or ratio. Within the set of rational numbers, several subsets exist that are referenced throughout the mathematics topics. Counting numbers are the first numbers learned as a child. Counting numbers consist of 1,2,3,4, and so on. Whole numbers include all counting numbers and zero (0,1,2,3,4,...). Integers include counting numbers, their opposites, and zero (...,-3,-2,-1,0,1,2,3,...). Rational numbers are inclusive of integers, fractions, and decimals that terminate, or end (1.7, 0.04213) or repeat ($0.136\overline{5}$).

When comparing or ordering numbers, the numbers should be written in the same format (decimal or fraction), if possible. For example, $\sqrt{49}$, 7.3, and $\frac{15}{2}$ are easier to order if each one is converted to a decimal, such as 7, 7.3, and 7.5 (converting fractions and decimals is covered in the following section). A number line is used to order and compare the numbers. Any number that is to the right of another number is greater than that number. Conversely, a number positioned to the left of a given number is less than that number.

Converting Between Fractions, Decimals, and Percent

To convert a fraction to a decimal, the numerator is divided by the denominator. For example, $\frac{3}{8}$ can be converted to a decimal by dividing 3 by 8 ($\frac{3}{8} = 0.375$). To convert a decimal to a fraction, the decimal point is dropped and the value is written as the numerator. The denominator is the place value farthest to the right with a digit other than zero. For example, to convert .48 to a fraction, the numerator is 48 and the denominator is 100 (the digit 8 is in the hundredths place). Therefore, .48 = $\frac{48}{100}$. Fractions should be written in the simplest form, or reduced. To reduce a fraction, the numerator and denominator are divided by the largest common factor. In the previous example, 48 and 100 are both divisible by 4. Dividing the numerator and denominator by 4 results in a reduced fraction of $\frac{12}{25}$.

To convert a decimal to a percent, the number is multiplied by 100. To convert .13 to a percent, .13 is multiplied by 100 to get 13 percent. To convert a fraction to a percent, the fraction is converted to a decimal and then multiplied by 100. For example, $\frac{1}{5}$ = .20 and .20 multiplied by 100 produces 20 percent.

To convert a percent to a decimal, the value is divided by 100. For example, 125 percent is equal to 1.25 ($\frac{125}{100}$). To convert a percent to a fraction, the percent sign is dropped and the value is written as the numerator with a denominator of 100. For example, 80% = $\frac{80}{100}$. This fraction can be reduced ($\frac{80}{100} = \frac{4}{5}$).

Understanding Proportional Relationships and Percent

Applying Ratios and Unit Rates
A *ratio* is a comparison of two quantities that represent separate groups. For example, if a recipe calls for 2 eggs for every 3 cups of milk, this is expressed as a ratio. Ratios can be written three ways:

- With the word "to"
- Using a colon
- As a fraction.

In the previous example, the ratio of eggs to cups of milk is written as 2 to 3, 2:3, or $\frac{2}{3}$. When writing ratios, the order is very important. The ratio of eggs to cups of milk is not the same as the ratio of cups of milk to eggs, 3:2.

In simplest form, both quantities of a ratio should be written as integers. These should also be reduced just as a fraction is reduced. For example, 5:10 is reduced to 1:2. Given a ratio where one or both quantities are expressed as a decimal or fraction, multiply both by the same number to produce integers. To write the ratio $\frac{1}{3}$ to 2 in simplest form, both quantities are multiplied by 3. The resulting ratio is 1 to 6.

A problem involving ratios may give a comparison between two groups. The problem may then provide a total and ask for a part, or provide a part and ask for a total. Consider the following: The ratio of boys to girls in the 11th grade class is 5:4. If there are a total of 270 11th grade students, how many are girls? The total number of *ratio pieces* should be determined first. The total number of 11th grade students is divided into 9 pieces. The ratio of boys to total students is 5:9, and the ratio of girls to total students is 4:9. Knowing the total number of students, the number of girls is determined by setting up a proportion:

$$\frac{4}{9} = \frac{x}{270}$$

A rate is a ratio comparing two quantities expressed in different units. A unit rate is a ratio in which the second quantity is one unit. Rates often include the word *per*. Examples include miles per hour, beats per minute, and price per pound. The word per is represented with a / symbol or abbreviated with the letter *p* and units abbreviated. For example, miles per hour is written as mi/h. When given a rate that is not in its simplest form (the second quantity is not one unit), both quantities are divided by the value of the second quantity. If 99 heartbeats were recorded in $1\frac{1}{2}$ minutes, both quantities are divided by $1\frac{1}{2}$ to determine the heart rate of 66 beats per minute.

Percent

The word *percent* means per hundred. Similar to a unit rate in which the second quantity is always one unit, a percent is a rate where the second quantity is always 100 units. If the results of a poll state that 47 percent of people support a given policy, this indicates that 47 out of every 100 individuals polled were in support. In other words, 47 per 100 support the policy. If an upgraded model of a car costs 110 percent of the cost of the base model, for every $100 that is spent for the base model, $110 must be spent to purchase the upgraded model. In other words, the upgraded model costs $110 per $100 for the cost of the base model.

When dealing with percentages, the numbers can be evaluated as a value in hundredths. For example, 15 percent is expressed as fifteen hundredths and is written as $\frac{15}{100}$ or 0.15.

Unit-Rate Problems

A rate is a ratio in which two terms are in different units. When rates are expressed as a quantity of one, they are considered *unit rates*. To determine a unit rate, the first quantity is divided by the second. Knowing a unit rate makes calculations easier than simply having a rate. For example, suppose a 3 pound bag of onions costs $1.77. To calculate the price of 5 pounds of onions, a proportion could show:

$$\frac{3}{1.77} = \frac{5}{x}$$

However, by knowing the unit rate, the value of pounds of onions is multiplied by the unit price. The unit price is calculated:

$$\$1.77/3lb = \$0.59/lb$$

Multiplying the weight of the onions by the unit price yields:

$$5lb \times \frac{\$0.59}{lb} = \$2.95$$

The *lb.* units cancel out.

Similar to unit-rate problems, *unit conversions* appear in real-world scenarios including cooking, measurement, construction, and currency. Given the conversion rate, unit conversions are written as a fraction (ratio) and multiplied by a quantity in one unit to convert it to the corresponding unit. To determine how many minutes are in $3\frac{1}{2}$ hours, the conversion rate of 60 minutes to 1 hour is written as $\frac{60\ min}{1h}$.

Multiplying the quantity by the conversion rate results in:

$$3\frac{1}{2}h \times \frac{60\ min}{1h} = 210\ min$$

(The h unit is canceled.) To convert a quantity in minutes to hours, the fraction for the conversion rate is flipped to cancel the min unit. To convert 195 minutes to hours, $195min \times \frac{1h}{60\ min}$ is multiplied. The result is $\frac{195h}{60}$ which reduces to:

$$3\frac{1}{4}h$$

Converting units may require more than one multiplication. The key is to set up conversion rates so that units cancel each other out and the desired unit is left. To convert 3.25 yards to inches, given that 1yd = 3ft and 12in = 1ft, the calculation is performed by multiplying:

$$3.25\ yd \times \frac{3ft}{1yd} \times \frac{12in}{1ft}$$

The yd and ft units will cancel, resulting in 117in.

Using Proportional Relationships
A proportion is a statement consisting of two equal ratios. Proportions will typically give three of four quantities and require solving for the missing value. The key to solving proportions is to set them up properly. Consider the following: 7 gallons of gas costs $14.70. How many gallons can you get for $20? The information is written as equal ratios with a variable representing the missing quantity:

$$\left(\frac{gallons}{cost} = \frac{gallons}{cost}\right): \frac{7}{14.70} = \frac{x}{20}$$

To solve for x, the proportion is cross-multiplied. This means the numerator of the first ratio is multiplied by the denominator of the second, and vice versa. The resulting products are shown equal to each other. Cross-multiplying results in $(7)(20) = (14.7)(x)$. By solving the equation for x (see the algebra content), the answer is that 9.5 gallons of gas may be purchased for $20.

Percent problems can also be solved by setting up proportions. Examples of common percent problems are:

   a. What is 15% of 25?
   b. What percent of 45 is 3?
   c. 5 is $\frac{1}{2}$% of what number?

Setting up the proper proportion is made easier by following the format:

$$\frac{is}{of} = \frac{percent}{100}$$

A variable is used to represent the missing value. The proportions for each of the three examples are set up as follows:

a. $\dfrac{x}{25} = \dfrac{15}{100}$

b. $\dfrac{3}{45} = \dfrac{x}{100}$

c. $\dfrac{5}{x} = \dfrac{\frac{1}{2}}{100}$

By cross-multiplying and solving the resulting equation for the variable, the missing values are determined to be:

a. 3.75

b. $6.\overline{6}\%$

c. 1,000

Basic Concepts of Number Theory

Prime and Composite Numbers

Whole numbers are classified as either prime or composite. A *prime number* can only be divided evenly by itself and one. For example, the number 11 can only be divided evenly by 11 and one; therefore, 11 is a prime number. A helpful way to visualize a prime number is to use concrete objects and try to divide them into equal piles. If dividing 11 coins, the only way to divide them into equal piles is to create 1 pile of 11 coins or to create 11 piles of 1 coin each. Other examples of prime numbers include 2, 3, 5, 7, 13, 17, and 19.

A *composite number* is any whole number that is not a prime number. A composite number is a number that can be divided evenly by one or more numbers other than itself and one. For example, the number 6 can be divided evenly by 2 and 3. Therefore, 6 is a composite number. If dividing 6 coins into equal piles, the possibilities are 1 pile of 6 coins, 2 piles of 3 coins, 3 piles of 2 coins, or 6 piles of 1 coin. Other examples of composite numbers include 4, 8, 9, 10, 12, 14, 15, 16, 18, and 20.

To determine if a number is a prime or composite number, the number is divided by every whole number greater than one and less than its own value. If it divides evenly by any of these numbers, then the number is composite. If it does not divide evenly by any of these numbers, then the number is prime. For example, when attempting to divide the number 5 by 2, 3, and 4, none of these numbers divide evenly. Therefore, 5 must be a prime number.

Factors and Multiples of Numbers

The *factors* of a number are all integers that can be multiplied by another integer to produce the given number. For example, 2 is multiplied by 3 to produce 6. Therefore, 2 and 3 are both factors of 6. Similarly, $1 \times 6 = 6$ and $2 \times 3 = 6$, so 1, 2, 3, and 6 are all factors of 6. Another way to explain a factor is to say that a given number divides evenly by each of its factors to produce an integer. For example, 6 does not divide evenly by 5. Therefore, 5 is not a factor of 6.

Multiples of a given number are found by taking that number and multiplying it by any other whole number. For example, 3 is a factor of 6, 9, and 12. Therefore, 6, 9, and 12 are multiples of 3. The multiples of any number are an infinite list. For example, the multiples of 5 are 5, 10, 15, 20, and so on. This list continues without end. A list of multiples is used in finding the least common multiple, or LCM, for fractions when a common denominator is needed. The denominators are written down and their multiples listed until a common number is found in both lists. This common number is the LCM.

Prime factorization breaks down each factor of a whole number until only prime numbers remain. All composite numbers can be factored into prime numbers. For example, the prime factors of 12 are 2, 2, and 3 ($2 \times 2 \times 3 = 12$). To produce the prime factors of a number, the number is factored and any composite numbers are continuously factored until the result is the product of prime factors only. A factor tree, such as the one below, is helpful when exploring this concept.

Here is an example of a factorization tree:

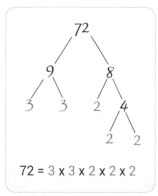

72 = 3 x 3 x 2 x 2 x 2

Determining the Reasonableness of Results

When solving math word problems, the solution obtained should make sense within the given scenario. The step of checking the solution will reduce the possibility of a calculation error or a solution that may be *mathematically* correct but not applicable in the real world. Consider the following scenarios:

A problem states that Lisa got 24 out of 32 questions correct on a test and asks to find the percentage of correct answers. To solve the problem, a student divided 32 by 24 to get 1.33, and then multiplied by 100 to get 133 percent. By examining the solution within the context of the problem, the student should recognize that getting all 32 questions correct will produce a perfect score of 100 percent. Therefore, a score of 133 percent with 8 incorrect answers does not make sense and the calculations should be checked.

A problem states that the maximum weight on a bridge cannot exceed 22,000 pounds. The problem asks to find the maximum number of cars that can be on the bridge at one time if each car weighs 4,000 pounds. To solve this problem, a student divided 22,000 by 4,000 to get an answer of 5.5. By examining the solution within the context of the problem, the student should recognize that although the calculations are mathematically correct, the solution does not make sense. Half of a car on a bridge is not possible, so the student should determine that a maximum of 5 cars can be on the bridge at the same time.

Mental Math Estimation

Once a result is determined to be logical within the context of a given problem, the result should be evaluated by its nearness to the expected answer. This is performed by approximating given values to perform mental math. Numbers should be rounded to the nearest value possible to check the initial results.

Consider the following example: A problem states that a customer is buying a new sound system for their home. The customer purchases a stereo for $435, 2 speakers for $67 each, and the necessary cables for $12. The customer chooses an option that allows him to spread the costs over equal payments for 4 months. How much will the monthly payments be?

After making calculations for the problem, a student determines that the monthly payment will be $145.25. To check the accuracy of the results, the student rounds each cost to the nearest ten (440 + 70 + 70 + 10) and determines that the total is approximately $590. Dividing by 4 months gives an approximate monthly payment of $147.50. Therefore, the student can conclude that the solution of $145.25 is very close to what should be expected.

When rounding, the place-value that is used in rounding can make a difference. Suppose the student had rounded to the nearest hundred for the estimation. The result ($400 + 100 + 100 + 0 = 600; 600 \div 4 = 150$) will show that the answer is reasonable, but not as close to the actual value as rounding to the nearest ten.

Algebra

Adding, Subtracting, Multiplying, and Factoring Linear Expressions

Algebraic expressions look similar to equations, but they do not include the equal sign. Algebraic expressions are comprised of numbers, variables, and mathematical operations. Some examples of algebraic expressions are $8x + 7y - 12z$, $3a^2$, and $5x^3 - 4y^4$.

Algebraic expressions consist of variables, numbers, and operations. A term of an expression is any combination of numbers and/or variables, and terms are separated by addition and subtraction. For example, the expression $5x^2 - 3xy + 4 - 2$ consists of 4 terms: $5x^2$, -3xy, 4y, and -2. Note that each term includes its given sign (+ or −). The variable part of a term is a letter that represents an unknown quantity. The coefficient of a term is the number by which the variable is multiplied. For the term 4y, the variable is y and the coefficient is 4. Terms are identified by the power (or exponent) of its variable.

A number without a variable is referred to as a constant. If the variable is to the first power (x^1 or simply x), it is referred to as a linear term. A term with a variable to the second power (x^2) is quadratic and a term to the third power (x^3) is cubic. Consider the expression $x^3 + 3x - 1$. The constant is -1. The linear term is 3x. There is no quadratic term. The cubic term is x^3.

An algebraic expression can also be classified by how many terms exist in the expression. Any like terms should be combined before classifying. A monomial is an expression consisting of only one term. Examples of monomials are: 17, 2x, and $-5ab^2$. A binomial is an expression consisting of two terms separated by addition or subtraction. Examples include $2x - 4$ and $-3y^2 + 2y$. A trinomial consists of 3 terms. For example, $5x^2 - 2x + 1$ is a trinomial.

Algebraic expressions and equations can be used to represent real-life situations and model the behavior of different variables. For example, $2x + 5$ could represent the cost to play games at an arcade. In this case, 5 represents the price of admission to the arcade and 2 represents the cost of each game played. To calculate the total cost, use the number of games played for x, multiply it by 2, and add 5.

Adding and Subtracting Linear Algebraic Expressions

An algebraic expression is simplified by combining like terms. A term is a number, variable, or product of a number, and variables separated by addition and subtraction. For the algebraic expression $3x^2 - 4x + 5 - 5x^2 + x - 3$, the terms are $3x^2$, -4x, 5, -5x^2, x, and -3. Like terms have the same variables raised to the same powers (exponents). The like terms for the previous example are $3x^2$ and -5x^2, -4x and x, 5 and -3. To combine like terms, the coefficients (numerical factor of the term including sign) are added and the variables and their powers are kept the same. Note that if a coefficient is not written, it is an implied coefficient of 1 ($x = 1x$). The previous example will simplify to:

$$-2x^2 - 3x + 2$$

When adding or subtracting algebraic expressions, each expression is written in parenthesis. The negative sign is distributed when necessary, and like terms are combined. Consider the following:

$$\text{add } 2a + 5b - 2 \text{ to } a - 2b + 8c - 4$$

The sum is set as follows:

$$(a - 2b + 8c - 4) + (2a + 5b - 2)$$

In front of each set of parentheses is an implied positive one, which, when distributed, does not change any of the terms. Therefore, the parentheses are dropped and like terms are combined:

$$a - 2b + 8c - 4 + 2a + 5b - 2$$

$$3a + 3b + 8c - 6$$

Consider the following problem:

$$\text{Subtract } 2a + 5b - 2 \text{ from } a - 2b + 8c - 4$$

The difference is set as follows:

$$(a - 2b + 8c - 4) - (2a + 5b - 2)$$

The implied one in front of the first set of parentheses will not change those four terms. However, distributing the implied -1 in front of the second set of parentheses will change the sign of each of those three terms:

$$a - 2b + 8c - 4 - 2a - 5b + 2$$

Combining like terms yields the simplified expression:

$$-a - 7b + 8c - 2$$

Distributive Property

The **distributive property** states that multiplying a sum (or difference) by a number produces the same result as multiplying each value in the sum (or difference) by the number and adding (or subtracting) the products. Using mathematical symbols, the distributive property states $a(b + c) = ab + ac$. The expression $4(3 + 2)$ is simplified using the order of operations. Simplifying inside the parenthesis first produces 4×5, which equals 20.

The expression $4(3 + 2)$ can also be simplified using the distributive property:

$$4(3 + 2)$$

$$4 \times 3 + 4 \times 2$$

$$12 + 8$$

$$20$$

Consider the following example: $4(3x - 2)$. The expression cannot be simplified inside the parenthesis because $3x$ and -2 are not like terms, and therefore cannot be combined. However, the expression can be simplified by using the distributive property and multiplying each term inside of the parenthesis by the term outside of the parenthesis: $12x - 8$. The resulting equivalent expression contains no like terms, so it cannot be further simplified.

Consider the expression:

$$(3x + 2y + 1) - (5x - 3) + 2(3y + 4)$$

Again, there are no like terms, but the distributive property is used to simplify the expression. Note there is an implied one in front of the first set of parentheses and an implied -1 in front of the second set of parentheses. Distributing the one, -1, and 2 produces:

$$1(3x) + 1(2y) + 1(1) - 1(5x) - 1(-3) + 2(3y) + 2(4)$$

$$3x + 2y + 1 - 5x + 3 + 6y + 8$$

This expression contains like terms that are combined to produce the simplified expression:

$$-2x + 8y + 12$$

Algebraic expressions are tested to be equivalent by choosing values for the variables and evaluating both expressions (see 2.A.4). For example, $4(3x - 2)$ and $12x - 8$ are tested by substituting 3 for the variable x and calculating to determine if equivalent values result.

Evaluating Algebraic Expressions

To evaluate the expression, the given values for the variables are substituted (or replaced) and the expression is simplified using the order of operations. Parenthesis should be used when substituting. Consider the following: Evaluate $a - 2b + ab$ for $a = 3$ and $b = -1$.

To evaluate, any variable a is replaced with 3 and any variable b with -1, producing:

$$(3) - 2(-1) + (3)(-1)$$

Next, the order of operations is used to calculate the value of the expression, which is 2.

Here's another example:

$$\text{Evaluate } a - 2b + ab \; for \; a = 3 \text{ and } b = -1$$

To evaluate an expression, the given values should be substituted for the variables and simplified using the order of operations. In this case:

$$(3) - 2(-1) + (3)(-1)$$

Parentheses are used when substituting.

Given an algebraic expression, students may be asked to simplify the expression. For example:

Simplify $5x^2 - 10x + 2 - 8x^2 + x - 1$.

Simplifying algebraic expressions requires combining like terms. A term is a number, variable, or product of a number and variables separated by addition and subtraction. The terms in the above expressions are: $5x^2, -10x, 2, -8x^2, x$, and -1. Like terms have the same variables raised to the same powers (exponents). To combine like terms, the coefficients (numerical factor of the term including sign) are added, while the variables and their powers are kept the same. The example above simplifies to:

$$-3x^2 - 9x + 1$$

Let's try two more.

Evaluate $\frac{1}{2}x^2 - 3, x = 4$.

The first step is to substitute in 4 for x in the expression:

$$\frac{1}{2}(4)^2 - 3$$

Then, the order of operations is used to simplify.

The exponent comes first, $\frac{1}{2}(16) - 3$, then the multiplication $8 - 3$, and then, after subtraction, the solution is 5.

Evaluate $4|5 - x| + 2y, x = 4, y = -3$.

The first step is to substitute 4 in for x and -3 in for y in the expression:

$$4|5 - 4| + 2(-3)$$

Then, the absolute value expression is simplified, which is:

$$|5 - 4| = |1| = 1$$

The expression is $4(1) + 2(-3)$ which can be simplified using the order of operations.

First is the multiplication, $4 + (-6)$; then addition yields an answer of -2.

Creating Algebraic Expressions

A linear expression is a statement about an unknown quantity expressed in mathematical symbols. The statement "five times a number added to forty" can be expressed as $5x + 40$. A linear equation is a statement in which two expressions (at least one containing a variable) are equal to each other. The statement "five times a number added to forty is equal to ten" can be expressed as $5x + 40 = 10$.

Real world scenarios can also be expressed mathematically. Suppose a job pays its employees $300 per week and $40 for each sale made. The weekly pay is represented by the expression $40x + 300$ where x is the number of sales made during the week.

Consider the following scenario: Bob had $20 and Tom had $4. After selling 4 ice cream cones to Bob, Tom has as much money as Bob. The cost of an ice cream cone is an unknown quantity and can be represented by a variable (x). The amount of money Bob has after his purchase is four times the cost of an ice cream cone subtracted from his original $20 → $20 - 4x$. The amount of money Tom has after his sale is four times the cost of an ice cream cone added to his original $4 → $4x + 4$. After the sale, the amount of money that Bob and Tom have are equal → $20 - 4x = 4x + 4$.

When expressing a verbal or written statement mathematically, it is key to understand words or phrases that can be represented with symbols. The following are examples:

Symbol	Phrase
$+$	added to, increased by, sum of, more than
$-$	decreased by, difference between, less than, take away
x	multiplied by, 3 (4, 5 . . .) times as large, product of
$\div$	divided by, quotient of, half (third, etc.) of
$=$	is, the same as, results in, as much as
$x, t, n, etc.$	a number, unknown quantity, value of

Adding, Subtracting, Multiplying, Dividing, and Factoring Polynomials

An expression of the form ax^n, where n is a non-negative integer, is called a **monomial** because it contains one term. A sum of monomials is called a **polynomial**. For example, $-4x^3 + x$ is a polynomial, while $5x^7$ is a monomial. A function equal to a polynomial is called a **polynomial function**.

The monomials in a polynomial are also called the **terms** of the polynomial.

The constants that precede the variables are called **coefficients**.

The highest value of the exponent of x in a polynomial is called the **degree** of the polynomial. So, $-4x^3 + x$ has a degree of 3, while $-2x^5 + x^3 + 4x + 1$ has a degree of 5. When multiplying polynomials, the degree of the result will be the sum of the degrees of the two polynomials being multiplied.

Addition and subtraction operations can be performed on polynomials with like terms. **Like terms** refers to terms that have the same variable and exponent. The two following polynomials can be added together by collecting like terms:

$$(x^2 + 3x - 4) + (4x^2 - 7x + 8)$$

The x^2 terms can be added as $x^2 + 4x^2 = 5x^2$. The x terms can be added as $3x + -7x = -4x$, and the constants can be added as $-4 + 8 = 4$. The following expression is the result of the addition:

$$5x^2 - 4x + 4$$

Let's try another:

$$(-2x^5 + x^3 + 4x + 1) + (-4x^3 + x)$$

$$-2x^5 + (1-4)x^3 + (4+1)x + 1$$

$$-2x^5 - 3x^3 + 5x + 1$$

Likewise, subtraction of polynomials is performed by subtracting coefficients of like powers of x. So,

$$(-2x^5 + x^3 + 4x + 1) - (-4x^3 + x)$$

$$-2x^5 + (1+4)x^3 + (4-1)x + 1$$

$$-2x^5 + 5x^3 + 3x + 1$$

To multiply two polynomials, multiply each term of the first polynomial by each term of the second polynomial and add the results. For example:

$$(4x^2 + x)(-x^3 + x)$$

$$4x^2(-x^3) + 4x^2(x) + x(-x^3) + x(x)$$

$$-4x^5 + 4x^3 - x^4 + x^2$$

In the case where each polynomial has two terms, like in this example, some students find it helpful to remember this as multiplying the First terms, then the Outer terms, then the Inner terms, and finally the Last terms, with the mnemonic FOIL. For longer polynomials, the multiplication process is the same, but there will be, of course, more terms, and there is no common mnemonic to remember each combination.

Factors for polynomials are similar to factors for integers—they are numbers, variables, or polynomials that, when multiplied together, give a product equal to the polynomial in question. One polynomial is a factor of a second polynomial if the second polynomial can be obtained from the first by multiplying by a third polynomial.

$6x^6 + 13x^4 + 6x^2$ can be obtained by multiplying together $(3x^4 + 2x^2)(2x^2 + 3)$. This means $2x^2 + 3$ and $3x^4 + 2x^2$ are factors of $6x^6 + 13x^4 + 6x^2$.

In general, finding the factors of a polynomial can be tricky. However, there are a few types of polynomials that can be factored in a straightforward way.

If a certain monomial divides each term of a polynomial, it can be factored out:

$$x^2 + 2xy + y^2 = (x+y)^2$$

$$x^2 - 2xy + y^2 = (x-y)^2$$

$$x^2 - y^2 = (x+y)(x-y)$$

$$x^3 + y^3 = (x+y)(x^2 - xy + y^2)$$

$$x^3 - y^3 = (x-y)(x^2 + xy + y^2)$$

$$x^3 + 3x^2y + 3xy^2 + y^3 = (x+y)^3$$

$$x^3 - 3x^2y + 3xy^2 - y^3 = (x-y)^3$$

These rules can be used in many combinations with one another. For example, the expression $3x^3 - 24$ factors to:

$$3(x^3 - 8) = 3(x - 2)(x^2 + 2x + 4)$$

When factoring polynomials, a good strategy is to multiply the factors to check the result.

Let's try another example:

$$4x^3 + 16x^2 = 4x^2(x + 4).$$

$$x^2 + 2xy + y^2 = (x + y)^2 \text{ or } x^2 - 2xy + y^2 = (x - y)^2$$

$$x^2 - y^2 = (x + y)(x - y)$$

$$x^3 + y^3 = (x + y)(x^2 - xy + y^2)$$

$$x^3 - y^3 = (x - y)(x^2 + xy + y^2)$$

$$x^3 + 3x^2y + 3xy^2 + y^3 = (x + y)^3 \text{ and } x^3 - 3x^2y + 3xy^2 - y^3 = (x - y)^3$$

It sometimes can be necessary to rewrite the polynomial in some clever way before applying the above rules. Consider the problem of factoring $x^4 - 1$. This does not immediately look like any of the cases for which there are rules. However, it's possible to think of this polynomial as $x^4 - 1 = (x^2)^2 - (1^2)^2$, and now apply the third rule in the above list to simplify this:

$$(x^2)^2 - (1^2)^2$$

$$(x^2 + 1^2)(x^2 - 1^2)$$

$$(x^2 + 1)(x^2 - 1)$$

Creating Polynomials from Written Descriptions

Polynomials that represent mathematical or real-world problems can also be created from written descriptions, much like algebraic expressions. For example, polynomials might be created when working with formulas. Formulas are mathematical expressions that define the value of one quantity, given the value of one or more different quantities. Formulas look like equations because they contain variables, numbers, operators, and an equal sign. All formulas are equations but not all equations are formulas. A formula must have more than one variable. For example, $2x + 7 = y$ is an equation and a formula (it relates the unknown quantities x and y). However, $2x + 7 = 3$ is an equation but not a formula (it only expresses the value of the unknown quantity x).

Formulas are typically written with one variable alone (or isolated) on one side of the equal sign. This variable can be thought of as the **subject** in that the formula is stating the value of the subject in terms of the relationship between the other variables. Consider the distance formula: $distance = rate \times time$ or $d = rt$. The value of the subject variable d (distance) is the product of the variable r and t (rate and time). Given the rate and time, the distance traveled can easily be determined by substituting the values into the formula and evaluating.

The formula $P = 2l + 2w$ expresses how to calculate the perimeter of a rectangle (P) given its length (l) and width (w). To find the perimeter of a rectangle with a length of 3ft and a width of 2ft, these values are substituted into the formula for *l* and *w*: $P = 2(3ft) + 2(2ft)$. Following the order of operations, the perimeter is determined to be 10ft. When working with formulas such as these, including units is an important step.

Given a formula expressed in terms of one variable, the formula can be manipulated to express the relationship in terms of any other variable. In other words, the formula can be rearranged to change which variable is the *subject*. To solve for a variable of interest by manipulating a formula, the equation may be solved as if all other variables were numbers. The same steps for solving are followed, leaving operations in terms of the variables instead of calculating numerical values. For the formula $P = 2l + 2w$, the perimeter is the subject expressed in terms of the length and width. To write a formula to calculate the width of a rectangle, given its length and perimeter, the previous formula relating the three variables is solved for the variable *w*. If *P* and *l* were numerical values, this is a two-step linear equation solved by subtraction and division. To solve the equation $P = 2l + 2w$ for *w*, $2l$ is first subtracted from both sides:

$$P - 2l = 2w$$

Then both sides are divided by 2:

$$\frac{P - 2l}{2} = w$$

Test questions may involve creating a polynomial based on a formula. For example, using the perimeter of a rectangle formula, a problem may ask for the perimeter of a rectangle with a length of $2x + 12$ and a width of $x + 1$. Using the formula $P = 2l + 2w$, the perimeter would then be:

$$P = 2(2x + 12) + 2(x + 1)$$

This equals:

$$4x + 24 + 2x + 2 = 6x + 26$$

The area of the same rectangle, which uses the formula $A = l \times w$, would be:

$$A = (2x + 12)(x + 1)$$

$$2x^2 + 2x + 12x + 12$$

$$2x^2 + 14x + 12$$

Adding, Subtracting, Multiplying, Dividing Rational Expressions

A fraction, or ratio, wherein each part is a polynomial, defines **rational expressions**. Some examples include $\frac{2x+6}{x}$, $\frac{1}{x^2-4x+8}$, and $\frac{z^2}{x+5}$. Exponents on the variables are restricted to whole numbers, which means roots and negative exponents are not included in rational expressions.

Rational expressions can be transformed by factoring. For example, the expression $\frac{x^2-5x+6}{(x-3)}$ can be rewritten by factoring the numerator to obtain:

$$\frac{(x - 3)(x - 2)}{(x - 3)}$$

102

Therefore, the common binomial $(x - 3)$ can cancel so that the simplified expression is:

$$\frac{(x - 2)}{1} = (x - 2)$$

Additionally, other rational expressions can be rewritten to take on different forms. Some may be factorable in themselves, while others can be transformed through arithmetic operations. Rational expressions are closed under addition, subtraction, multiplication, and division by a nonzero expression. **Closed** means that if any one of these operations is performed on a rational expression, the result will still be a rational expression. The set of all real numbers is another example of a set closed under all four operations.

Adding and subtracting rational expressions is based on the same concepts as adding and subtracting simple fractions. For both concepts, the denominators must be the same for the operation to take place. For example, here are two rational expressions:

$$\frac{x^3 - 4}{(x - 3)} + \frac{x + 8}{(x - 3)}$$

Since the denominators are both $(x - 3)$, the numerators can be combined by collecting like terms to form:

$$\frac{x^3 + x + 4}{(x - 3)}$$

If the denominators are different, they need to be made common (the same) by using the **Least Common Denominator (LCD)**. Each denominator needs to be factored, and the LCD contains each factor that appears in any one denominator the greatest number of times it appears in any denominator. The original expressions need to be multiplied by a form of 1 such as 5/5 or x-2/x-2, which will turn each denominator into the LCD. This process is like adding fractions with unlike denominators. It is also important when working with rational expressions to define what value of the variable makes the denominator zero. For this particular value, the expression is undefined.

Multiplication of rational expressions is performed like multiplication of fractions. The numerators are multiplied; then, the denominators are multiplied. The final fraction is then simplified. The expressions are simplified by factoring and cancelling out common terms. In the following example, the numerator of the second expression can be factored first to simplify the expression before multiplying:

$$\frac{x^2}{(x - 4)} \times \frac{x^2 - x - 12}{2}$$

$$\frac{x^2}{(x - 4)} \times \frac{(x - 4)(x + 3)}{2}$$

The $(x - 4)$ on the top and bottom cancel out:

$$\frac{x^2}{1} \times \frac{(x + 3)}{2}$$

Then multiplication is performed, resulting in:

$$\frac{x^3 + 3x^2}{2}$$

Dividing rational expressions is similar to the division of fractions, where division turns into multiplying by a reciprocal. Thus, the following expression can be rewritten as a multiplication problem:

$$\frac{x^2 - 3x + 7}{x - 4} \div \frac{x^2 - 5x + 3}{x - 4}$$

$$\frac{x^2 - 3x + 7}{x - 4} \times \frac{x - 4}{x^2 - 5x + 3}$$

The $x - 4$ cancels out, leaving:

$$\frac{x^2 - 3x + 7}{x^2 - 5x + 3}$$

The final answers should always be completely simplified. If a function is composed of a rational expression, the zeros of the graph can be found from setting the polynomial in the numerator as equal to zero and solving. The values that make the denominator equal to zero will either exist on the graph as a **hole** or a **vertical asymptote**.

A **complex fraction** is a fraction in which the numerator and denominator are themselves fractions, of the form:

$$\frac{\left(\frac{a}{b}\right)}{\left(\frac{c}{d}\right)}$$

These can be simplified by following the usual rules for the order of operations, or by remembering that dividing one fraction by another is the same as multiplying by the reciprocal of the divisor. This means that any complex fraction can be rewritten using the following form:

$$\frac{\left(\frac{a}{b}\right)}{\left(\frac{c}{d}\right)} = \frac{a}{b} \times \frac{d}{c}$$

The following problem is an example of solving a complex fraction:

$$\frac{\left(\frac{5}{4}\right)}{\left(\frac{3}{8}\right)} = \frac{5}{4} \times \frac{8}{3} = \frac{40}{12} = \frac{10}{3}$$

Writing an Expression from a Written Description

When expressing a verbal or written statement mathematically, it is vital to understand words or phrases that can be represented with symbols. The following are examples:

Symbol	Phrase
+	Added to; increased by; sum of; more than
−	Decreased by; difference between; less than; take away
×	Multiplied by; 3(4,5…) times as large; product of
÷	Divided by; quotient of; half (third, etc.) of
=	Is; the same as; results in; as much as; equal to
x,t,n, etc.	A number; unknown quantity; value of; variable

Addition and subtraction are **inverse operations**. Adding a number and then subtracting the same number will cancel each other out, resulting in the original number, and vice versa. For example, $8 + 7 - 7 = 8$ and $137 - 100 + 100 = 137$. Similarly, multiplication and division are inverse operations. Therefore, multiplying by a number and then dividing by the same number results in the original number, and vice versa. For example, $8 \times 2 \div 2 = 8$ and $12 \div 4 \times 4 = 12$. Inverse operations are used to work backwards to solve problems. In the case that 7 and a number add to 18, the inverse operation of subtraction is used to find the unknown value ($18 - 7 = 11$). If a school's entire 4th grade was divided evenly into 3 classes each with 22 students, the inverse operation of multiplication is used to determine the total students in the grade ($22 \times 3 = 66$). Additional scenarios involving inverse operations are included in the tables below.

Recall that a rational expression is a fraction where the numerator and denominator are both polynomials. Some examples of rational expressions include the following: $\frac{4x^3y^5}{3z^4}$, $\frac{4x^3+3x}{x^2}$, and $\frac{x^2+7x+10}{x+2}$. Since these refer to expressions and not equations, they can be simplified but not solved. Using the rules in the previous Exponents and Roots sections, some rational expressions with monomials can be simplified. Other rational expressions such as the last example, $\frac{x^2+7x+10}{x+2}$, take more steps to be simplified. First, the polynomial on top can be factored from $x^2 + 7x + 10$ into $(x + 5)(x + 2)$. Then the common factors can be canceled, and the expression can be simplified to $(x + 5)$.

Consider this problem as an example of using rational expressions. Reggie wants to lay sod in his rectangular backyard. The length of the yard is given by the expression $4x + 2$ and the width is unknown. The area of the yard is $20x + 10$. Reggie needs to find the width of the yard. Knowing that the area of a rectangle is length multiplied by width, an expression can be written to find the width: $\frac{20x+10}{4x+2}$, area divided by length. Simplifying this expression by factoring out 10 on the top and 2 on the bottom leads to this expression:

$$\frac{10(2x + 1)}{2(2x + 1)}$$

By cancelling out the $2x + 1$, that results in $\frac{10}{2} = 5$. The width of the yard is found to be 5 by simplifying a rational expression.

Using Linear Equations to Solve Real-World Problems

Linear relationships describe the way two quantities change with respect to each other. The relationship is defined as linear because a line is produced if all the sets of corresponding values are graphed on a coordinate grid. When expressing the linear relationship as an equation, the equation is often written in the form $y = mx + b$ (slope-intercept form) where m and b are numerical values and x and y are variables (for example, $y = 5x + 10$). Given a linear equation and the value of either variable (x or y), the value of the other variable can be determined.

Imagine the following problem: The sum of a number and 5 is equal to -8 times the number.

To find this unknown number, a simple equation can be written to represent the problem. Key words such as difference, equal, and times are used to form the following equation with one variable: $n + 5 = -8n$. When solving for n, opposite operations are used. First, n is subtracted from $-8n$ across the equals sign, resulting in $5 = -9n$. Then, -9 is divided on both sides, leaving $n = -\frac{5}{9}$. This solution can be graphed on the number line with a dot as shown below:

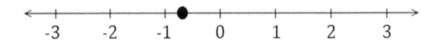

Suppose a teacher is grading a test containing 20 questions with 5 points given for each correct answer, adding a curve of 10 points to each test. This linear relationship can be expressed as the equation $y = 5x + 10$ where x represents the number of correct answers and y represents the test score. To determine the score of a test with a given number of correct answers, the number of correct answers is substituted into the equation for x and evaluated. For example, for 10 correct answers, 10 is substituted for x: $y = 5(10) + 10 \rightarrow y = 60$. Therefore, 10 correct answers will result in a score of 60. The number of correct answers needed to obtain a certain score can also be determined. To determine the number of correct answers needed to score a 90, 90 is substituted for y in the equation (y represents the test score) and solved: $90 = 5x + 10 \rightarrow 80 = 5x \rightarrow 16 = x$. Therefore, 16 correct answers are needed to score a 90.

Linear relationships may be represented by a table of 2 corresponding values. Certain tables may determine the relationship between the values and predict other corresponding sets. Consider the table below, which displays the money in a checking account that charges a monthly fee:

Month	0	1	2	3	4
Balance	$210	$195	$180	$165	$150

An examination of the values reveals that the account loses $15 every month (the month increases by one and the balance decreases by 15). This information can be used to predict future values. To determine what the value will be in month 6, the pattern can be continued, and it can be concluded that the balance will be $120. To determine which month the balance will be $0, $210 is divided by $15 (since the balance decreases $15 every month), resulting in month 14.

Solving a System of Two Linear Equations

A **system of equations** is a group of equations that have the same variables or unknowns. These equations can be linear, but they are not always so. Finding a solution to a system of equations means finding the values of the variables that satisfy each equation. For a linear system of two equations and two variables, there could be a single solution, no solution, or infinitely many solutions.

A single solution occurs when there is one value for x and y that satisfies the system. This would be shown on the graph where the lines cross at exactly one point. When there is no solution, the lines are parallel and do not ever cross. With infinitely many solutions, the equations may look different, but they are the same line. One equation will be a multiple of the other, and on the graph, they lie on top of each other.

The process of elimination can be used to solve a system of equations. For example, the following equations make up a system:

$$x + 3y = 10 \text{ and } 2x - 5y = 9$$

Immediately adding these equations does not eliminate a variable, but it is possible to change the first equation by multiplying the whole equation by -2. This changes the first equation to

$$-2x - 6y = -20$$

The equations can be then added to obtain $-11y = -11$. Solving for y yields $y = 1$. To find the rest of the solution, 1 can be substituted in for y in either original equation to find the value of $x = 7$. The solution to the system is (7, 1) because it makes both equations true, and it is the point in which the lines intersect. If the system is **dependent**—having infinitely many solutions—then both variables will cancel out when the elimination method is used, resulting in an equation that is true for many values of x and y. Since the system is dependent, both equations can be simplified to the same equation or line.

A system can also be solved using **substitution.** This involves solving one equation for a variable and then plugging that solved equation into the other equation in the system. This equation can be solved for one variable, which can then be plugged in to either original equation and solved for the other variable. For example, $x - y = -2$ and $3x + 2y = 9$ can be solved using substitution. The first equation can be solved for x, where $x = -2 + y$. Then it can be plugged into the other equation:

$$3(-2 + y) + 2y = 9$$

Solving for y yields:

$$-6 + 3y + 2y = 9$$

That shows that $y = 3$. If $y = 3$, then $x = 1$.

This solution can be checked by plugging in these values for the variables in each equation to see if it makes a true statement.

Finally, a solution to a system of equations can be found graphically. The solution to a linear system is the point or points where the lines cross. The values of x and y represent the coordinates (x, y) where the lines intersect. Using the same system of equation as above, they can be solved for y to put them in slope-intercept form, $y = mx + b$. These equations become $y = x + 2$ and $y = -\frac{3}{2}x + 4.5$. The slope is the coefficient of x, and the y-intercept is the constant value.

This system with the solution is shown below:

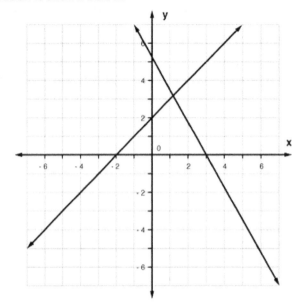

If the lines intersect, the point of intersection is the solution to the system. Every point on a line represents an ordered pair that makes its equation true. The ordered pair represented by this point of intersection lies on both lines and therefore makes both equations true. This ordered pair should be checked by substituting its values into both of the original equations of the system. Note that given a system of equations and an ordered pair, the ordered pair can be determined to be a solution or not by checking it in both equations.

If, when graphed, the lines representing the equations of a system do not intersect, then the two lines are parallel to each other or they are the same exact line. Parallel lines extend in the same direction without ever meeting. A system consisting of parallel lines has no solution. If the equations for a system represent the same exact line, then every point on the line is a solution to the system. In this case, there would be an infinite number of solutions. A system consisting of intersecting lines is referred to as independent; a system consisting of parallel lines is referred to as inconsistent; and a system consisting of coinciding lines is referred to as dependent.

Parallel Lines	**Intersecting Lines**	**Coincident Lines**
Inconsistent	Independent	Dependent

Matrices can also be used to solve systems of linear equations. Specifically, for systems, the coefficients of the linear equations in standard form are the entries in the matrix. Using the same system of linear equations as above, $x - y = -2$ and $3x + 2y = 9$, the matrix to represent the system is:

$$\begin{bmatrix} 1 & -1 \\ 3 & 2 \end{bmatrix} \begin{bmatrix} x \\ y \end{bmatrix} = \begin{bmatrix} -2 \\ 9 \end{bmatrix}$$

To solve this system using matrices, the inverse matrix must be found. For a general 2×2 matrix:

$$\begin{bmatrix} a & b \\ c & d \end{bmatrix}$$

The inverse matrix is found by the expression:

$$\frac{1}{ad - bc} \begin{bmatrix} d & -b \\ -c & a \end{bmatrix}$$

The inverse matrix for the system given above is:

$$\frac{1}{2 - -3} \begin{bmatrix} 2 & 1 \\ -3 & 1 \end{bmatrix} = \frac{1}{5} \begin{bmatrix} 2 & 1 \\ -3 & 1 \end{bmatrix}$$

The next step in solving is to multiply this identity matrix by the system matrix above. This is given by the following equation:

$$\frac{1}{5} \begin{bmatrix} 2 & 1 \\ -3 & 1 \end{bmatrix} \begin{bmatrix} 1 & -1 \\ 3 & 2 \end{bmatrix} \begin{bmatrix} x \\ y \end{bmatrix} = \begin{bmatrix} -2 \\ 9 \end{bmatrix} \begin{bmatrix} 2 & 1 \\ -3 & 1 \end{bmatrix} \frac{1}{5}$$

which simplifies to

$$\frac{1}{5} \begin{bmatrix} 5 & 0 \\ 0 & 5 \end{bmatrix} \begin{bmatrix} x \\ y \end{bmatrix} = \frac{1}{5} \begin{bmatrix} 5 \\ 15 \end{bmatrix}$$

Solving for the solution matrix, the answer is:

$$\begin{bmatrix} 1 & 0 \\ 0 & 1 \end{bmatrix} \begin{bmatrix} x \\ y \end{bmatrix} = \begin{bmatrix} 1 \\ 3 \end{bmatrix}$$

Since the first matrix is the identity matrix, the solution is $x = 1$ and $y = 3$.

Finding solutions to systems of equations is essentially finding what values of the variables make both equations true. It is finding the input value that yields the same output value in both equations. For functions $g(x)$ and $f(x)$, the equation $g(x) = f(x)$ means the output values are being set equal to each other. Solving for the value of x means finding the x-coordinate that gives the same output in both functions. For example, $f(x) = x + 2$ and $g(x) = -3x + 10$ is a system of equations. Setting $f(x) = g(x)$ yields the equation $x + 2 = -3x + 10$. Solving for x, gives the x-coordinate $x = 2$ where the two lines cross. This value can also be found by using a table or a graph. On a table, both equations can be given the same inputs, and the outputs can be recorded to find the point(s) where the lines cross. Any method of solving finds the same solution, but some methods are more appropriate for some systems of equations than others.

Solving Inequalities and Graphing the Answer on a Number Line

Linear inequalities and linear equations are both comparisons of two algebraic expressions. However, unlike equations in which the expressions are equal to each other, linear inequalities compare expressions that are unequal. Linear equations typically have one value for the variable that makes the statement true. Linear inequalities generally have an infinite number of values that make the statement true.

Linear inequalities are a concise mathematical way to express the relationship between unequal values. More specifically, they describe in what way the values are unequal. A value could be greater than ($>$); less than ($<$); greater than or equal to ($\geq$); or less than or equal to ($\leq$) another value. The statement "five times a number added to forty is more than sixty-five" can be expressed as $5x + 40 > 65$. Common words and phrases that express inequalities are:

Symbol	Phrase
$<$	is under, is below, smaller than, beneath
$>$	is above, is over, bigger than, exceeds
$\leq$	no more than, at most, maximum
$\geq$	no less than, at least, minimum

If a problem were to say, "The sum of a number and 5 is greater than -8 times the number," then an inequality would be used instead of an equation. Using key words again, *greater than* is represented by the symbol >. The inequality $n + 5 > -8n$ can be solved using the same techniques, resulting in $n < -\frac{5}{9}$. The only time solving an inequality differs from solving an equation is when a negative number is either multiplied by or divided by each side of the inequality. The sign must be switched in this case. For this example, the graph of the solution changes to the following graph because the solution represents all real numbers less than $-\frac{5}{9}$. Not included in this solution is $-\frac{5}{9}$ because it is a *less than* symbol, not *equal to*.

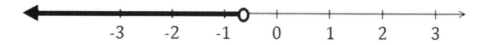

When solving a linear inequality, the solution is the set of all numbers that makes the statement true. The inequality $x + 2 \geq 6$ has a solution set of 4 and every number greater than 4 (4.0001, 5, 12, 107, etc.). Adding 2 to 4 or any number greater than 4 would result in a value that is greater than or equal to 6. Therefore, $x \geq 4$ would be the solution set.

Solution sets for linear inequalities often will be displayed using a number line. If a value is included in the set ($\geq$ or $\leq$), there is a shaded dot placed on that value and an arrow extending in the direction of the solutions. For a variable $>$ or $\geq$ a number, the arrow would point right on the number line (the direction where the numbers increase); and if a variable is $<$ or $\leq$ a number, the arrow would point left (where the numbers decrease). If the value is not included in the set ($>$ or $<$), an open circle on that value would be used with an arrow in the appropriate direction.

Observe this number line:

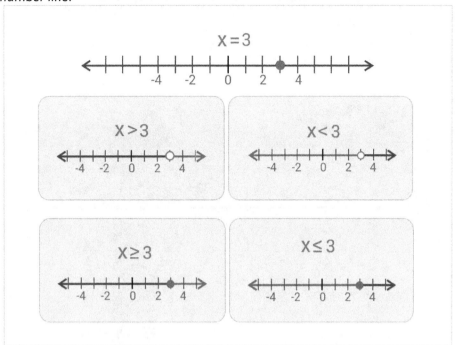

Students may be asked to write a linear inequality given a graph of its solution set. To do so, they should identify whether the value is included (shaded dot or open circle) and the direction in which the arrow is pointing.

In order to algebraically solve a linear inequality, the same steps should be followed as in solving a linear equation. The inequality symbol stays the same for all operations EXCEPT when dividing by a negative number. If dividing by a negative number while solving an inequality, the relationship reverses (the sign flips). Dividing by a positive does not change the relationship, so the sign stays the same. In other words, $>$ switches to $<$ and vice versa. An example is shown below.

Solve $-2(x + 4) \leq 22$

Distribute: $-2x - 8 \leq 22$

Add 8 to both sides: $-2x \leq 30$

Divide both sides by -2: $x \geq 15$

With a single equation in two variables, the solutions are limited only by the situation the equation represents. When two equations or inequalities are used, more constraints are added. For example, in a system of linear equations, there is often—although not always—only one answer. The point of intersection of two lines is the solution. For a system of inequalities, there are infinitely many answers.

The intersection of two solution sets gives the solution set of the system of inequalities. In the following graph, the darker shaded region is where two inequalities overlap. Any set of x and y found in that region satisfies both inequalities. The line with the positive slope is solid, meaning the values on that line are included in the solution.

111

The line with the negative slope is dotted, so the coordinates on that line are not included.

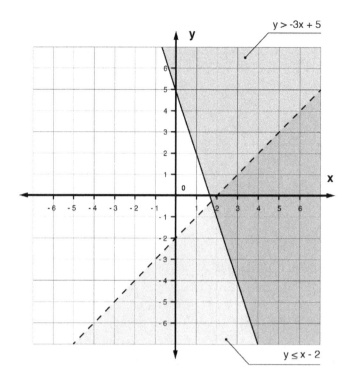

Quadratic Equations with One Variable

A **quadratic equation** can be written in the form $y = ax^2 + bx + c$. The u-shaped graph of a quadratic equation is called a **parabola**. The graph can either open up or open down (upside down u). The graph is symmetric about a vertical line, called the **axis of symmetry**. Corresponding points on the parabola are directly across from each other (same y-value) and are the same distance from the axis of symmetry (on either side). The axis of symmetry intersects the parabola at its **vertex**. The y-value of the vertex represents the minimum or maximum value of the function. If the graph opens up, the value of a in its equation is positive and the vertex represents the minimum of the function. If the graph opens down, the value of a in its equation is negative and the vertex represents the maximum of the function.

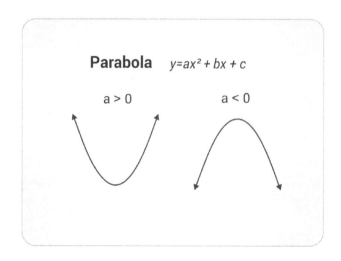

A quadratic equation can be written in the standard form: $y = ax^2 + bx + c$. It can be represented by a u-shaped graph called a parabola. For a quadratic equation where the value of a is positive, as the inputs increase, the outputs increase until a certain value (maximum of the function) is reached. As inputs increase past the value that corresponds with the maximum output, the relationship reverses and the outputs decrease. For a quadratic equation where a is negative, as the inputs increase, the outputs (1) decrease, (2) reach a maximum, and (3) then increase.

Consider a ball thrown straight up into the air. As time passes, the height of the ball increases until it reaches its maximum height. After reaching the maximum height, as time increases, the height of the ball decreases (it is falling toward the ground). This relationship can be expressed as a quadratic equation where time is the input (x) and the height of the ball is the output (y).

Equations with one variable (linear equations) can be solved using the addition principle and multiplication principle. If $a = b$, then $a + c = b + c$, and $ac = bc$. Given the equation $2x - 3 = 5x + 7$, the first step is to combine the variable terms and the constant terms. Using the principles, expressions can be added and subtracted onto and off both sides of the equals sign, so the equation turns into $-10 = 3x$. Dividing by 3 on both sides through the multiplication principle with $c = \frac{1}{3}$ results in the final answer of $x = \frac{-10}{3}$.

However, this same process cannot be used to solve nonlinear equations, including quadratic equations. Quadratic equations have a higher degree than linear ones (2 versus 1) and are not solved by simply using opposite operations. When an equation has a degree of 2, completing the square is an option. For example, the quadratic equation $x^2 - 6x + 2 = 0$ can be rewritten by completing the square. The goal of completing the square is to get the equation into the form $(x - p)^2 = q$. Using the example, the constant term 2 first needs to be moved over to the opposite side by subtracting. Then, the square can be completed by adding 9 to both sides, which is the square of half of the coefficient of the middle term $-6x$. The current equation is $x^2 - 6x + 9 = 7$. The left side can be factored into a square of a binomial, resulting in $(x - 3)^2 = 7$. To solve for x, the square root of both sides should be taken, resulting in $(x - 3) = \pm\sqrt{7}$, and $x = 3 \pm \sqrt{7}$.

Other ways of solving quadratic equations include graphing, factoring, and using the quadratic formula. The equation $y = x^2 - 4x + 3$ can be graphed on the coordinate plane, and the solutions can be observed where it crosses the x-axis. The graph will be a parabola that opens up with two solutions at 1 and 3.

If quadratic equations take the form $ax^2 - b = 0$, then the equation can be solved by adding b to both sides and dividing by a to get:

$$x^2 = \frac{b}{a} \text{ or } x = \pm\sqrt{\frac{b}{a}}$$

Note that this is actually two separate solutions, unless b happens to be 0.

If a quadratic equation has no constant—so that it takes the form $ax^2 + bx = 0$—then the x can be factored out to get $x(ax + b) = 0$. Then, the solutions are $x = 0$, together with the solutions to $ax + b = 0$. Both factors x and $(ax + b)$ can be set equal to zero to solve for x because one of those values must be zero for their product to equal zero. For an equation $ab = 0$ to be true, either $a = 0$, or $b = 0$.

A given quadratic equation $x^2 + bx + c$ can be factored into $(x + A)(x + B)$, where $A + B = b$, and $AB = c$. Finding the values of A and B can take time, but such a pair of numbers can be found by guessing and checking. Looking at the positive and negative factors for c offers a good starting point.

For example, in $x^2 - 5x + 6$, the factors of 6 are 1, 2, and 3. Now,$(-2)(-3) = 6$, and $-2 - 3 = -5$. In general, however, this may not work, in which case another approach may need to be used.

A quadratic equation of the form $x^2 + 2xb + b^2 = 0$ can be factored into $(x + b)^2 = 0$. Similarly, $x^2 - 2xy + y^2 = 0$ factors into $(x - y)^2 = 0$.

The first method of completing the square can be used in finding the second method, the quadratic formula. It can be used to solve any quadratic equation. This formula may be the longest method for solving quadratic equations and is commonly used as a last resort after other methods are ruled out.

It can be helpful in memorizing the formula to see where it comes from, so here are the steps involved.

The most general form for a quadratic equation is:

$$ax^2 + bx + c = 0$$

First, dividing both sides by a leaves us with:

$$x^2 + \frac{b}{a}x + \frac{c}{a} = 0$$

To complete the square on the left-hand side, c/a can be subtracted on both sides to get:

$$x^2 + \frac{b}{a}x = -\frac{c}{a}$$

$(\frac{b}{2a})^2$ is then added to both sides.

This gives:

$$x^2 + \frac{b}{a}x + (\frac{b}{2a})^2 = (\frac{b}{2a})^2 - \frac{c}{a}$$

The left can now be factored and the right-hand side simplified to give:

$$(x + \frac{b}{2a})^2 = \frac{b^2 - 4ac}{4a}$$

Taking the square roots gives:

$$x + \frac{b}{2a} = \pm \frac{\sqrt{b^2 - 4ac}}{2a}$$

Solving for x yields the quadratic formula:

$$x = \frac{-b \pm \sqrt{b^2 - 4ac}}{2a}$$

It isn't necessary to remember how to get this formula but memorizing the formula itself is the goal.

If an equation involves taking a root, then the first step is to move the root to one side of the equation and everything else to the other side. That way, both sides can be raised to the index of the radical in order to remove it, and solving the equation can continue.

Geometry

Side Lengths of Shapes When Given the Area or Perimeter

The **perimeter** of a polygon is the distance around the outside of the two-dimensional figure or the sum of the lengths of all the sides. Perimeter is a one-dimensional measurement and is therefore expressed in linear units such as centimeters (*cm*), feet (*ft*), and miles (*mi*). The perimeter (*P*) of a figure can be calculated by adding together each of the sides.

Properties of certain polygons allow that the perimeter may be obtained by using formulas. A regular polygon is one in which all sides have equal length and all interior angles have equal measures, such as a square and an equilateral triangle. To find the perimeter of a regular polygon, the length of one side is multiplied by the number of sides.

A rectangle consists of two sides called the length (*l*), which have equal measures, and two sides called the width (*w*), which have equal measures. Therefore, the perimeter (*P*) of a rectangle can be expressed as $P = l + l + w + w$. This can be simplified to produce the following formula to find the perimeter of a rectangle: $P = 2l + 2w$ or $P = 2(l + w)$.

The perimeter of a square is measured by adding together all of the sides. Since a square has four equal sides, its perimeter can be calculated by multiplying the length of one side by 4. Thus, the formula is $P = 4 \times s$, where *s* equals one side. For example, the following square has side lengths of 5 meters:

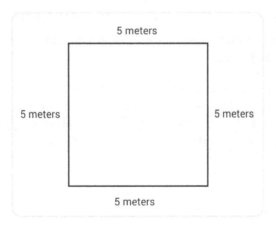

The perimeter is 20 meters because 4 times 5 is 20.

Like a square, a rectangle's perimeter is measured by adding together all of the sides. But as the sides are unequal, the formula is different. A rectangle has equal values for its lengths (long sides) and equal values for its widths (short sides), so the perimeter formula for a rectangle is:

$$P = l + l + w + w = 2l + 2w$$

l equals length
w equals width

115

Consider the following problem:

The total perimeter of a rectangular garden is 36m. If the length of each side is 12m, what is the width?

The formula for the perimeter of a rectangle is $P = 2L + 2W$, where P is the perimeter, L is the length, and W is the width. The first step is to substitute all of the data into the formula:

$$36 = 2(12) + 2W$$

Simplify by multiplying 2×12:

$$36 = 24 + 2W$$

Simplify this further by subtracting 24 on each side, which gives:

$$36 - 24 = 24 - 24 + 2W$$

$$12 = 2W$$

Divide by 2:

$$6 = W$$

The width is 6m. Remember to test this answer by substituting this value into the original formula:

$$36 = 2(12) + 2(6)$$

A triangle's perimeter is measured by adding together the three sides, so the formula is $P = a + b + c$, where $a, b,$ and c are the values of the three sides. The area is calculated by multiplying the length of the base times the height times ½, so the formula is $A = \frac{1}{2} \times b \times h = \frac{bh}{2}$. The base is the bottom of the triangle, and the height is the distance from the base to the peak. If a problem asks to calculate the area of a triangle, it will provide the base and height.

A circle's perimeter—also known as its circumference—is measured by multiplying the diameter (the straight line measured from one end to the direct opposite end of the circle) by π, so the formula is $\pi \times d$. This is sometimes expressed by the formula $C = 2 \times \pi \times r$, where r is the radius of the circle. These formulas are equivalent, as the radius equals half of the diameter.

Missing side lengths can be determined using subtraction. For example, if you are told that a triangle has a perimeter of 34 inches and that one side is 12 inches, another side is 16 inches, and the third side is unknown, you can calculate the length of that unknown side by setting up the following subtraction problem:

$$34\ inches = 12\ inches + 16\ inches + x$$

$$34\ inches = 28\ inches + x$$

$$6\ inches = x$$

Therefore, the missing side length is 6 inches.

Area and Perimeter of Two-Dimensional Shapes

As mentioned, the **perimeter** of a polygon is the distance around the outside of the two-dimensional figure. Perimeter is a one-dimensional measurement and is therefore expressed in linear units such as centimeters (*cm*), feet (*ft*), and miles (*mi*). The perimeter (*P*) of a figure can be calculated by adding together each of the sides.

Properties of certain polygons allow that the perimeter may be obtained by using formulas. A rectangle consists of two sides called the length (*l*), which have equal measures, and two sides called the width (*w*), which have equal measures. Therefore, the perimeter (*P*) of a rectangle can be expressed as:

$$P = l + l + w + w$$

This can be simplified to produce the following formula to find the perimeter of a rectangle:

$$P = 2l + 2w \text{ or } P = 2(l + w)$$

A regular polygon is one in which all sides have equal length and all interior angles have equal measures, such as a square and an equilateral triangle. To find the perimeter of a regular polygon, the length of one side is multiplied by the number of sides. For example, to find the perimeter of an equilateral triangle with a side of length of 4 feet, 4 feet is multiplied by 3 (number of sides of a triangle). The perimeter of a regular octagon (8 sides) with a side of length of $\frac{1}{2}$ cm is:

$$\frac{1}{2} cm \times 8 = 4cm$$

The **area** of a polygon is the number of square units needed to cover the interior region of the figure. Area is a two-dimensional measurement. Therefore, area is expressed in square units, such as square centimeters (cm^2), square feet (ft^2), or square miles (mi^2). Regarding the area of a rectangle with sides of length *x* and *y*, the area is given by xy. For a triangle with a base of length *b* and a height of length *h*, the area is $\frac{1}{2}bh$. To find the area (*A*) of a parallelogram, the length of the base (*b*) is multiplied by the length of the height (*h*) $\rightarrow A = b \times h$. Similar to triangles, the height of the parallelogram is measured from one base to the other at a 90° angle (or perpendicular).

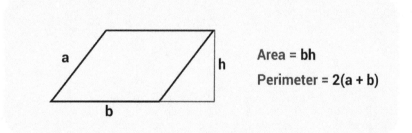

117

The area of a trapezoid can be calculated using the formula: $A = \frac{1}{2} \times h(b_1 + b_2)$, where h is the height and b_1 and b_2 are the parallel bases of the trapezoid.

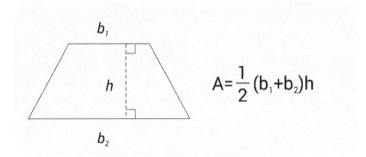

The area of a regular polygon can be determined by using its perimeter and the length of the **apothem**. The apothem is a line from the center of the regular polygon to any of its sides at a right angle. (Note that the perimeter of a regular polygon can be determined given the length of only one side.) The formula for the area (A) of a regular polygon is:

$$A = \frac{1}{2} \times a \times P$$

where a is the length of the apothem and P is the perimeter of the figure.

Consider the following regular pentagon:

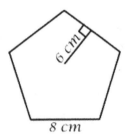

To find the area, the perimeter (P) is calculated first: $8cm \times 5 \rightarrow P = 40cm$. Then the perimeter and the apothem are used to find the area (A):

$$A = \frac{1}{2} \times a \times P$$

$$A = \frac{1}{2} \times (6cm) \times (40cm)$$

$$A = 120cm^2$$

Note that the unit is:

$$cm^2 \rightarrow cm \times cm = cm^2$$

The area of irregular polygons is found by decomposing, or breaking apart, the figure into smaller shapes. When the area of the smaller shapes is determined, the area of the smaller shapes will produce the area of the original figure when added together. Consider the example below:

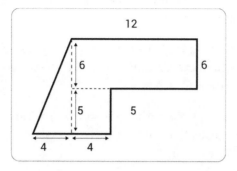

The irregular polygon is decomposed into two rectangles and a triangle. The area of the large rectangles ($A = l \times w \rightarrow A = 12 \times 6$) is 72 square units. The area of the small rectangle is 20 square units:

$$A = 4 \times 5$$

The area of the triangle:

$$A = \frac{1}{2} \times b \times h$$

$$A = \frac{1}{2} \times 4 \times 11$$

22 square units

The sum of the areas of these figures produces the total area of the original polygon:

$$A = 72 + 20 + 22$$

A = 114 square units

The perimeter (P) of the figure below is calculated by: $P = 9m + 5m + 4m + 6m + 8m \rightarrow P = 32\ m$.

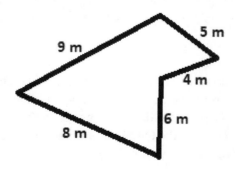

Area, Circumference, Radius, and Diameter of a Circle

A **circle** can be defined as the set of all points that are the same distance (known as the **radius**, *r*) from a single point (known as the **center** of the circle). The center has coordinates (h, k), and any point on the circle can be labelled with coordinates (x, y).

The **circumference** of a circle is the distance traveled by following the edge of the circle for one complete revolution, and the length of the circumference is given by $2\pi r$, where *r* is the radius of the circle. The formula for circumference is $C = 2\pi r$.

The area of a circle is calculated through the formula $A = \pi \times r^2$. The test will indicate either to leave the answer with π attached or to calculate to the nearest decimal place, which means multiplying by 3.14 for π.

Given two points on the circumference of a circle, the path along the circle between those points is called an **arc** of the circle. For example, the arc between *B* and *C* is denoted by a thinner line:

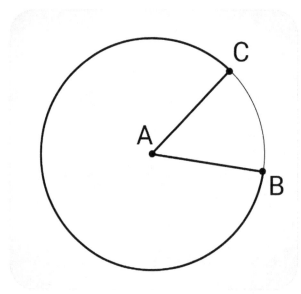

The length of the path along an arc is called the **arc length**. If the circle has radius *r*, then the arc length is given by multiplying the measure of the angle in radians by the radius of the circle.

Pythagorean Theorem

The Pythagorean theorem is an important result in geometry. It states that for right triangles, the sum of the squares of the two shorter sides will be equal to the square of the longest side (also called the **hypotenuse**). The longest side will always be the side opposite to the 90° angle. If this side is called *c*, and the other two sides are *a* and *b*, then the Pythagorean theorem states that $c^2 = a^2 + b^2$. Since lengths are always positive, this also can be written as:

$$c = \sqrt{a^2 + b^2}$$

A diagram to show the parts of a triangle using the Pythagorean theorem is below.

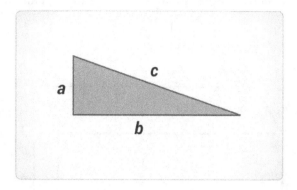

As an example of the theorem, suppose that Shirley has a rectangular field that is 5 feet wide and 12 feet long, and she wants to split it in half using a fence that goes from one corner to the opposite corner. How long will this fence need to be? To figure this out, note that this makes the field into two right triangles, whose hypotenuse will be the fence dividing it in half. Therefore, the fence length will be given by $\sqrt{5^2 + 12^2} = \sqrt{169} = 13$ feet long.

Volume and Surface Area of Three-Dimensional Shapes

Geometry in three dimensions is similar to geometry in two dimensions. The main new feature is that three points now define a unique **plane** that passes through each of them. Three-dimensional objects can be made by putting together two-dimensional figures in different surfaces. Below, some of the possible three-dimensional figures will be provided, along with formulas for their volumes and surface areas.

Volume is the measurement of how much space an object occupies, like how much space is in the cube. Volume questions will ask how much of something is needed to completely fill the object. The most common surface area and volume questions deal with spheres, cubes, and rectangular prisms.

Surface area of a three-dimensional figure refers to the number of square units needed to cover the entire surface of the figure. This concept is similar to using wrapping paper to completely cover the outside of a box. For example, if a triangular pyramid has a surface area of 17 square inches (written $17in^2$), it will take 17 squares, each with sides one inch in length, to cover the entire surface of the pyramid. Surface area is also measured in square units.

A **rectangular prism** is a box whose sides are all rectangles meeting at 90° angles. Such a box has three dimensions: length, width, and height. If the length is x, the width is y, and the height is z, then the volume is given by $V = xyz$.

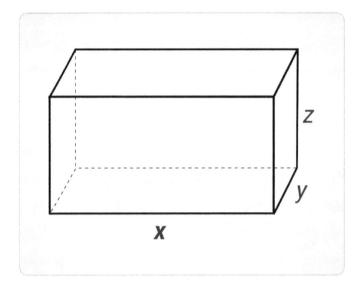

The **surface area** will be given by computing the surface area of each rectangle and adding them together. There is a total of six rectangles. Two of them have sides of length x and y, two have sides of length y and z, and two have sides of length x and z. Therefore, the total surface area will be given by:

$$SA = 2xy + 2yz + 2xz$$

A **cube** is a special type of rectangular solid in which its length, width, and height are the same. If this length is s, then the formula for the volume of a cube is $V = s \times s \times s$. The surface area of a cube is $SA = 6s^2$.

A **rectangular pyramid** is a figure with a rectangular base and four triangular sides that meet at a single vertex. If the rectangle has sides of length x and y, then the volume will be given by $V = \frac{1}{3}xyh$.

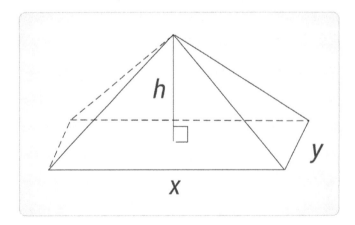

Many three-dimensional figures (solid figures) can be represented by nets consisting of rectangles and triangles. The surface area of such solids can be determined by adding the areas of each of its faces and bases. Finding the surface area using this method requires calculating the areas of rectangles and triangles. To find the area (A) of a rectangle, the length (l) is multiplied by the width (w) → $A = l \times w$. The area of a rectangle with a length of 8cm and a width of 4cm is calculated: $A = (8cm) \times (4cm) \rightarrow A = 32cm^2$.

To calculate the area (A) of a triangle, the product of $\frac{1}{2}$, the base (b), and the height (h) is found:

$$A = \frac{1}{2} \times b \times h$$

Note that the height of a triangle is measured from the base to the vertex opposite of it forming a right angle with the base. The area of a triangle with a base of 11cm and a height of 6cm is calculated:

$$A = \frac{1}{2} \times (11cm) \times (6cm)$$

$$A = 33cm^2$$

Consider the following triangular prism, which is represented by a net consisting of two triangles and three rectangles.

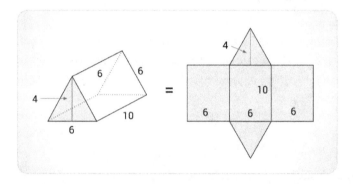

The surface area of the prism can be determined by adding the areas of each of its faces and bases. The surface area (SA) = area of triangle + area of triangle + area of rectangle + area of rectangle + area of rectangle.

$$SA = \left(\frac{1}{2} \times b \times h\right) + \left(\frac{1}{2} \times b \times h\right) + (l \times w) + (l \times w) + (l \times w)$$

$$SA = \left(\frac{1}{2} \times 6 \times 4\right) + \left(\frac{1}{2} \times 6 \times 4\right) + (6 \times 10) + (6 \times 10) + (6 \times 10)$$

$$SA = (12) + (12) + (60) + (60) + (60)$$

$$SA = 204 \; square \; units$$

A **sphere** is a set of points all of which are equidistant from some central point. It is like a circle, but in three dimensions. The volume of a sphere of radius r is given by:

$$V = \frac{4}{3}\pi r^3$$

The surface area is given by $A = 4\pi r^2$.

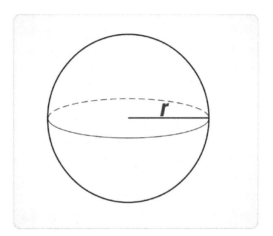

The volume of a **cylinder** is then found by adding a third dimension onto the circle. Volume of a cylinder is calculated by multiplying the area of the base (which is a circle) by the height of the cylinder. Doing so results in the equation $V = \pi r^2 h$. The volume of a **cone** is $\frac{1}{3}$ of the volume of a cylinder. Therefore, the formula for the volume of a **cone** is:

$$\frac{1}{3}\pi r^2 h$$

Solving Three-Dimensional Problems
Three-dimensional objects can be simplified into related two-dimensional shapes to solve problems. This simplification can make problem-solving a much easier experience. An isometric representation of a three-dimensional object can be completed so that important properties (e.g., shape, relationships of faces and surfaces) are noted. Edges and vertices can be translated into two-dimensional objects as well.

Consider this three-dimensional object that's been partitioned into two-dimensional representations of its faces:

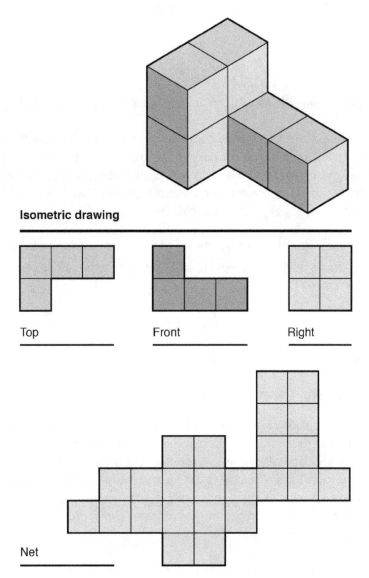

The net represents the sum of the three different faces. Depending on the problem, using a smaller portion of the given shape may be helpful, by simplifying the steps necessary to solve.

Many objects in the real world consist of three-dimensional shapes such as prisms, cylinders, and spheres. Surface area problems involve quantifying the outside area of such a three-dimensional object, and volume problems involve quantifying how much space the object takes up. Surface area of a prism is the sum of the areas, which is simplified into $SA = 2A + Bh$, where A is the area of the base, B is the perimeter of the base, and h is the height of the prism. The volume of the same prism is $V = Ah$.

The surface area of a cylinder is equal to the sum of the areas of each end and the side, which is:

$$SA = 2\pi rh + 2\pi r^2$$

and its volume is:

$$V = \pi r^2 h$$

Finally, the surface area of a sphere is $SA = 4\pi r^2$, and its volume is $V = \frac{4}{3}\pi r^3$.

An example when one of these formulas should be used would be when calculating how much paint is needed for the outside of a house. In this scenario, surface area must be used. The sum of all individual areas of each side of the house must be found. Also, when calculating how much water a cylindrical tank can hold, a volume formula is used. Therefore, the amount of water that a cylindrical tank that is 8 feet tall with a radius of 3 feet is $\pi \times 3^2 \times 8 = 226.1$ cubic feet.

The formula used to calculate the volume of a cone is $\frac{1}{3}\pi r^2 h$. Essentially, the area of the base of the cone is multiplied by the cone's height. In a real-life example where the radius of a cone is 2 meters and the height of a cone is 5 meters, the volume of the cone is calculated by utilizing the formula:

$$\frac{1}{3}\pi 2^2 \times 5$$

After substituting 3.14 for π, the volume is 20.9 m^3.

Graphical Data Including Graphs, Tables, and More

A set of data can be visually displayed in various forms allowing for quick identification of characteristics of the set. **Histograms**, such as the one shown below, display the number of data points (vertical axis) that fall into given intervals (horizontal axis) across the range of the set. The histogram below displays the heights of black cherry trees in a certain city park. Each rectangle represents the number of trees with heights between a given five-point span. For example, the furthest bar to the right indicates that two trees are between 85 and 90 feet. Histograms can describe the center, spread, shape, and any unusual characteristics of a data set.

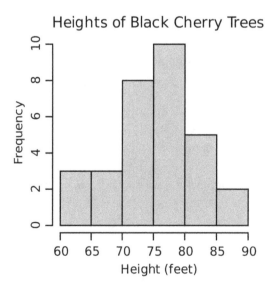

A **box plot**, also called a **box-and-whisker plot**, divides the data points into four groups and displays the five-number summary for the set, as well as any outliers. The five-number summary consists of:

- The lower extreme: the lowest value that is not an outlier
- The higher extreme: the highest value that is not an outlier
- The median of the set: also referred to as the second quartile or Q_2
- The first quartile or Q_1: the median of values below Q_2
- The third quartile or Q_3: the median of values above Q_2

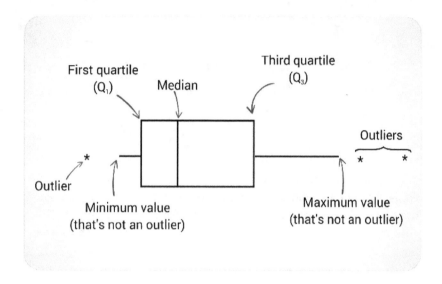

Suppose the box plot displays IQ scores for 12th grade students at a given school. The five-number summary of the data consists of: lower extreme (67); upper extreme (127); Q_2 or median (100); Q_1 (91); Q_3 (108); and outliers (135 and 140). Although all data points are not known from the plot, the points are divided into four quartiles each, including 25% of the data points. Therefore, 25% of students scored between 67 and 91, 25% scored between 91 and 100, 25% scored between 100 and 108, and 25% scored between 108 and 127. These percentages include the normal values for the set and exclude the outliers. This information is useful when comparing a given score with the rest of the scores in the set.

A **scatter plot** is a mathematical diagram that visually displays the relationship or connection between two variables. The independent variable is placed on the *x*-axis, or horizontal axis, and the dependent variable is placed on the *y*-axis, or vertical axis. When visually examining the points on the graph, if the points model a linear relationship, or a **line of best-fit** can be drawn through the points with the points relatively close on either side, then a correlation exists. If the line of best-fit has a positive slope (rises from left to right), then the variables have a positive correlation. If the line of best-fit has a negative slope (falls from left to right), then the variables have a negative correlation. If a line of best-fit cannot be drawn, then no correlation exists. A positive or negative correlation can be categorized as strong or weak, depending on how closely the points are graphed around the line of best-fit.

Consider this display of correlations:

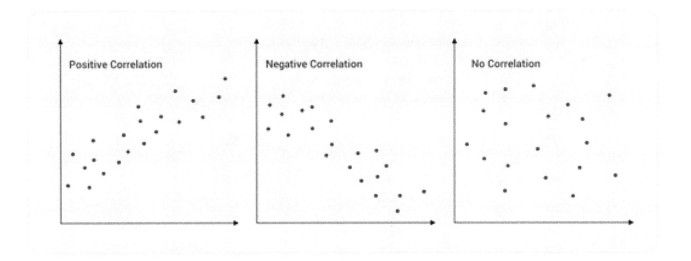

Like a scatter plot, a **line graph** compares variables that change continuously, typically over time. Paired data values (ordered pair) are plotted on a coordinate grid with the *x*- and *y*-axis representing the variables. A line is drawn from each point to the next, going from left to right. The line graph below displays cell phone use for given years (two variables) for men, women, and both sexes (three data sets).

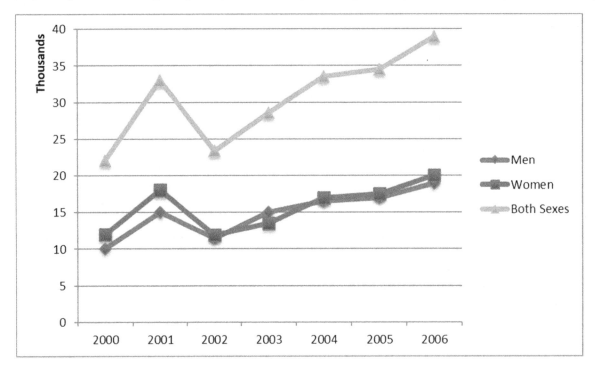

A **line plot**, also called **dot plot**, displays the frequency of data (numerical values) on a number line. To construct a line plot, a number line is used that includes all unique data values. It is marked with x's or dots above the value the number of times that the value occurs in the data set.

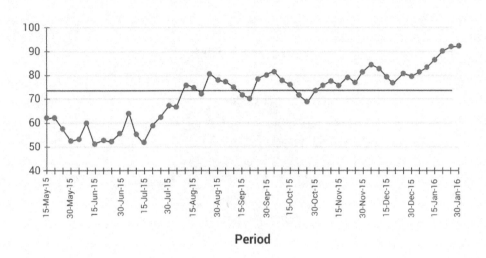

A **bar graph** is a diagram in which the quantity of items within a specific classification is represented by the height of a rectangle. Each type of classification is represented by a rectangle of equal width. Here is an example of a bar graph:

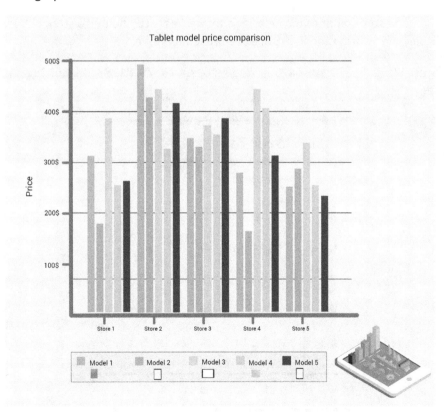

A **circle graph**, also called a **pie chart**, shows categorical data with each category representing a percentage of the whole data set. To make a circle graph, the percent of the data set for each category must be determined. To do so, the frequency of the category is divided by the total number of data points and converted to a percent. For example, if 80 people were asked what their favorite sport is and 20 responded basketball, basketball makes up 25% of the data ($\frac{20}{80}$ =.25=25%). Each category in a data set is represented by a slice of the circle proportionate to its percentage of the whole.

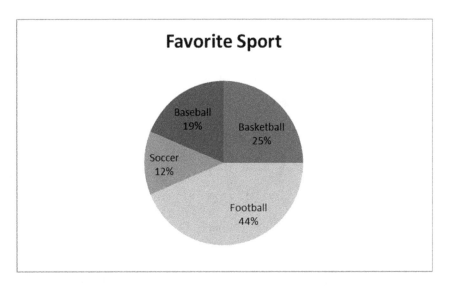

A **stem-and-leaf plot** is a method of displaying sets of data by organizing the numbers by their stems (usually the tens digit) and the different leaf values (usually the ones digit).

For example, to organize a number of movie critic's ratings, as listed below, a stem and leaf plot could be utilized to display the information in a more condensed manner.

Movie critic scores: 47, 52, 56, 59, 61, 64, 66, 68, 68, 70, 73, 75, 79, 81, 83, 85, 86, 88, 88, 89, 90, 90, 91, 93, 94, 96, 96, 99.

	Movie Ratings
4	7
5	2 6 9
6	1 4 6 8 8
7	0 3 5 9
8	1 3 5 6 8 8 9
9	0 0 1 3 4 6 6 9
Key	6 │ 1 represents 61

Looking at this stem and leaf plot, it is easy to ascertain key features of the data set. For example, what is the range of the data in the stem-and-leaf plot?

Using this method, it is easier to visualize the distribution of the scores and answer the question pertaining to the range of scores, which is $99 - 47 = 52$.

A **tally chart** is a diagram in which tally marks are utilized to represent data. Tally marks are a means of showing a quantity of objects within a specific classification. Here is an example of a tally chart:

Number of days with rain	Number of weeks
0	II
1	HHT
2	HHT
3	HHT
4	HHT HHT HHT IIII
5	HHT I
6	HHT I
7	IIII

Data is often recorded using fractions, such as half a mile, and understanding fractions is critical because of their popular use in real-world applications. Also, it is extremely important to label values with their units when using data. For example, regarding length, the number 2 is meaningless unless it is attached to a unit. Writing 2 cm shows that the number refers to the length of an object.

Mean, Median, Mode, and Range

Suppose that X is a set of data points $(x_1, x_2, x_3, \ldots x_n)$ and some description of the general properties of this data need to be found.

The first property that can be defined for this set of data is the **mean**. To find the mean, add up all the data points, then divide by the total number of data points. This can be expressed using **summation notation** as:

$$\bar{X} = \frac{x_1 + x_2 + x_3 + \cdots + x_n}{n} = \frac{1}{n}\sum_{i=1}^{n} x_i$$

For example, suppose that in a class of 10 students, the scores on a test were 50, 60, 65, 65, 75, 80, 85, 85, 90, 100. Therefore, the average test score will be:

$$\frac{1}{10}(50 + 60 + 65 + 65 + 75 + 80 + 85 + 85 + 90 + 100) = 75.5$$

The mean is a useful number if the distribution of data is normal (more on this later), which roughly means that the frequency of different outcomes has a single peak and is roughly equally distributed on both sides of that peak. However, it is less useful in some cases where the data might be split or where there are some outliers. **Outliers** are data points that are far from the rest of the data. For example, suppose there are 90 employees and 10 executives at a company. The executives make $1000 per hour, and the employees make $10 per hour. Therefore, the average pay rate will be:

$$\frac{1000 \times 10 + 10 \times 90}{100} = 109$$

or $109 per hour

In this case, this average is not very descriptive.

Another useful measurement is the **median**. In a data set X consisting of data points $x_1, x_2, x_3, \ldots x_n$, the median is the point in the middle. The middle refers to the point where half the data comes before it and half comes after, when the data is recorded in numerical order. If n is odd, then the median is:

$$x_{\frac{n+1}{2}}$$

If n is even, it is defined as:

$$\frac{1}{2}\left(x_{\frac{n}{2}} + x_{\frac{n}{2}+1}\right)$$

the mean of the two data points closest to the middle of the data points. In the previous example of test scores, the two middle points are 75 and 80. Since there is no single point, the average of these two scores needs to be found. The average is:

$$\frac{75 + 80}{2} = 77.5$$

The median is generally a good value to use if there are a few outliers in the data. It prevents those outliers from affecting the "middle" value as much as when using the mean.

Since an outlier is a data point that is far from most of the other data points in a data set, this means an outlier also is any point that is far from the median of the data set. The outliers can have a substantial effect on the mean of a data set, but usually do not change the median or mode, or do not change them by a large quantity. For example, consider the data set (3, 5, 6, 6, 6, 8). This has a median of 6 and a mode of 6, with a mean of $\frac{34}{6} \approx 5.67$. Now, suppose a new data point of 1000 is added so that the data set is now (3, 5, 6, 6, 6, 8, 1000). This does not change the median or mode, which are both still 6. However, the average is now $\frac{1034}{7}$, which is approximately 147.7. In this case, the median and mode will be better descriptions for most of the data points.

The reason for outliers in a given data set is a complicated problem. It is sometimes the result of an error by the experimenter, but often they are perfectly valid data points that must be taken into consideration.

One additional measure to define for X is the **mode**. This is the data point that appears more frequently. If two or more data points all tie for the most frequent appearance, then each of them is considered a mode. In the case of the test scores, where the numbers were 50, 60, 65, 65, 75, 80, 85, 85, 90, 100, there are two modes: 65 and 85.

The **first quartile** of a set of data X refers to the largest value from the first ¼ of the data points. In practice, there are sometimes slightly different definitions that can be used, such as the median of the first half of the data points (excluding the median itself if there are an odd number of data points). The term also has a slightly different use: when it is said that a data point lies in the first quartile, it means it is less than or equal to the median of the first half of the data points. Conversely, if it lies *at* the first quartile, then it is equal to the first quartile.

When it is said that a data point lies in the **second quartile**, it means it is between the first quartile and the median.

The **third quartile** refers to data that lies between ½ and ¾ of the way through the data set. Again, there are various methods for defining this precisely, but the simplest way is to include all of the data that lie between the median and the median of the top half of the data.

Data that lies in the **fourth quartile** refers to all of the data above the third quartile.

Percentiles may be defined in a similar manner to quartiles. Generally, this is defined in the following manner:

If a data point lies *in* the n-th percentile, this means it lies in the range of the first *n*% of the data.

If a data point lies *at* the *n*-th percentile, then it means that *n*% of the data lies below this data point.

Given a data set X consisting of data points $(x_1, x_2, x_3, \dots x_n)$, the **variance of X** is defined to be:

$$\frac{\sum_{i=1}^{n}(x_i - \bar{X})^2}{n}$$

This means that the variance of X is the average of the squares of the differences between each data point and the mean of X. In the formula, $\bar{X}$ is the mean of the values in the data set, and x_i represents each individual value in the data set. The sigma notation indicates that the sum should be found with n being the number of values to add together. $i = 1$ means that the values should begin with the first value.

Given a data set X consisting of data points $(x_1, x_2, x_3, \dots x_n)$, the **standard deviation of X** is defined to be

$$s_x = \sqrt{\frac{\sum_{i=1}^{n}(x_i - \bar{X})^2}{n}}$$

In other words, the standard deviation is the square root of the variance.

Both the variance and the standard deviation are measures of how much the data tend to be spread out. When the standard deviation is low, the data points are mostly clustered around the mean. When the standard deviation is high, this generally indicates that the data are quite spread out, or else that there are a few substantial outliers.

As a simple example, compute the standard deviation for the data set (1, 3, 3, 5). First, compute the mean, which will be:

$$\frac{1 + 3 + 3 + 5}{4} = \frac{12}{4} = 3$$

Now, find the variance of X with the formula:

$$\sum_{i=1}^{4}(x_i - \bar{X})^2 = (1 - 3)^2 + (3 - 3)^2 + (5 - 3)^2$$

$$-2^2 + 0^2 + 0^2 + 2^2 = 8$$

Therefore, the variance is $\frac{8}{4} = 2$. Taking the square root, the standard deviation will be $\sqrt{2}$.

Note that the standard deviation only depends upon the mean, not upon the median or mode(s). Generally, if there are multiple modes that are far apart from one another, the standard deviation will be high. A high standard deviation does not always mean there are multiple modes, however.

Describing a Set of Data

A set of data can be described in terms of its center, spread, shape and any unusual features. The center of a data set can be measured by its mean, median, or mode. The spread of a data set refers to how far the data points are from the center (mean or median). The spread can be measured by the range or the quartiles and interquartile range. A data set with data points clustered around the center will have a small spread. A data set covering a wide range will have a large spread.

When a data set is displayed as a **histogram** or frequency distribution plot, the shape indicates if a sample is normally distributed, symmetrical, or has measures of skewness or kurtosis. When graphed, a data set with a **normal distribution** will resemble a bell curve.

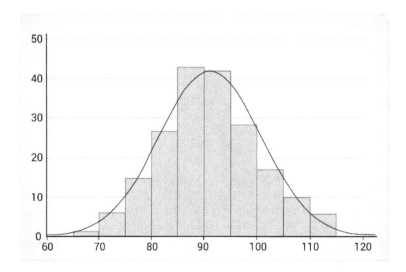

If the data set is symmetrical, each half of the graph when divided at the center is a mirror image of the other. If the graph has fewer data points to the right, the data is **skewed right**. If it has fewer data points to the left, the data is **skewed left**.

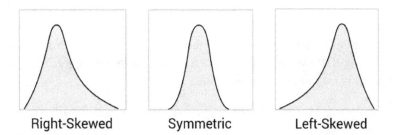

Right-Skewed   Symmetric   Left-Skewed

Kurtosis is a measure of whether the data is heavy-tailed with a high number of outliers, or light-tailed with a low number of outliers.

A description of a data set should include any unusual features such as gaps or outliers. A **gap** is a span within the range of the data set containing no data points. An **outlier** is a data point with a value either extremely large or extremely small when compared to the other values in the set.

Counting Techniques

The **addition rule** for probabilities states that the probability of A or B happening is:

$$P(A \cup B) = P(A) + P(B) - P(A \cap B)$$

Note that the subtraction of $P(A \cap B)$ must be performed, or else it would result in double counting any outcomes that lie in both A and in B. For example, suppose that a 20-sided die is being rolled. Fred bets that the outcome will be greater than 10, while Helen bets that it will be greater than 4 but less than 15. What is the probability that at least one of them is correct?

We apply the rule:

$$P(A \cup B) = P(A) + P(B) - P(A \cap B)$$

where A is that outcome x is in the range $x > 10$, and B is that outcome x is in the range $4 < x < 15$.

$$P(A) = 10 \times \frac{1}{20} = \frac{1}{2}$$

$$P(B) = 10 \times \frac{1}{20} = \frac{1}{2}$$

$P(A \cap B)$ can be computed by noting that $A \cap B$ means the outcome x is in the range $10 < x < 15$, so

$$P(A \cap B) = 4 \times \frac{1}{20} = \frac{1}{5}$$

Therefore:

$$P(A \cup B) = P(A) + P(B) - P(A \cap B)$$

$$\frac{1}{2} + \frac{1}{2} - \frac{1}{5} = \frac{4}{5}$$

Note that in this particular example, we could also have directly reasoned about the set of possible outcomes $A \cup B$, by noting that this would mean that x must be in the range $5 \leq x$. However, this is not always the case, depending on the given information.

The **multiplication rule** for probabilities states the probability of A and B both happening is:

$$P(A \cap B) = P(A)P(B|A)$$

As an example, suppose that when Jamie wears black pants, there is a ½ probability that she wears a black shirt as well, and that she wears black pants ¾ of the time. What is the probability that she is wearing both a black shirt and black pants?

To figure this, use the above formula, where A will be "Jamie is wearing black pants," while B will be "Jamie is wearing a black shirt." It is known that $P(A)$ is ¾. It is also known that $P(B|A) = \frac{1}{2}$. Multiplying the two, the probability that she is wearing both black pants and a black shirt is:

$$P(A)P(B|A) = \frac{3}{4} \times \frac{1}{2} = \frac{3}{8}$$

Probability of an Event

Given a set of possible outcomes X, a **probability distribution** of X is a function that assigns a probability to each possible outcome. If the outcomes are $(x_1, x_2, x_3, \ldots x_n)$, and the probability distribution is p, then the following rules are applied.

- $0 \leq p(x_i) \leq 1$, for any i.

- $\sum_{i=1}^{n} p(x_i) = 1$.

In other words, the probability of a given outcome must be between zero and 1, while the total probability must be 1.

If $p(x_i)$ is constant, then this is called a **uniform probability distribution**, and $p(x_i) = \frac{1}{n}$. For example, on a six-sided die, the probability of each of the six outcomes will be $\frac{1}{6}$.

If seeking the probability of an outcome occurring in some specific range A of possible outcomes, written $P(A)$, add up the probabilities for each outcome in that range. For example, consider a six-sided die, and figure the probability of getting a 3 or lower when it is rolled. The possible rolls are 1, 2, 3, 4, 5, and 6. So, to get a 3 or lower, a roll of 1, 2, or 3 must be completed. The probabilities of each of these is $\frac{1}{6}$, so add these to get:

$$p(1) + p(2) + p(3) = \frac{1}{6} + \frac{1}{6} + \frac{1}{6} = \frac{1}{2}$$

An outcome occasionally lies within some range of possibilities B, and the probability that the outcomes also lie within some set of possibilities A needs to be figured. This is called a **conditional probability**. It is written as $P(A|B)$, which is read "the probability of A given B." The general formula for computing conditional probabilities is:

$$P(A|B) = \frac{P(A \cap B)}{P(B)}$$

However, when dealing with uniform probability distributions, simplify this a bit. Write $|A|$ to indicate the number of outcomes in A. Then, for uniform probability distributions, write:

$$P(A|B) = \frac{|A \cap B|}{|B|}$$

(recall that $A \cap B$ means "A intersect B," and consists of all of the outcomes that lie in both A and B)

This means that all possible outcomes do not need to be known. To see why this formula works, suppose that the set of outcomes X is $(x_1, x_2, x_3, \dots x_n)$, so that $|X| = n$. Then, for a uniform probability distribution:

$$P(A) = \frac{|A|}{n}$$

However, this means:

$$(A|B) = \frac{P(A \cap B)}{P(B)} = \frac{\frac{|A \cap B|}{n}}{\frac{|B|}{n}} = \frac{|A \cap B|}{|B|}$$

since the n's cancel out.

For example, suppose a die is rolled and it is known that it will land between 1 and 4. However, how many sides the die has is unknown. Figure the probability that the die is rolled higher than 2. To figure this, $P(3)$ or $P(4)$ does not need to be determined, or any of the other probabilities, since it is known that a fair die has a uniform probability distribution. Therefore, apply the formula $\frac{|A \cap B|}{|B|}$. So, in this case B is (1, 2, 3, 4) and $A \cap B$ is (3, 4). Therefore:

$$\frac{|A \cap B|}{|B|} = \frac{2}{4} = \frac{1}{2}$$

Conditional probability is an important concept because, in many situations, the likelihood of one outcome can differ radically depending on how something else comes out. The probability of passing a test given that one has studied all of the material is generally much higher than the probability of passing a test given that one has not studied at all. The probability of a person having heart trouble is much lower if that person exercises regularly. The probability that a college student will graduate is higher when his or her SAT scores are higher, and so on. For this reason, there are many people who are interested in conditional probabilities.

Note that in some practical situations, changing the order of the conditional probabilities can make the outcome very different. For example, the probability that a person with heart trouble has exercised regularly is quite different than the probability that a person who exercises regularly will have heart trouble. The probability of a person receiving a military-only award, given that he or she is or was a soldier, is generally not very high, but the probability that a person being or having been a soldier, given that he or she received a military-only award, is 1.

However, in some cases, the outcomes do not influence one another this way. If the probability of A is the same regardless of whether B is given; that is, if $P(A|B) = P(A)$, then A and B are considered **independent**. In this case:

$$P(A|B) = \frac{P(A \cap B)}{P(B)} = P(A)$$

so $P(A \cap B) = P(A)P(B)$. In fact, if $P(A \cap B) = P(A)P(B)$, it can be determined that $P(A|B) = P(A)$ and $P(A|B) = P(B)$ by working backward. Therefore, B is also independent of A.

An example of something being independent can be seen in rolling dice. In this case, consider a red die and a green die. It is expected that when the dice are rolled, the outcome of the green die should not depend in any way on the outcome of the red die. Or, to take another example, if the same die is rolled repeatedly, then the next number rolled should not depend on which numbers have been rolled previously. Similarly, if a coin is flipped, then the next flip's outcome does not depend on the outcomes of previous flips.

This can sometimes be counter-intuitive, since when rolling a die or flipping a coin, there can be a streak of surprising results. If, however, it is known that the die or coin is fair, then these results are just the result of the fact that over long periods of time, it is very likely that some unlikely streaks of outcomes will occur. Therefore, avoid making the mistake of thinking that when considering a series of independent outcomes, a particular outcome is "due to happen" simply because a surprising series of outcomes has already been seen.

There is a second type of common mistake that people tend to make when reasoning about statistical outcomes: the idea that when something of low probability happens, this is surprising. It would be surprising that something with low probability happened after just one attempt. However, with so much happening all at once, it is easy to see at least something happen in a way that seems to have a very low probability. In fact, a lottery is a good example. The odds of winning a lottery are very small, but the odds that somebody wins the lottery each week are actually fairly high. Therefore, no one should be surprised when some low probability things happen.

A **simple event** consists of only one outcome. The most popular simple event is flipping a coin, which results in either heads or tails. A **compound event** results in more than one outcome and consists of more than one simple event. An example of a compound event is flipping a coin while tossing a die. The result is either heads or tails on the coin and a number from one to six on the die. The probability of a simple event is calculated by dividing the number of possible outcomes by the total number of outcomes. Therefore, the probability of obtaining heads on a coin is $\frac{1}{2}$, and the probability of rolling a 6 on a die is $\frac{1}{6}$. The probability of compound events is calculated using the basic idea of the probability of simple events. If the two events are independent, the probability of one outcome is equal to the product of the probabilities of each simple event. For example, the probability of obtaining heads on a coin and rolling a 6 is equal to $\frac{1}{2} \times \frac{1}{6} = \frac{1}{12}$. The probability of either A or B occurring is equal to the sum of the probabilities minus the probability that both A and B will occur. Therefore, the probability of obtaining either heads on a coin or rolling a 6 on a die is:

$$\frac{1}{2} + \frac{1}{6} - \frac{1}{12} = \frac{7}{12}$$

The two events aren't mutually exclusive because they can happen at the same time. If two events are mutually exclusive, and the probability of both events occurring at the same time is zero, the probability of event A or B occurring equals the sum of both probabilities. An example of calculating the probability of two mutually exclusive events is determining the probability of pulling a king or a queen from a deck of cards. The two events cannot occur at the same time.

Math Questions

1. Which of the following numbers has the greatest value?
    a. 1.4378
    b. 1.07548
    c. 1.43592
    d. 0.89409

2. The value of 6×12 is the same as:
    a. $2 \times 4 \times 4 \times 2$
    b. $7 \times 4 \times 3$
    c. $6 \times 6 \times 3$
    d. $3 \times 3 \times 4 \times 2$

3. This chart indicates how many sales of CDs, vinyl records, and MP3 downloads occurred over the last year. Approximately what percentage of the total sales was from CDs?

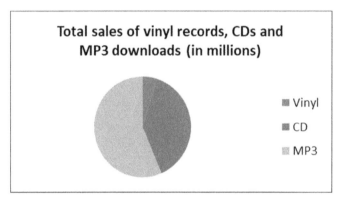

    a. 55%
    b. 25%
    c. 40%
    d. 5%

4. After a 20% sale discount, Frank purchased a new refrigerator for $850. How much did he save from the original price?
    a. $170
    b. $212.50
    c. $105.75
    d. $200

5. Which of the following is largest?
    a. 0.45
    b. 0.096
    c. 0.3
    d. 0.313

6. What is the value of *b* in this equation?

$$5b - 4 = 2b + 17$$

    a. 13
    b. 24
    c. 7
    d. 21

7. A school has 15 teachers and 20 teaching assistants. They have 200 students. What is the ratio of faculty to students?
    a. 3:20
    b. 4:17
    c. 3:2
    d. 7:40

8. Express the solution to the following problem in decimal form:

$$\frac{3}{5} \times \frac{7}{10} \div \frac{1}{2}$$

    a. 0.042
    b. 84%
    c. 0.84
    d. 0.42

9. A student gets an 85% on a test with 20 questions. How many answers did the student solve correctly?
    a. 15
    b. 16
    c. 17
    d. 18

10. If Sarah reads at an average rate of 21 pages in four nights, how long will it take her to read 140 pages?
    a. 6 nights
    b. 26 nights
    c. 8 nights
    d. 27 nights

11. Alan currently weighs 200 pounds, but he wants to lose weight to get down to 175 pounds. What is this difference in kilograms? (1 pound is approximately equal to 0.45 kilograms.)
    a. 9 kg
    b. 11.25 kg
    c. 78.75 kg
    d. 90 kg

12. Johnny earns $2334.50 from his job each month. He pays $1437 for monthly expenses. Johnny is planning a vacation in 3 months' time that he estimates will cost $1750 total. How much will Johnny have left over from three months' of saving once he pays for his vacation?

    a. $948.50

    b. $584.50

    c. $852.50

    d. $942.50

13. What is $\frac{420}{98}$ rounded to the nearest integer?

    a. 3

    b. 4

    c. 5

    d. 6

14. Solve the following:

$$4 \times 7 + (25 - 21)^2 \div 2$$

    a. 512

    b. 36

    c. 60.5

    d. 22

15. The total perimeter of a rectangle is 36 cm. If the length of each side is 12 cm, what is the width?

    a. 3 cm

    b. 12 cm

    c. 6 cm

    d. 8 cm

16. Dwayne has received the following scores on his math tests: 78, 92, 83, 97. What score must Dwayne get on his next math test to have an overall average of at least 90?

    a. 89

    b. 98

    c. 95

    d. 100

17. What is the overall median of Dwayne's current scores: 78, 92, 83, 97?

    a. 19

    b. 85

    c. 83

    d. 87.5

18. Solve the following:

$$\left(\sqrt{36} \times \sqrt{16}\right) - 3^2$$

    a. 30

    b. 21

    c. 15

    d. 13

19. In Jim's school, there are 3 girls for every 2 boys. There are 650 students in total. Using this information, how many students are girls?

    a. 260

    b. 130

    c. 65

    d. 390

20. What is the solution to $4 \times 7 + (25 - 21)^2 \div 2$?

    a. 512

    b. 36

    c. 60.5

    d. 22

21. Kimberley earns $10 an hour babysitting, and after 10 p.m., she earns $12 an hour, with the amount paid being rounded to the nearest hour accordingly. On her last job, she worked from 5:30 p.m. to 11 p.m. In total, how much did Kimberley earn on her last job?

    a. $45

    b. $57

    c. $62

    d. $42

22. Solve this equation:

$$9x + x - 7 = 16 + 2x$$

    a. $x = -4$

    b. $x = 3$

    c. $x = \dfrac{9}{8}$

    d. $x = \dfrac{23}{8}$

23. Arrange the following numbers from least to greatest value:

$0.85, \dfrac{4}{5}, \dfrac{2}{3}, \dfrac{91}{100}$

    a. $0.85, \dfrac{4}{5}, \dfrac{2}{3}, \dfrac{91}{100}$

    b. $\dfrac{4}{5}, 0.85, \dfrac{91}{100}, \dfrac{2}{3}$

    c. $\dfrac{2}{3}, \dfrac{4}{5}, 0.85, \dfrac{91}{100}$

    d. $0.85, \dfrac{91}{100}, \dfrac{4}{5}, \dfrac{2}{3}$

24. Keith's bakery had 252 customers go through its doors last week. This week, that number increased to 378. Express this increase as a percentage.

    a. 26%

    b. 50%

    c. 35%

    d. 12%

25. If $4x - 3 = 5$, then $x =$
    a. 1
    b. 2
    c. 3
    d. 4

26. Simplify the following fraction:

$$\frac{\frac{5}{7}}{\frac{9}{11}}$$

    a. $\frac{55}{63}$

    b. $\frac{7}{1000}$

    c. $\frac{13}{15}$

    d. $\frac{5}{11}$

27. The following graph compares the various test scores of the top three students in each of these teacher's classes. Based on the graph, which teacher's students had the lowest range of test scores?

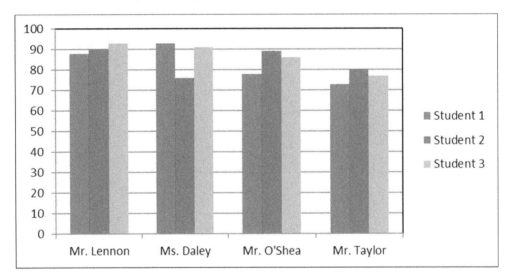

    a. Mr. Lennon
    b. Mr. O'Shea
    c. Mr. Taylor
    d. Ms. Daley

28. Bernard can make $80 per day. If he needs to make $300 and only works full days, how many days will this take?

    a. 2
    b. 3
    c. 4
    d. 5

29. Using the following diagram, calculate the total circumference, rounding to the nearest decimal place:

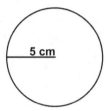

    a. 25.0 cm
    b. 15.7 cm
    c. 78.5 cm
    d. 31.4 cm

30. Which measure for the center of a small sample set would be most affected by outliers?
    a. Mean
    b. Median
    c. Mode
    d. None of the above

31. A line that travels from the bottom-left of a graph to the upper-right of the graph indicates what kind of relationship between a predictor and a dependent variable?
    a. Positive
    b. Negative
    c. Exponential
    d. Logarithmic

32. How many kilometers is 4382 feet?
    a. 1.336 kilometers
    b. 14,376 kilometers
    c. 1.437 kilometers
    d. 13,336 kilometers

33. Which of the following is the best description of the relationship between Y and X?
     a. The data has normal distribution.
     b. X and Y have a negative relationship.
     c. No relationship
     d. X and Y have a positive relationship.

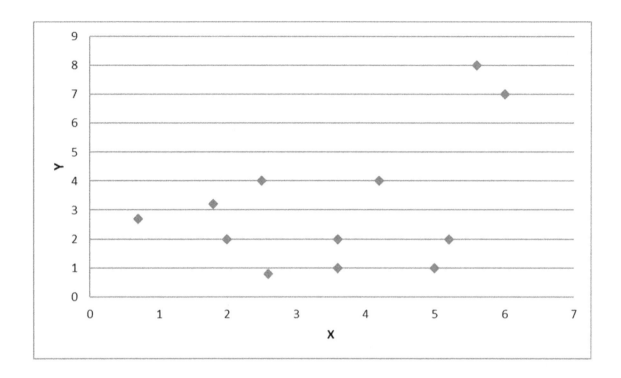

34. What is the slope of this line?

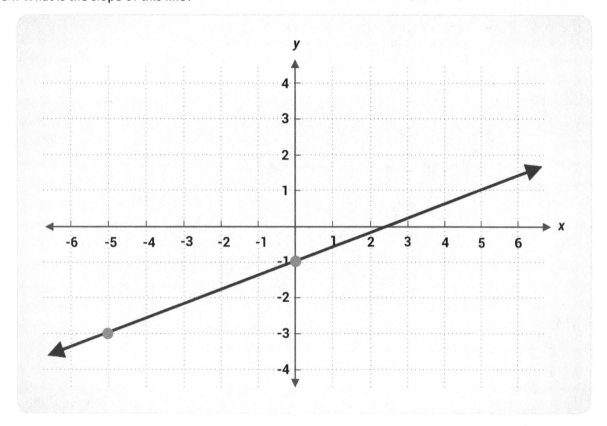

a. 2

b. $\frac{5}{2}$

c. $\frac{1}{2}$

d. $\frac{2}{5}$

35. What is the perimeter of the figure below? Note that the solid outer line is the perimeter.

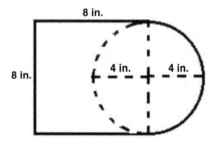

a. 48.565 in
b. 36.565 in
c. 39.78 in
d. 39.565 in

36. Which of the following equations best represents the problem below?

The width of a rectangle is 2 centimeters less than the length. If the perimeter of the rectangle is 44 centimeters, then what are the dimensions of the rectangle?

a. $2l + 2(l - 2) = 44$
b. $l + 2) + (l + 2) + l = 48$
c. $l \times (l - 2) = 44$
d. $(l + 2) + (l + 2) + l = 44$

37. Which of the following is the result of simplifying the expression: $\frac{4a^{-1}b^3}{a^4b^{-2}} * \frac{3a}{b}$?
   a. $12a^3b^5$
   b. $12\frac{b^4}{a^4}$
   c. $\frac{12}{a^4}$
   d. $7\frac{b^4}{a}$

38. What is the product of two irrational numbers?
   a. Irrational
   b. Rational
   c. Irrational or rational
   d. Complex and imaginary

39. The graph shows the position of a car over a 10-second time interval. Which of the following is the correct interpretation of the graph for the interval 1 to 3 seconds?

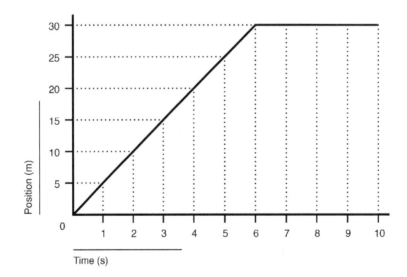

a. The car remains in the same position.
b. The car is traveling at a speed of 5m/s.
c. The car is traveling up a hill.
d. The car is traveling at 5mph.

40. How is the number -4 classified?
    a. Real, rational, integer, whole, natural
    b. Real, rational, integer, natural
    c. Real, rational, integer
    d. Real, irrational

41. $4\frac{1}{3} + 3\frac{3}{4} =$
    a. $6\frac{5}{12}$

    b. $8\frac{1}{12}$

    c. $8\frac{2}{3}$

    d. $7\frac{7}{12}$

42. Five of six numbers have a sum of 25. The average of all six numbers is 6. What is the sixth number?
    a. 8
    b. 10
    c. 11
    d. 12

43. 4.67 miles is equivalent to how many kilometers to three significant digits?
    a. 7.514 km
    b. 7.51 km
    c. 2.90 km
    d. 2.902 km

44. If $\frac{5}{2} \div \frac{1}{3} = n$, then n is between:
    a. 5 and 7
    b. 7 and 9
    c. 9 and 11
    d. 3 and 5

45. A closet is filled with red, blue, and green shirts. If $\frac{1}{3}$ of the shirts are green and $\frac{2}{5}$ are red, what fraction of the shirts are blue?
    a. $\frac{4}{15}$

    b. $\frac{1}{5}$

    c. $\frac{7}{15}$

    d. $\frac{1}{2}$

46. Shawna buys $2\frac{1}{2}$ gallons of paint. If she uses $\frac{1}{3}$ of it on the first day, how much does she have left?

    a. $1\frac{5}{6}$ gallons

    b. $1\frac{1}{2}$ gallons

    c. $1\frac{2}{3}$ gallons

    d. 2 gallons

47. How will $\frac{4}{5}$ be written as a percent?
    a. 40%
    b. 125%
    c. 90%
    d. 80%

48. What are all the factors of 12?
    a. 12, 24, 36
    b. 1, 2, 4, 6, 12
    c. 12, 24, 36, 48
    d. 1, 2, 3, 4, 6, 12

49. At the beginning of the day, Xavier has 20 apples. At lunch, he meets his sister Emma and gives her half of his apples. After lunch, he stops by his neighbor Jim's house and gives him 6 of his apples. He then uses ¾ of his remaining apples to make an apple pie for dessert at dinner. At the end of the day, how many apples does Xavier have left?
    a. 4
    b. 6
    c. 2
    d. 1

50. How will the number 847.89632 be written if rounded to the nearest hundredth?
    a. 847.90
    b. 900
    c. 847.89
    d. 847.896

51. What is the value of the sum of $\frac{1}{3}$ and $\frac{2}{5}$?

    a. $\frac{3}{8}$

    b. $\frac{11}{15}$

    c. $\frac{11}{30}$

    d. $\frac{4}{5}$

52. Add and express in reduced form $5/12 + 4/9$.

    a. $\frac{9}{17}$

    b. $\frac{1}{3}$

    c. $\frac{31}{36}$

    d. $\frac{3}{5}$

53. Divide and reduce $\frac{4}{13} \div \frac{27}{169}$.

    a. $\frac{52}{27}$

    b. $\frac{51}{27}$

    c. $\frac{52}{29}$

    d. $\frac{51}{29}$

54. Express as a reduced mixed number $\frac{54}{15}$.

    a. $3\frac{3}{5}$

    b. $3\frac{1}{15}$

    c. $3\frac{3}{54}$

    d. $3\frac{1}{54}$

Answer Explanations

1. A: Compare each numeral after the decimal point to figure out which overall number is greatest. In answers A (1.43785) and C (1.43592), both have the same tenths (4) and hundredths (3). However, the thousandths is greater in answer A (7), so A has the greatest value overall.

2. D: By grouping the four numbers in the answer into factors of the two numbers of the question (6 and 12), it can be determined that $(3 \times 2) \times (4 \times 3) = 6 \times 12$. Alternatively, each of the answer choices could be prime factored or multiplied out and compared to the original value. 6×12 has a value of 72 and a prime factorization of $2^3 \times 3^2$. The answer choices respectively have values of 64, 84, 108, 72, and 144 and prime factorizations of 2^6, $2^2 \times 3 \times 7$, $2^2 \times 3^3$, and $2^3 \times 3^2$, so answer D is the correct choice.

3. C: The sum total percentage of a pie chart must equal 100%. Since the CD sales take up less than half of the chart and more than a quarter (25%), it can be determined to be 40% overall. This can also be measured with a protractor. The angle of a circle is 360°. Since 25% of 360 would be 90° and 50% would be 180°, the angle percentage of CD sales falls in between; therefore, it would be answer C.

4. B: Since $850 is the price *after* a 20% discount, $850 represents 80% of the original price. To determine the original price, set up a proportion with the ratio of the sale price (850) to original price (unknown) equal to the ratio of sale percentage:

$$\frac{850}{x} = \frac{80}{100}$$

(where x represents the unknown original price)

To solve a proportion, cross multiply the numerators and denominators and set the products equal to each other: $(850)(100) = (80)(x)$. Multiplying each side results in the equation $85,000 = 80x$.

To solve for x, divide both sides by 80: $\frac{85,000}{80} = \frac{80x}{80}$, resulting in x=1062.5. Remember that x represents the original price. Subtracting the sale price from the original price ($1062.50 − $850) indicates that Frank saved $212.50.

5. A: To figure out which is largest, look at the first non-zero digits. Answer B's first nonzero digit is in the hundredths place. The other three all have nonzero digits in the tenths place, so it must be A, C, or D. Of these, A has the largest first nonzero digit.

6. C: To solve for the value of b, both sides of the equation need to be equalized.

Start by cancelling out the lower value of -4 by adding 4 to both sides:

$$5b - 4 = 2b + 17$$

$$5b - 4 + 4 = 2b + 17 + 4$$

$$5b = 2b + 21$$

The variable *b* is the same on each side, so subtract the lower 2b from each side:

$$5b = 2b + 21$$

$$5b - 2b = 2b + 21 - 2b$$

$$3b = 21$$

Then divide both sides by 3 to get the value of *b*:

$$3b = 21$$

$$\frac{3b}{3} = \frac{21}{3}$$

$$b = 7$$

7. D: The total faculty is $15 + 20 = 35$. So, the ratio is 35:200. Then, divide both of these numbers by 5, since 5 is a common factor to both, with a result of 7:40.

8. C: The first step in solving this problem is expressing the result in fraction form. Separate this problem first by solving the division operation of the last two fractions. When dividing one fraction by another, invert or flip the second fraction and then multiply the numerator and denominator.

$$\frac{7}{10} \times \frac{2}{1} = \frac{14}{10}$$

Next, multiply the first fraction with this value:

$$\frac{3}{5} \times \frac{14}{10} = \frac{42}{50}$$

Decimals are expressions of 1 or 100%, so multiply both the numerator and denominator by 2 to get the fraction as an expression of 100.

$$\frac{42}{50} \times \frac{2}{2} = \frac{84}{100}$$

In decimal form, this would be expressed as 0.84.

9. C: 85% of a number means that number should be multiplied by 0.85: $0.85 \times 20 = \frac{85}{100} \times \frac{20}{1}$, which can be simplified to $\frac{17}{20} \times \frac{20}{1} = 17$. The answer is *C*.

10. D: This problem can be solved by setting up a proportion involving the given information and the unknown value. The proportion is:

$$\frac{21\ pages}{4\ nights} = \frac{140\ pages}{x\ nights}$$

Solving the proportion by cross-multiplying, the equation becomes $21x = 4 \times 140$, where $x = 26.67$. Since it is not an exact number of nights, the answer is rounded up to 27 nights. Twenty-six nights would not give Sarah enough time.

11. B: Using the conversion rate, multiply the projected weight loss of 25 lb by $0.45\ \frac{kg}{lb}$ to get the amount in kilograms (11.25 kg).

12. D: First, subtract $1437 from $2334.50 to find Johnny's monthly savings; this equals $897.50. Then, multiply this amount by 3 to find out how much he will have (in three months) before he pays for his vacation: this equals $2692.50. Finally, subtract the cost of the vacation ($1750) from this amount to find how much Johnny will have left: $942.50.

13. B: Dividing by 98 can be approximated by dividing by 100, which would mean shifting the decimal point of the numerator to the left by 2. The result is 4.2 which rounds to 4.

14. B: To solve this correctly, keep in mind the order of operations with the mnemonic PEMDAS (Please Excuse My Dear Aunt Sally). This stands for Parentheses, Exponents, Multiplication, Division, Addition, Subtraction. Taking it step by step, solve the parentheses first:

$$4 \times 7 + (4)^2 \div 2$$

Then, apply the exponent:

$$4 \times 7 + 16 \div 2$$

Multiplication and division are both performed next:

$$28 + 8 = 36$$

15. C: The formula for the perimeter of a rectangle is P=2L+2W, where P is the perimeter, L is the length, and W is the width. The first step is to substitute all of the data into the formula:

$$36 = 2(12) + 2W$$

Simplify by multiplying 2x12:

$$36 = 24 + 2W$$

Simplifying this further by subtracting 24 on each side, which gives:

$$36 - 24 = 24 - 24 + 2W$$

$$12 = 2W$$

Divide by 2:

$$6 = W$$

The width is 6 cm. Remember to test this answer by substituting this value into the original formula: $36 = 2(12) + 2(6)$.

16. D: To find the average of a set of values, add the values together and then divide by the total number of values. In this case, include the unknown value of what Dwayne needs to score on his next test, in order to solve it.

$$\frac{78 + 92 + 83 + 97 + x}{5} = 90$$

Add the unknown value to the new average total, which is 5. Then multiply each side by 5 to simplify the equation, resulting in:

$$78 + 92 + 83 + 97 + x = 450$$

$$350 + x = 450$$

$$x = 100$$

Dwayne would need to get a perfect score of 100 in order to get an average of at least 90.

Test this answer by substituting back into the original formula.

$$\frac{78 + 92 + 83 + 97 + 100}{5} = 90$$

17. D: For an even number of total values, the *median* is calculated by finding the *mean* or average of the two middle values once all values have been arranged in ascending order from least to greatest. In this case, $(92 + 83) \div 2$ would equal the median 87.5, answer *D*.

18. C: Follow the *order of operations* in order to solve this problem. Solve the parentheses first, and then follow the remainder as usual: $(6 \times 4) - 9$

This equals $24 - 9$ or 15, answer *C*.

19. D: Three girls for every two boys can be expressed as a ratio: 3:2. This can be visualized as splitting the school into 5 groups: 3 girl groups and 2 boy groups. The number of students which are in each group can be found by dividing the total number of students by 5:

650 divided by 5 equals 1 part, or 130 students per group

To find the total number of girls, multiply the number of students per group (130) by how the number of girl groups in the school (3). This equals 390, answer *D*.

20. B: To solve this correctly, keep in mind the order of operations with the mnemonic PEMDAS (Please Excuse My Dear Aunt Sally). This stands for Parentheses, Exponents, Multiplication, Division, Addition, Subtraction. Taking it step by step, solve the parentheses first:

$$4 \times 7 + (4)^2 \div 2$$

Then, apply the exponent:

$$4 \times 7 + 16 \div 2$$

Multiplication and division are both performed next:

$$28 + 8 = 36$$

21. C: Kimberley worked 4.5 hours at the rate of $10/h and 1 hour at the rate of $12/h. The problem states that her pay is rounded to the nearest hour, so the 4.5 hours would round up to 5 hours at the rate of $10/h. $(5h)(\$10/h) + (1h)(\$12/h) = \$50 + \$12 = \$62$.

22. D:

$9x + x - 7 = 16 + 2x$	Combine $9x$ and x.
$10x - 7 = 16 + 2x$	
$10x - 7 + 7 = 16 + 2x + 7$	Add 7 to both sides to remove (-7).
$10x = 23 + 2x$	
$10x - 2x = 23 + 2x - 2x$	Subtract 2x from both sides to move it to the other side of the equation.
$8x = 23$	
$\dfrac{8x}{8} = \dfrac{23}{8}$	Divide by 8 to get x by itself.
$x = \dfrac{23}{8}$	

23. C: The first step is to depict each number using decimals. $\frac{91}{100} = 0.91$

Multiplying both the numerator and denominator of $\frac{4}{5}$ by 20 makes it $\frac{80}{100}$ or 0.80; the closest approximation of $\frac{2}{3}$ would be $\frac{66}{100}$ or 0.66 recurring. Rearrange each expression in ascending order, as found in answer *C*.

24. B: First, calculate the difference between the larger value and the smaller value.

$$378 - 252 = 126$$

To calculate this difference as a percentage of the original value, and thus calculate the percentage *increase*, divide 126 by 252, then multiply by 100 to reach the percentage = 50%, answer *B*.

25. B: Add 3 to both sides to get $4x = 8$. Then divide both sides by 4 to get $x = 2$.

26. A: First simplify the larger fraction by separating it into two. When dividing one fraction by another, remember to *invert* the second fraction and multiply the two as follows:

$$\frac{5}{7} \times \frac{11}{9}$$

The resulting fraction $\frac{55}{63}$ cannot be simplified further, so this is the answer to the problem.

27. A: To calculate the range in a set of data, subtract the highest value with the lowest value. In this graph, the range of Mr. Lennon's students is 5, which can be seen physically in the graph as having the smallest difference compared with the other teachers between the highest value and the lowest value.

28. C: 300/80 =30/8 = 15/4 =3.75. But Bernard is only working full days, so he will need to work 4 days, since 3 days is not sufficient.

29. D: To calculate the circumference of a circle, use the formula $2\pi r$, where r equals the radius or half of the diameter of the circle and $\pi = 3.14 \dots$. Substitute the given information, $2\pi 5 = 31.4 \dots$, answer D.

30. A: Mean. An outlier is a data value that's either far above or below the majority of values in a sample set. The mean is the average of all values in the set. In a small sample, a very high or low number could greatly change the average. The median is the middle value when arranged from lowest to highest. Outliers would have no more of an effect on the median than any other value. Mode is the value that repeats most often in a set. Assuming that the same outlier doesn't repeat, outliers would have no effect on the mode of a sample set.

31. A: This vector indicates a positive relationship. A negative relationship would show points traveling from the top-left of the graph to the bottom-right. Exponential and logarithmic functions aren't linear (don't create a straight line), so these options could have been immediately eliminated.

32. A: The conversion can be obtained by setting up and solving the following equation:

$$4382 \, ft \, \times \frac{.3048 \, m}{1 \, ft} \times \frac{1 \, km}{1000 \, m} = 1.336 \, km$$

33. C: There is no verifiable relationship between the two variables. While it may seem to have somewhat of a positive correlation because of the last two data points: (5.6,8) and (6,7), you must also take into account the two data points before those (5,1) and (5.2, 2) that have low Y values despite high X values. Data with a normal distribution (Choice A) has an arc to it. This data does not.

34. D: The slope is given by the change in *y* divided by the change in *x*. Specifically, it's:

$$slope = \frac{y_2 - y_1}{x_2 - x_1}$$

The first point is (-5,-3) and the second point is (0,-1). Work from left to right when identifying coordinates. Thus the point on the left is point 1 (-5,-3) and the point on the right is point 2 (0,-1).

Now we need to just plug those numbers into the equation:

$$slope = \frac{-1 - (-3)}{0 - (-5)}$$

It can be simplified to:

$$slope = \frac{-1 + 3}{0 + 5}$$

$$slope = \frac{2}{5}$$

35. B: The figure is composed of three sides of a square and a semicircle. The sides of the square are simply added: $8 + 8 + 8 = 24 \ inches$. The circumference of a circle is found by the equation C = 2πr. The radius is 4 in, so the circumference of the circle is 25.13 in. Only half of the circle makes up the outer border of the figure (part of the perimeter) so half of 25.13 in is 12.565 in. Therefore, the total perimeter is: $24 \ in + 12.565 \ in = 36.565 \ in$. The other answer choices use the incorrect formula or fail to include all of the necessary sides.

36. A: The first step is to determine the unknown, which is in terms of the length, l.

The second step is to translate the problem into the equation using the perimeter of a rectangle, $P = 2l + 2w$. The width is the length minus 2 centimeters. The resulting equation is $2l + 2(l - 2) = 44$. The equation can be solved as follows:

$2l + 2l - 4 = 44$	Apply the distributive property on the left side of the equation
$4l - 4 = 44$	Combine like terms on the left side of the equation
$4l = 48$	Add 4 to both sides of the equation
$l = 12$	Divide both sides of the equation by 4

The length of the rectangle is 12 centimeters. The width is the length minus 2 centimeters, which is 10 centimeters. Checking the answers for length and width forms the following equation:

$$44 = 2(12) + 2(10)$$

The equation can be solved using the order of operations to form a true statement: $44 = 44$.

37. B: To simplify the given equation, the first step is to make all exponents positive by moving them to the opposite place in the fraction. This expression becomes $\frac{4b^3b^2}{a^1a^4} \times \frac{3a}{b}$. Then the rules for exponents can be used to simplify. Multiplying the same bases means the exponents can be added. Dividing the same bases means the exponents are subtracted.

38. C: The product of two irrational numbers can be rational or irrational. Sometimes, the irrational parts of the two numbers cancel each other out, leaving a rational number. For example, $\sqrt{2} \times \sqrt{2} = 2$ because the roots cancel each other out. Technically, the product of two irrational numbers can be complex because complex numbers can have either the real or imaginary part (in this case, the imaginary part) equal zero and still be considered a complex number. However, Choice D is incorrect because the product of two irrational numbers is not an imaginary number so saying the product is complex *and* imaginary is incorrect.

39. B: The car is traveling at a speed of five meters per second. On the interval from one to three seconds, the position changes by fifteen meters. By making this change in position over time into a rate, the speed becomes ten meters in two seconds or five meters in one second.

40. C: The number negative four is classified as a real number because it exists and is not imaginary. It is rational because it does not have a decimal that never ends. It is an integer because it does not have a fractional component. The next classification would be whole numbers, for which negative four does not qualify because it is negative. Although -4 could technically be considered a complex number because complex numbers can have either the real or imaginary part equal zero and still be considered a complex number, Choice *D* is wrong because -4 is not considered an irrational number because it does not have a never-ending decimal component.

41. B: $4\frac{1}{3} + 3\frac{3}{4} = 4 + 3 + \frac{1}{3} + \frac{3}{4} = 7 + \frac{1}{3} + \frac{3}{4}$

Adding the fractions gives:

$$\frac{1}{3} + \frac{3}{4} = \frac{4}{12} + \frac{9}{12} = \frac{13}{12} = 1 + \frac{1}{12}$$

Thus:

$$7 + \frac{1}{3} + \frac{3}{4} = 7 + 1 + \frac{1}{12} = 8\frac{1}{12}$$

42. C: The average is calculated by adding all six numbers, then dividing by 6. The first five numbers have a sum of 25. If the total divided by 6 is equal to 6, then the total itself must be 36. The sixth number must be 36 − 25 = 11.

43. B: The answer choices for this question are tricky. Converting to kilometers from miles will yield the choice 7.514 when using the conversion 1 mile = 1.609 km. However, because the value in miles is written to three significant figures, the answer choice should also yield a value in three significant figures, making 7.51 km the correct answer. Choices *C* and *D* could seem correct if someone flipped the conversion upside-down—that is, if they divided by 1.609 instead of multiplied by it.

$$4.67mi \times \frac{1.609km}{1mi} = 7.514 \ or \ 7.51$$

44. B: $\frac{5}{2} \div \frac{1}{3} = \frac{5}{2} \times \frac{3}{1} = \frac{15}{2} = 7.5$.

45. A: The total fraction taken up by green and red shirts will be:

$$\frac{1}{3} + \frac{2}{5} = \frac{5}{15} + \frac{6}{15} = \frac{11}{15}$$

The remaining fraction is:

$$1 - \frac{11}{15} = \frac{15}{15} - \frac{11}{15} = \frac{4}{15}$$

46. C: If she has used 1/3 of the paint, she has 2/3 remaining. $2\frac{1}{2}$ gallons are the same as $\frac{5}{2}$ gallons. The calculation is:

$$\frac{2}{3} \times \frac{5}{2} = \frac{5}{3} = 1\frac{2}{3} \text{gallons}$$

47. D: 80%. To convert a fraction to a percent, the fraction is first converted to a decimal. To do so, the numerator is divided by the denominator: $4 \div 5 = 0.8$. To convert a decimal to a percent, the number is multiplied by 100: $0.8 \times 100 = 80\%$.

48. D: 1, 2, 3, 4, 6, 12. A given number divides evenly by each of its factors to produce an integer (no decimals). The number 5, 7, 8, 9, 10, 11 (and their opposites) do not divide evenly into 12. Therefore, these numbers are not factors.

49. D: This problem can be solved using basic arithmetic. Xavier starts with 20 apples, then gives his sister half, so 20 divided by 2.

$$\frac{20}{2} = 10$$

He then gives his neighbor 6, so 6 is subtracted from 10.

$$10 - 6 = 4$$

Lastly, he uses ¾ of his apples to make an apple pie, so to find remaining apples, the first step is to subtract ¾ from one and then multiply the difference by 4.

$$\left(1 - \frac{3}{4}\right) \times 4 = ?$$

$$\left(\frac{4}{4} - \frac{3}{4}\right) \times 4 = ?$$

$$\left(\frac{1}{4}\right) \times 4 = 1$$

50. A: 847.90. The hundredth place value is located two digits to the right of the decimal point (the digit 9). The digit to the right of the place value is examined to decide whether to round up or keep the digit. In this case, the digit 6 is 5 or greater so the hundredth place is rounded up. When rounding up, if the digit to be increased is a 9, the digit to its left is increased by one and the digit in the desired place value is made a zero. Therefore, the number is rounded to 847.90.

51. B: $\frac{11}{15}$. Fractions must have like denominators to be added. The least common multiple of the denominators 3 and 5 is found. The LCM is 15, so both fractions should be changed to equivalent fractions with a denominator of 15. To determine the numerator of the new fraction, the old numerator is multiplied by the same number by which the old denominator is multiplied to obtain the new denominator. For the fraction $\frac{1}{3}$, 3 multiplied by 5 will produce 15. Therefore, the numerator is multiplied by 5 to produce the new numerator $\left(\frac{1 \times 5}{3 \times 5} = \frac{5}{15}\right)$. For the fraction $\frac{2}{5}$, multiplying both the numerator and denominator by 3 produces $\frac{6}{15}$. When fractions have like denominators, they are added by adding the numerators and keeping the denominator the same: $\frac{5}{15} + \frac{6}{15} = \frac{11}{15}$.

52. C: 31/36

Set up the problem and find a common denominator for both fractions.

$$\frac{5}{12} + \frac{4}{9}$$

Multiply each fraction across by 1 to convert to a common denominator.

$$\frac{5}{12} \times \frac{3}{3} + \frac{4}{9} \times \frac{4}{4}$$

Once over the same denominator, add across the top. The total is over the common denominator.

$$\frac{15 + 16}{36} = \frac{31}{36}$$

53. A: 52/27

Set up the division problem.

$$\frac{4}{13} \div \frac{27}{169}$$

Flip the second fraction and multiply.

$$\frac{4}{13} \times \frac{169}{27}$$

Simplify and reduce with cross multiplication.

$$\frac{4}{1} \times \frac{13}{27}$$

Multiply across the top and across the bottom to solve.

$$\frac{4 \times 13}{1 \times 27} = \frac{52}{27}$$

54. A: $3\frac{3}{5}$

Divide.

$$15\overline{)54} \\ \underline{-45} \\ 9$$

with 3 above.

The result is $3\frac{9}{15}$.

Reduce the remainder for the final answer.

$$3\frac{3}{5}$$

Science

General Biology

Biology is the study of living organisms and the processes that are vital for life. Scientists who study biology study these organisms on a cellular level, individually or as populations, and look at the effects they have on their surrounding environment.

Water

Most cells are primarily composed of water and live in water-rich environments. Since water is such a familiar substance, it is easy to overlook its unique properties. Chemically, water is made up of two hydrogen atoms bonded to one oxygen atom by covalent bonds. The three atoms join to make a V-shaped molecule. Water is a polar molecule, meaning it has an unevenly distributed overall charge due to an unequal sharing of electrons. Due to oxygen's electronegativity and its more substantial positively charged nucleus, hydrogen's electrons are pulled closer to the oxygen. This causes the hydrogen atoms to have a slight positive charge and the oxygen atom to have a slight negative charge. In a glass of water, the molecules constantly interact and link for a fraction of a second due to intermolecular bonding between the slightly positive hydrogen atoms of one molecule and the slightly negative oxygen of a different molecule. These weak intermolecular bonds are called **hydrogen bonds**.

Water has several important qualities, including: cohesive and adhesive behaviors, temperature moderation ability, expansion upon freezing, and diverse use as a solvent.

Cohesion is the interaction of many of the same molecules. In water, cohesion occurs when there is hydrogen bonding between water molecules. Water molecules use this bonding ability to attach to each other and can work against gravity to transport dissolved nutrients to the top of a plant. A network of water-conducting cells can push water from the roots of a plant up to the leaves. Adhesion is the linking of two different substances. Water molecules can form a weak hydrogen bond with, or adhere to, plant cell walls to help fight gravity. The cohesive behavior of water also causes surface tension. If a glass of water is slightly overfull, water can still stand above the rim. This is because of the unique bonding of water molecules at the surface—they bond to each other and to the molecules below them, making it seem like it is covered with an impenetrable film. A raft spider could actually walk across a small body of water due to this surface tension.

Another important property of water is its ability to moderate temperature. Water can moderate the temperature of air by absorbing or releasing stored heat into the air. Water has the distinctive capability of being able to absorb or release large quantities of stored heat while undergoing only a small change in temperature. This is because of the relatively high **specific heat** of water, where specific heat is the amount of heat it takes for one gram of a material to change its temperature by 1 degree Celsius. The specific heat of water is one calorie per gram per degree Celsius, meaning that for each gram of water, it takes one calorie of heat to raise or lower the temperature of water by 1 degree Celsius.

When the temperature of water is reduced to freezing levels, water displays another interesting property: It expands instead of contracts. Most liquids become denser as they freeze because the molecules move around slower and stay closer together. Water molecules, however, form hydrogen bonds with each other as they move together. As the temperature lowers and they begin to move slower, these bonds become harder to break apart. When water freezes into ice, molecules are frozen with hydrogen bonds between them and they take up about 10 percent more volume than in their liquid state. The fact that ice is less dense than water is what makes ice float to the top of a glass of water.

Lastly, the **polarity** of water molecules makes it a versatile solvent. **Ionic compounds**, such as salt, are made up of positively- and negatively-charged atoms, called **cations** and **anions**, respectively. Cations and anions are easily dissolved in water because of their individual attractions to the slight positive charge of the hydrogen atoms or the slight negative charge of the oxygen atoms in water molecules. Water molecules separate the individually charged atoms and shield them from each other so they don't bond to each other again, creating a homogenous solution of the cations and anions. Nonionic compounds, such as sugar, have polar regions, so are easily dissolved in water. For these compounds, the water molecules form hydrogen bonds with the polar regions (hydroxyl groups) to create a homogenous solution. Any substance that is attracted to water is termed **hydrophilic**. Substances that repel water are termed **hydrophobic**.

Biological Molecules

Basic units of organic compounds are often called **monomers**. Repeating units of linked monomers are called **polymers**. The most important large molecules, or polymers, found in all living things can be divided into four categories: carbohydrates, lipids, proteins, and nucleic acids. This may be surprising since there is so much diversity in the outward appearance and physical abilities of living things present on Earth. Carbon (C), hydrogen (H), oxygen (O), nitrogen (N), sulfur (S), and phosphorus (P) are the major elements of most biological molecules. Carbon is a common backbone of large molecules because of its ability to form four covalent bonds.

Carbohydrates

Carbohydrates consist of sugars and polymers of sugars. The simplest sugars are **monosaccharides**, which have the empirical formula of CH_2O. The formula for the monosaccharide glucose, for example, is $C_6H_{12}O_6$. Glucose is an important molecule for cellular respiration, the process of cells extracting energy by breaking bonds through a series of reactions. The individual atoms are then used to rebuild new small molecules. **Polysaccharides** are made up of a few hundred to a few thousand monosaccharides linked together. These larger molecules have two major functions. The first is that they can be stored as starches, such as **glycogen**, and then broken down later for energy. Secondly, they may be used to form strong materials, such as **cellulose**, which is the firm wall that encloses plant cells, and **chitin**, the carbohydrate insects use to build exoskeletons.

Use this chart to better understand the classification of carbs:

Classification of Carbs

Monosaccharides

| Trioses | Tetroses | Pentoses | Hexoses or Heptoses |

Lipids

Lipids are a class of biological molecules that are **hydrophobic**, meaning they don't mix well with water. They are mostly made up of large chains of carbon and hydrogen atoms, termed **hydrocarbon chains**. When lipids mix with water, the water molecules bond to each other and exclude the lipids because they are unable to form bonds with the long hydrocarbon chains. The three most important types of lipids are fats, phospholipids, and steroids.

Fats are made up of two types of smaller molecules: glycerol and fatty acids. **Glycerol** is a chain of three carbon atoms, with a **hydroxyl group** attached to each carbon atom. A hydroxyl group is made up of an oxygen and hydrogen atom bonded together. **Fatty acids** are long hydrocarbon chains that have a backbone of sixteen or eighteen carbon atoms. The carbon atom on one end of the fatty acid is part of a **carboxyl group.** A carboxyl group is a carbon atom that uses two of its four bonds to bond to one oxygen atom (double bond) and uses another one of its bonds to link to a hydroxyl group.

Fats are made by joining three fatty acid molecules and one glycerol molecule.

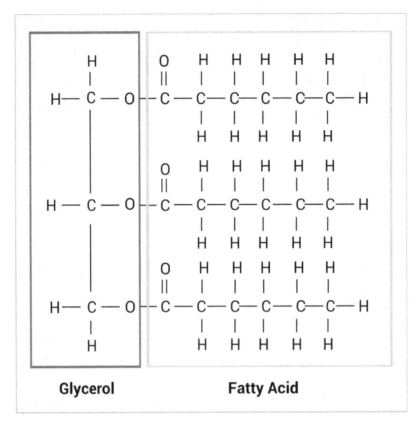

Glycerol   **Fatty Acid**

Phospholipids are made of two fatty acid molecules linked to one glycerol molecule. A **phosphate group** is attached to a third hydroxyl group of the glycerol molecule. A phosphate group consists of a phosphate atom connected to four oxygen atoms and has an overall negative charge.

Phospholipids have an interesting structure because their fatty acid tails are hydrophobic, but their phosphate group heads are hydrophilic. When phospholipids mix with water, they create double-layered structures, called **bilayers,** that shield their hydrophobic regions from water molecules. Cell membranes are made of phospholipid bilayers, which allow the cells to mix with aqueous solutions outside and inside, while forming a protective barrier and a semi-permeable membrane around the cell.

Steroids are lipids that consist of four fused carbon rings. The different chemical groups that attach to these rings are what make up the many types of steroids. **Cholesterol** is a common type of steroid found in animal cell membranes. Steroids are mixed in between the phospholipid bilayer and help maintain the structure of the membrane and aids in cell signaling.

Proteins

Proteins are essential for most all functions in living beings. The term *protein* is derived from the Greek word *proteios*, meaning *first* or *primary*. All proteins are made from a set of twenty amino acids that are linked in unbranched polymers. The combinations are numerous, which accounts for the diversity of proteins. Amino acids are linked by peptide bonds, while polymers of amino acids are called **polypeptides**. These polypeptides, either individually or in linked combination with each other, fold up to form coils of biologically-functional molecules, called proteins.

There are four levels of protein structure: primary, secondary, tertiary, and quaternary. The **primary structure** is the sequence of amino acids, similar to the letters in a long word. The **secondary structure** is beta sheets, or alpha helices, formed by hydrogen bonding between the polar regions of the polypeptide backbone. **Tertiary structure** is the overall shape of the molecule that results from the interactions between the side chains linked to the polypeptide backbone. **Quaternary structure** is the overall protein structure that occurs when a protein is made up of two or more polypeptide chains.

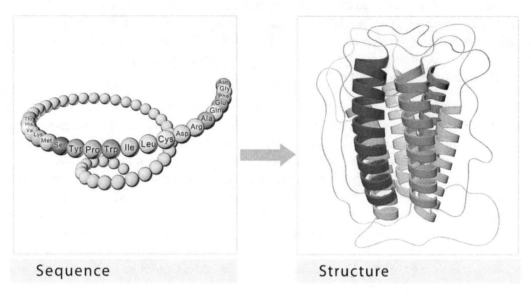

Sequence   Structure

Nucleic Acids

Nucleic acids can also be called **polynucleotides** because they are made up of chains of monomers called **nucleotides.** Nucleotides consist of a five-carbon sugar, a nitrogen-containing base, and a phosphate group. There are two types of nucleic acids: **deoxyribonucleic acid (DNA)** and **ribonucleic acid (RNA)**. Both DNA and RNA enable living organisms to pass on their genetic information and complex components to subsequent generations. While DNA is made up of two strands of nucleotides coiled together in a double-helix structure, RNA is made up of a single strand of nucleotides that folds onto itself.

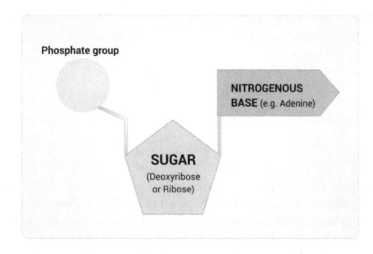

Metabolism

Metabolism is the set of chemical processes that occur within a cell for the maintenance of life. It includes both the synthesizing and breaking down of substances. A metabolic pathway begins with a molecule and ends with a specific product after going through a series of reactions, often involving an enzyme at each step. An **enzyme** is a protein that aids in the reaction. **Catabolic pathways** are metabolic pathways in which energy is released by complex molecules being broken down into simpler molecules. Contrast to catabolic pathways are **anabolic pathways**, which use energy to build complex molecules out of simple molecules. With cell metabolism, remember the **first law of thermodynamics**: Energy can be transformed, but it cannot be created or destroyed. Therefore, the energy released in a cell by a catabolic pathway is used up in anabolic pathways.

The reactions that occur within metabolic pathways are classified as either exergonic reactions or endergonic reactions. **Exergonic reactions** end in a release of free energy, while **endergonic reactions** absorb free energy from its surroundings. **Free energy** is the portion of energy in a system, such as a living cell, that can be used to perform work, such as a chemical reaction. It is denoted as the capital letter G and the change in free energy from a reaction or set of reactions is denoted as delta G (ΔG). When reactions do not require an input of energy, they are said to occur spontaneously. Exergonic reactions are considered spontaneous because they result in a negative delta G ($-\Delta G$), where the products of the reaction have less free energy within them than the reactants. Endergonic reactions require an input of energy and result in a positive delta G ($+\Delta G$), with the products of the reaction containing more free energy than the individual reactants. When a system no longer has free energy to do work, it has reached **equilibrium**. Since cells always work, they are no longer alive if they reach equilibrium.

Cells balance their energy resources by using the energy from exergonic reactions to drive endergonic reactions forward, a process called **energy coupling**. **Adenosine triphosphate**, or ATP, is a molecule that is an immediate source of energy for cellular work. When it is broken down, it releases energy used in endergonic reactions and anabolic pathways. ATP breaks down into adenosine diphosphate, or ADP, and a separate phosphate group, releasing energy in an exergonic reaction. As ATP is used up by reactions, it is also regenerated by having a new phosphate group added onto the ADP products within the cell in an endergonic reaction.

Enzymes are special proteins that help speed up metabolic reactions and pathways. They do not change the overall free energy release or consumption of reactions; they just make the reactions occur more quickly as it lowers the activation energy required. Enzymes are designed to act only on specific substrates. Their physical shape fits snugly onto their matched substrates, so enzymes only speed up reactions that contain the substrates to which they are matched.

The Cell

Cells are the basic structural and functional unit of all organisms. They are the smallest unit of matter that is living. While there are many single-celled organisms, most biological organisms are more complex and made up of many different types of cells. There are two distinct types of cells: prokaryotic and eukaryotic. **Prokaryotic cells** include bacteria, while **eukaryotic cells** include animal and plant cells. Both types of cells are enclosed by a cell membrane, which is selectively permeable. Selective permeability means essentially that it is a gatekeeper, allowing certain molecules and ions in and out, and keeping unwanted ones at bay, at least until they are ready for use. Both contain ribosomes, which are complexes that make protein inside the cell, and DNA. One major difference is that the DNA in eukaryotic cells are enclosed in a membrane-bound **nucleus**, where in prokaryotic cells, DNA is in the **nucleoid**, a region that is not enclosed by a membrane. Another major difference is that eukaryotic cells contain **organelles,** which are membrane-enclosed structures, each with a specific function, while prokaryotic cells do not have organelles.

Organelles Found in Eukaryotic Cells

The following cell organelles are found in both animal and plant cells unless otherwise noted:

Nucleus: The nucleus consists of three parts: nuclear envelope, nucleolus, and chromatin. The **nuclear envelope** is the double membrane that surrounds the nucleus and separates its contents from the rest of the cell. It is porous so substances can pass back and forth between the nucleus and the other parts of the cell. It is also continuous, with the endoplasmic reticulum that is present within the cytosol of the cell. The **nucleolus** is in charge of producing ribosomes. **Chromosomes are comprised of tightly coiled proteins, RNA, and DNA and are collectively called chromatin.**

Endoplasmic Reticulum (ER): The ER is a network of membranous sacs and tubes responsible for membrane synthesis and other metabolic and synthetic activities of the cell. There are two types of ER, rough and smooth. Rough ER is lined with ribosomes and is the location of protein synthesis. This provides a separate compartment for site-specific protein synthesis and is important for the intracellular transport of proteins. Smooth ER does not contain ribosomes and is the location of lipid synthesis.

Flagellum: The flagellum is found in protists and animal cells. It is a cluster of microtubules projected out of the plasma membrane and aids in cell motility.

Centrosome: The centrosome is the area of the cell where microtubules are created and organized for mitosis. Each centrosome contains two **centrioles.**

Cytoskeleton: The cytoskeleton in animal cells is made up of microfilaments, intermediate filaments, and microtubules. In plant cells, the cytoskeleton is made up of only microfilaments and microtubules. These structures reinforce the cell's shape and aid in cell movements.

Microvilli: Microvilli are found only in animal cells. They are protrusions in the cell membrane that increase the cell's surface area. They have a variety of functions, including absorption, secretion, and cellular adhesion.

Peroxisome: A peroxisome contains enzymes that are involved in many of the cell's metabolic functions, one of the most important being the breakdown of fatty acid chains. It produces hydrogen peroxide as a by-product of these processes and then converts the hydrogen peroxide to water.

Mitochondrion: The mitochondrion, considered the cell's powerhouse, is one of the most important structures for maintaining regular cell function. It is where cellular respiration occurs and where most of the cell's ATP is generated.

Lysosome: Lysosomes are found exclusively in animal cells. They are responsible for digestion and can hydrolyze macromolecules.

Golgi Apparatus: The Golgi apparatus is responsible for synthesizing, modifying, sorting, transporting, and secreting cell products. Because of its large size, it was one of the first organelles studied in detail.

Ribosomes: Ribosomes are found either free in the cytosol, bound to the rough ER, or bound to the nuclear envelope. They are also found in prokaryotes. Ribosomes make up a complex that forms proteins within the cell.

Plasmodesmata: Found only in plant cells, plasmodesmata are cytoplasmic channels, or tunnels, that go through the cell wall and connect the cytoplasm of adjacent cells.

Chloroplast: Chloroplasts are found in protists, such as algae and plant cells. It is responsible for photosynthesis, which is the process of converting sunlight to chemical energy that is stored and used later to drive cellular activities.

Central Vacuole: A central vacuole is found only in plant cells, and is responsible for storage, breakdown of waste products, and hydrolysis of macromolecules.

Plasma Membrane: The plasma membrane is a phospholipid bilayer that encloses the cell. It is also found in prokaryotes.

Cell Wall: Cell walls are present in fungi, plant cells, and some protists. The cell wall is made up of strong fibrous substances, including cellulose (plants), chitin (fungi) and other polysaccharides, and protein. It is a layer outside of the plasma membrane that protects the cell from mechanical damage and helps maintain the cell's shape.

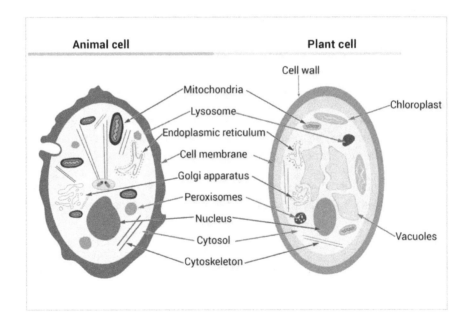

Cellular Respiration

Cellular respiration is a set of metabolic processes that converts energy from nutrients into ATP. Respiration can either occur aerobically, using oxygen, or anaerobically, without oxygen. While prokaryotic cells carry out respiration in the cytosol, most of the respiration in eukaryotic cells occurs in the mitochondria.

Aerobic Respiration

There are three main steps in aerobic cellular respiration: glycolysis, the citric acid cycle (also known as the Krebs cycle), and oxidative phosphorylation. **Glycolysis** is an essential metabolic pathway that converts glucose to pyruvate and allows for cellular respiration to occur. It does not require oxygen to be present. Glucose is a common molecule used for energy production in cells. During glycolysis, two three-carbon sugars are generated from the splitting of a glucose molecule. These smaller sugars are then converted into pyruvate molecules via oxidation and atom rearrangement. Glycolysis requires two ATP molecules to drive the process forward, but the end product of the process has four ATP molecules, for a net production of two ATP molecules. Also, two reduced nicotinamide adenine dinucleotide (NADH) molecules are created from when the electron carrier oxidized nicotinamide adenine dinucleotide (NAD+) peels off two electrons and a hydrogen atom.

In aerobically-respiring eukaryotic cells, the pyruvate molecules then enter the mitochondrion. Pyruvate is oxidized and converted into a compound called acetyl-CoA. This molecule enters the **citric acid cycle** to begin the process of aerobic respiration.

The citric acid cycle has eight steps. Remember that glycolysis produces two pyruvate molecules from each glucose molecule. Each pyruvate molecule oxidizes into a single acetyl-CoA molecule, which then enters the citric acid cycle. Therefore, two citric acid cycles can be completed and twice the number of ATP molecules are generated per glucose molecule.

Eight Steps of the Citric Acid Cycle

Step 1: Acetyl-CoA adds a two-carbon acetyl group to an oxaloacetate molecule and produces one citrate molecule.

Step 2: Citrate is converted to its isomer isocitrate by removing one water molecule and adding a new water molecule in a different configuration.

Step 3: Isocitrate is oxidized and converted to α-ketoglutarate. A carbon dioxide (CO_2) molecule is released and one NAD+ molecule is converted to NADH.

Step 4: α-Ketoglutarate is converted to succinyl-CoA. Another carbon dioxide molecule is released and another NAD+ molecule is converted to NADH.

Step 5: Succinyl-CoA becomes succinate by the addition of a phosphate group to the cycle. The oxygen molecule of the phosphate group attaches to the succinyl-CoA molecule and the CoA group is released. The rest of the phosphate group transfers to a guanosine diphosphate (GDP) molecule, converting it to guanosine triphosphate (GTP). GTP acts similarly to ATP and can actually be used to generate an ATP molecule at this step.

Step 6: Succinate is converted to fumarate by losing two hydrogen atoms. The hydrogen atoms join a flavin adenine dinucleotide (FAD) molecule, converting it to $FADH_2$, which is a hydroquinone form.

Step 7: A water molecule is added to the cycle and converts fumarate to malate.

Step 8: Malate is oxidized and converted to oxaloacetate. One lost hydrogen atom is added to an NAD molecule to create NADH. The oxaloacetate generated here then enters back into step one of the cycle.

At the end of glycolysis and the citric acid cycles, four ATP molecules have been generated. The NADH and $FADH_2$ molecules are used as energy to drive the next step of oxidative phosphorylation.

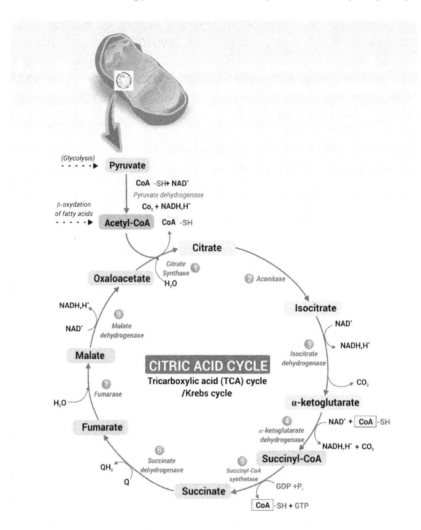

Oxidative Phosphorylation

Oxidative phosphorylation includes two steps: the electron transport chain and chemiosmosis. The inner mitochondrial membrane has four protein complexes, sequenced I to IV, used to transport protons and electrons through the inner mitochondrial matrix. Two electrons and a proton (H+) are passed from each NADH and $FADH_2$ to these channel proteins, pumping the hydrogen ions to the inner-membrane space using energy from the high-energy electrons to create a concentration gradient. NADH and $FADH_2$ also drop their high-energy electrons to the electron transport chain. NAD+ and FAD molecules in the mitochondrial matrix return to the Krebs cycle to pick up materials for the next delivery. From here, two processes happen simultaneously:

1. **Electron Transport Chain:** In addition to complexes I to IV, there are two mobile electron carriers present in the inner mitochondrial membrane, called **ubiquinone** and **cytochrome C.** At the end of this transport chain, electrons are accepted by an O_2 molecule in the matrix, and water is formed with the addition of two hydrogen atoms from chemiosmosis.

2. **Chemiosmosis:** This occurs in an ATP synthase complex that sits next to the four electron transporting complexes. ATP synthase uses **facilitated diffusion** (passive transport) to deliver protons across the concentration gradient from the inner mitochondrial membrane to the matrix. As the protons travel, the ATP synthase protein physically spins, and the kinetic energy generated is invested into phosphorylation of ADP molecules to generate ATP. Oxidative phosphorylation produces twenty-six to twenty-eight ATP molecules, bringing the total number of ATP generated through glycolysis and cellular respiration to thirty to thirty-two molecules.

Anaerobic Respiration

Some organisms do not live in oxygen-rich environments and must find alternate methods of respiration. Anaerobic respiration occurs in certain prokaryotic organisms. They utilize an electron transport chain similar to the aerobic respiration pathway; however, the terminal acceptor molecule is an electronegative substance that is not O_2. Some bacteria, for example, use the sulfate ion (SO_4^{2-}) as the final electron accepting molecule and the resulting byproduct is hydrogen sulfide (H_2S) instead of water.

Muscle cells that reach anaerobic threshold go through lactic acid respiration, while yeasts go through alcohol fermentation. Both processes only make two ATP.

Photosynthesis

Photosynthesis is the process of converting light energy into chemical energy that is then stored in sugar and other organic molecules. It can be divided into two stages: the light-dependent reactions and the Calvin cycle. In plants, the photosynthetic process takes place in the chloroplast. Inside the chloroplast are membranous sacs, called **thylakoids**. Chlorophyll is a green pigment that lives in the thylakoid membranes and absorbs the light energy, starting the process of photosynthesis. The **Calvin cycle** takes place in the **stroma,** or inner space, of the chloroplasts. The complex series of reactions that take place in photosynthesis can be simplified into the following equation: $6CO_2 + 12H_2O$ + Light Energy $\rightarrow C_6H_{12}O_6 + 6O_2 + 6H_2O$. Basically, carbon dioxide and water mix with light energy inside the chloroplast to produce organic molecules, oxygen, and water. Note that water is on both sides of the equation. Twelve water molecules are consumed during this process and six water molecules are newly formed as byproducts.

The Light Reactions

During the **light reactions**, chlorophyll molecules absorb light energy, or solar energy. In the thylakoid membrane, chlorophyll molecules, together with other small molecules and proteins, form photosystems, which are made up of a reaction-center complex surrounded by a light-harvesting complex. In the first step of photosynthesis, the light-harvesting complex from photosystem II (PSII) absorbs a photon from light, passes the photon from one pigment molecule to another within itself, and then transfers it to the reaction-center complex. Inside the reaction-center complex, the energy from the photon enables a special pair of chlorophyll *a* molecules to release two electrons. These two electrons are then accepted by a primary electron acceptor molecule. Simultaneously, a water molecule is split into two hydrogen atoms, two electrons and one oxygen atom. The two electrons are transferred one by one to the chlorophyll *a* molecules, replacing their released electrons. The released electrons are then transported down an electron transport chain by attaching to the electron carrier plastoquinone (Pq), a cytochrome complex, and then a protein called plastocyanin (Pc) before they reach photosystem I (PS I). As the electrons pass through the cytochrome complex, protons are pumped into the thylakoid space, providing the concentration gradient that will eventually travel through ATP synthase to make

ATP (like in aerobic respiration). PS I absorbs photons from light, similar to PS II. However, the electrons that are released from the chlorophyll *a* molecules in PS I are replaced by the electrons coming down the electron transport chain (from PS II). A primary electron acceptor molecule accepts the released electrons in PS I and passes the electrons onto another electron transport chain involving the protein ferredoxin (Fd). In the final steps of the light reactions, electrons are transferred from Fd to Nicotinamide adenine dinucleotide phosphate (NADP+) with the help of the enzyme NADP+ reductase and NADPH is produced. The ATP and nicotinamide adenine dinucleotide phosphate-oxidase (NADPH) produced from the light reactions are used as energy to form organic molecules in the Calvin cycle.

The Calvin Cycle

There are three phases in the Calvin cycle: carbon fixation, reduction, and regeneration of the CO_2 acceptor. **Carbon fixation** is when the first carbon molecule is introduced into the cycle, when CO_2 from the air is absorbed by the chloroplast. Each CO_2 molecule enters the cycle and attaches to ribulose bisphosphate (RuBP), a five-carbon sugar. The enzyme RuBP carboxylase-oxygenase, also known as rubisco, catalyzes this reaction. Next, two three-carbon 3-phosphoglycerate sugar molecules are formed immediately from the splitting of the six-carbon sugar.

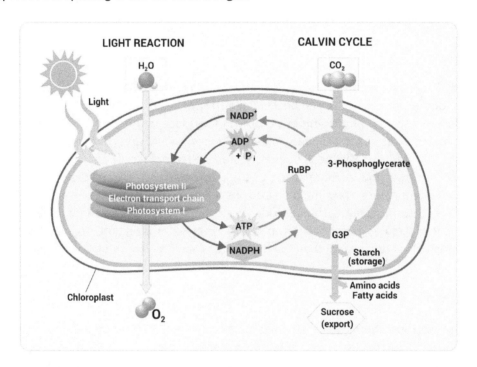

Next, during the **reduction** phase, an ATP molecule is reduced to ADP and the phosphate group attaches to 3-phosphoglycerate, forming 1,3-bisphosphoglycerate. An NADPH molecule then donates two high-energy electrons to the newly formed 1,3-bisphosphate, causing it to lose the phosphate group and become glyceraldehyde 3-phosphate (G3P), which is a high-energy sugar molecule. At this point in the cycle, one G3P molecule exits the cycle and is used by the plant. However, to regenerate RuBP molecules, which are the CO_2 acceptors in the cycle, five G3P molecules continue in the cycle. It takes three turns of the cycle and three CO_2 molecules entering the cycle to form one G3P molecule.

In the final phase of the Calvin cycle, three RuBP molecules are formed from the rearrangement of the carbon skeletons of five G3P molecules. It is a complex process that involves the reduction of three ATP molecules. At the end of the process, RuBP molecules are again ready to enter the first phase and accept CO_2 molecules.

Although the Calvin cycle is not dependent on light energy, both steps of photosynthesis usually occur during daylight, as the Calvin cycle is dependent upon the ATP and NADPH produced by the light reactions, because that energy can be invested into bonds to create high-energy sugars. The Calvin cycle invests nine ATP molecules and six NADPH molecules into every one molecule of G3P that it produces. The G3P that is produced can be used as the starting material to build larger organic compounds, such as glucose.

Cellular Reproduction

Cellular reproduction is the process that cells use to divide into two new cells. The ability of a multi-cellular organism to generate new cells to replace dying and damaged cells is vital for sustaining its life. There are two processes by which a cell can divide: mitosis and meiosis. In **mitosis,** the daughter cells produced from parental cell division are identical to each other and the parent. **Meiosis** produces genetically unique haploid cells due to two stages of cell division. Meiosis produces **haploid** cells, or **gametes** (sperm and egg cells), which only have one set of chromosomes. Humans are **diploid** because we have two sets of chromosomes – one from each parent. **Somatic** (body) cells are all diploid and are produced via mitosis.

Mitosis

Mitosis is the division of the genetic material in the nucleus of a cell, and is immediately followed by **cytokinesis**, which is the division of the cytoplasm of the cell. The two processes make up the mitotic phase of the cell cycle. Mitosis can be broken down into five stages: prophase, prometaphase, metaphase, anaphase, and telophase. Mitosis is preceded by **interphase**, where the cell spends the majority of its life while growing and replicating its DNA.

Prophase: During this phase, the mitotic spindles begin to form. They are made up of centrosomes and microtubules. As the microtubules lengthen, the centrosomes move farther away from each other. The nucleolus disappears and the chromatin fibers begin to coil up and form chromosomes. Two sister **chromatids**, which are two identical copies of one chromosome, are joined together at the centromere.

Prometaphase: The nuclear envelope begins to break down and the microtubules enter the nuclear area. Each pair of chromatin fibers develops a **kinetochore**, which is a specialized protein structure in the middle of the adjoined fibers. The chromosomes are further condensed.

Metaphase: The microtubules are stretched across the cell and the centrosomes are at opposite ends of the cell. The chromosomes align at the metaphase plate, which is a plane that is exactly between the two centrosomes. The centromere of each chromosome is attached to the kinetochore microtubules that are stretching from each centrosome to the metaphase plate.

Anaphase: The sister chromatids break apart, forming individual chromosomes. The two daughter chromosomes move to opposite ends of the cell. The microtubules shorten toward opposite ends of the cell as well. The cell elongates and, by the end of this phase, there is a complete set of chromosomes at each end of the cell.

Telophase: Two nuclei form at each end of the cell and nuclear envelopes begin to form around each nucleus. The nucleoli reappear and the chromosomes become less condensed. The microtubules are broken down by the cell and mitosis is complete.

Cytokinesis divides the cytoplasm by pinching off the cytoplasm, forming a cleavage furrow, and the two daughter cells then enter interphase, completing the cycle.

Plant cell mitosis is similar except that it lacks centromeres, and instead has a microtubule organizing center. Cytokinesis occurs with the formation of a cell plate.

Meiosis

Meiosis is a type of cell division in which the parent cell has twice as many sets of chromosomes as the daughter cells into which it divides. Although the first stage of meiosis involves the duplication of chromosomes, similar to that of mitosis, the parent cell in meiosis divides into four cells, as opposed to the two produced in mitosis.

Meiosis has the same phases as mitosis, except that they occur twice: once in meiosis I and again in meiosis II. The diploid parent has two sets of homologous chromosomes, one set from each parent. During meiosis I, each chromosome set goes through a process called **crossing over**, which jumbles up the genes on each chromatid. In anaphase one, the separated chromosomes are no longer identical and, once the chromosomes pull apart, each daughter cell is haploid (one set of chromosomes with two non-identical sister chromatids). Next, during meiosis II, the two intermediate daughter cells divide again, separating the chromatids, producing a total of four total haploid cells that each contains one set of chromosomes.

Genetics

Genetics is the study of heredity, which is the transmission of traits from one generation to the next, and hereditary variation. The chromosomes passed from parent to child contain hereditary information in the form of genes. Each gene has specific sequences of DNA that encode proteins, start pathways, and result in inherited traits. In the human life cycle, one haploid sperm cell joins one haploid egg cell to form a diploid cell. The diploid cell is the zygote, the first cell of the new organism, and from then on mitosis takes over and nine months later, there is a fully developed human that has billions of identical cells.

The monk Gregor Mendel is referred to as the father of genetics. In the 1860s, Mendel came up with one of the first models of inheritance, using peapods with different traits in the garden at his abbey to test his theory and develop his model. His model included three laws to determine which traits are inherited; his theories still apply today, after genetics has been studied more in depth.

> 1. The **Law of Dominance:** Each characteristic has two versions that can be inherited. The gene that encodes for the characteristic has two variations, or alleles, and one is dominant over the other.

> 2. The **Law of Segregation:** When two parent cells form daughter cells, the alleles segregate and each daughter cell only inherits one of the alleles from each parent.

> 3. The **Law of Independent Assortment:** Different traits are inherited independent of one another because in metaphase, the set of chromosomes line up in random fashion – mom's set of chromosomes do not line up all on the left or right, there is a random mix.

Dominant and Recessive Traits

Each gene has two **alleles**, one inherited from each parent. **Dominant alleles** are noted in capital letters (A) and **recessive alleles** are noted in lower case letters (a). There are three possible combinations of alleles among dominant and recessive alleles: AA, Aa (known as a heterozygote), and aa. Dominant alleles, when mixed with recessive alleles, will mask the recessive trait. The recessive trait would only appear as the phenotype when the allele combination is aa because a dominant allele is not present to mask it.

Although most genes follow the standard dominant/recessive rules, there are some genes that defy them. Examples include cases of co-dominance, multiple alleles, incomplete dominance, sex-linked traits, and polygenic inheritance.

In cases of **co-dominance**, both alleles are expressed equally. For example, blood type has three alleles: I^A, I^B, and i. I^A and I^B are both dominant to i, but co-dominant with each other. An $I^A I^B$ has AB blood. With incomplete dominance, the allele combination Aa actually makes a third phenotype. An example: certain flowers can be red (AA), white (aa), or pink (Aa).

Punnett Square

For simple genetic combinations, a **Punnett square** can be used to assess the phenotypes of subsequent generations. In a 2 x 2 cell square, one parent's alleles are set up in columns and the other parent's alleles are in rows. The resulting allele combinations are shown in the four internal cells.

Mutations

Genetic **mutations** occur when there is a permanent alteration in the DNA sequence that codes for a specific gene. They can be small, affecting only one base pair, or large, affecting many genes on a chromosome. Mutations are classified as either hereditary, which means they were also present in the parent gene, or acquired, meaning they occurred after the genes were passed down from the parents. Although mutations are not common, they are an important aspect of genetics and variation in the general population.

DNA

DNA is made of nucleotide and contains the genetic information of a living organism. It consists of two polynucleotide strands that are twisted and linked together in a double-helix structure. The polynucleotide strands are made up of four nitrogenous bases: adenine (A), thymine (T), guanine (G), and cytosine (C). Adenine and guanine are purines while thymine and cytosine are pyrimidines. These bases have specific pairings of A with T, and G with C. The bases are ordered so that these specific pairings will occur when the two polynucleotide strands coil together to form a DNA molecule. The two strands of DNA are described as antiparallel because one strand runs 5' → 3' while the other strand of the helix runs 3' → 5'.

Before chromosome replication and cell division can occur, DNA replication must happen in interphase. There are specific base pair sequences on DNA, called origins of replication, where DNA replication begins. The proteins that begin the replication process attach to this site and begin separating the two strands and creating a replication bubble. Each end of the bubble has a replication fork, which is a Y-shaped area of the DNA that is being unwound. Several types of proteins are important to the beginning of DNA replication. **Helicases** are enzymes responsible for untwisting the two strands at the replication fork. Single-strand binding proteins bind to the separated strands so that they do not join back together during the replication process. While part of the DNA is unwound, the remainder of the molecule becomes even more twisted in response. Topoisomerase enzymes help relieve this strain by breaking, untwisting, and rejoining the DNA strands.

Once the DNA strand is unwound, an initial primer chain of RNA from the enzyme primase is made to start replication. Replication of DNA can only occur in the 5' → 3' direction. Therefore, during replication, one strand of the DNA template creates the leading strand in the 5' → 3' direction and the other strand creates the lagging strand. While the leading strand is created efficiently and in one piece, the lagging strand is generated in fragments, called **Okazaki fragments**, then are pieced together to form a complete strand by DNA ligase. Following the primer chain of RNA, DNA polymerases are the enzymes responsible for extending the DNA chains by adding on base pairs.

Human Anatomy and Physiology

General Anatomy and Physiology of a Human

Anatomy may be defined as the structural makeup of an organism. The study of anatomy may be divided into microscopic/fine anatomy and macroscopic/gross anatomy. Fine anatomy concerns itself with viewing the features of the body with the aid of a microscope, while gross anatomy concerns itself with viewing the features of the body with the naked eye. *Physiology* refers to the functions of an organism and it examines the chemical or physical functions that help the body function appropriately.

Levels of Organization of the Human Body

All the parts of the human body are built of individual units called *cells*. Groups of similar cells are arranged into *tissues*, different tissues are arranged into *organs*, and organs working together form entire *organ systems*. The human body has twelve organ systems that govern circulation, digestion, immunity, hormones, movement, support, coordination, urination & excretion, reproduction (male and female), respiration, and general protection. Here are some of the systems of the body:

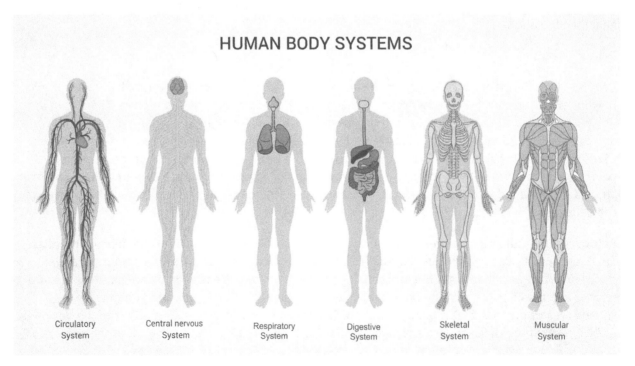

HUMAN BODY SYSTEMS

Circulatory System   Central nervous System   Respiratory System   Digestive System   Skeletal System   Muscular System

Body Cavities

The body is partitioned into different hollow spaces that house organs. The human body contains the following cavities:

- Cranial cavity: The cranial cavity is surrounded by the skull and contains organs such as the brain and pituitary gland.

- Thoracic cavity: The thoracic cavity is encircled by the sternum (breastbone) and ribs. It contains organs such as the lungs, heart, trachea (windpipe), esophagus, and bronchial tubes.

- Abdominal cavity: The abdominal cavity is separated from the thoracic cavity by the diaphragm. It contains organs such as the stomach, gallbladder, liver, small intestines, and large intestines. The abdominal organs are held in place by a membrane called the peritoneum.

- Pelvic cavity: The pelvic cavity is enclosed by the pelvis, or bones of the hip. It contains organs such as the urinary bladder, urethra, ureters, anus, and rectum. It contains the reproductive organs as well. In females, the pelvic cavity also contains the uterus.

- Spinal cavity: The spinal cavity is surrounded by the vertebral column. The vertebral column has five regions: cervical, thoracic, lumbar, sacral, and coccygeal. The spinal cord runs through the middle of the spinal cavity.

Human Tissues

Human tissues can be grouped into four categories:

Muscle: Muscle tissue supports the body and allows it to move, and muscles are special as their cells have the ability to contract. There are three distinct types of muscle tissue: skeletal, smooth, and cardiac. Skeletal muscle is voluntary, or under conscious control, and is usually attached to bones. Most body movement is directly caused by the contraction of skeletal muscle. Smooth muscle is typically involuntary, or not under conscious control, and may be found in blood vessels, the walls of hollow organs, and the urinary bladder. Cardiac muscle is involuntary and found in the heart, which helps propel blood throughout the body.

Nervous: Nervous tissue is unique in that it is able to coordinate information from sensory organs as well as communicate the proper behavioral responses. Neurons, or nerve cells, are the workhorses of the nervous system. They communicate via action potentials (electrical signals) and neurotransmitters (chemical signals).

Epithelial: Epithelial tissue covers the external surfaces of organs and lines many of the body's cavities. Epithelial tissue helps to protect the body from invasion by microbes (bacteria, viruses, parasites), fluid loss, and injury.

Epithelial cell shapes can be:

- Squamous: cells with a flat shape
- Cuboidal: cells with a cubed shape
- Columnar: cells shaped like a column

Epithelial cells can be arranged in four patterns:

- Simple: a type of epithelium composed solely from a single layer of cells
- Stratified: a type of epithelium composed of multiple layers of cells
- Pseudostratified: a type of epithelium which appears to be stratified but in reality consists of only one layer of cells
- Transitional: a type of epithelium noted for its ability to expand and contract

Connective: Connective tissue supports and connects the tissues and organs of the body. Connective tissue is composed of cells dispersed throughout a matrix which can be gel, liquid, protein fibers, or salts. The primary protein fibers in the matrix are collagen (for strength), elastin (for flexibility), and reticulum (for support). Connective tissue can be categorized as either *loose* or *dense*. Examples of connective tissue include bones, cartilage, ligaments, tendons, blood, and adipose (fat) tissue.

Three Primary Body Planes
A plane is an imaginary flat surface. The three primary planes of the human body are frontal, sagittal, and transverse. The frontal, or coronal, plane is a vertical plane that divides the body or organ into front (anterior) and back (posterior) portions. The sagittal, or lateral, plane is a vertical plane divides the body or organ into right and left sides. The transverse, or axial, plane is a horizontal plane that divides the body or organ into upper and lower portions. In medical imaging, computed tomography (CT) scans are oriented only in the transverse plane; while magnetic resonance imaging (MRI) scans may be oriented in any of the three planes.

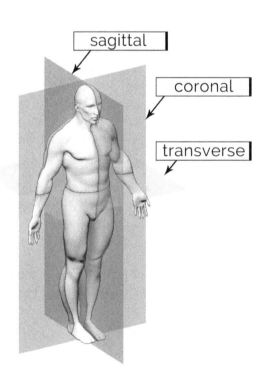

Terms of Direction

Medial refers to a structure being closer to the midline of the body. For example, the nose is medial to the eyes.

Lateral refers to a structure being farther from the midline of the body, and it is the opposite of *medial*. For example, the eyes are lateral to the nose.

Proximal refers to a structure or body part located near an attachment point. For example, the elbow is proximal to the wrist.

Distal refers to a structure or body part located far from an attachment point, and it is the opposite of *proximal*. For example, the wrist is distal to the elbow.

Anterior means toward the front in humans. For example, the lips are anterior to the teeth. The term *ventral* can be used in place of *anterior*.

Posterior means toward the back in humans, and it is the opposite of *anterior*. For example, the teeth are posterior to the lips. The term *dorsal* can be used in place of *posterior*.

Superior means above and refers to a structure closer to the head. For example, the head is superior to the neck. The terms *cephalic* or *cranial* may be used in place of *superior*.

Inferior means below and refers to a structure farther from the head, and it is the opposite of *superior*. For example, the neck is inferior to the head. The term *caudal* may be used in place of *inferior*.

Superficial refers to a structure closer to the surface. For example, the muscles are superficial because they are just beneath the surface of the skin.

Deep refers to a structure farther from the surface, and it is the opposite of *superficial*. For example, the femur is a deep structure lying beneath the muscles.

Body Regions

- Terms for general locations on the body include:
- Cervical: relating to the neck
- Clavicular: relating to the clavicle, or collarbone
- Ocular: relating to the eyes
- Acromial: relating to the shoulder
- Cubital: relating to the elbow
- Brachial: relating to the arm
- Carpal: relating to the wrist
- Thoracic : relating to the chest
- Abdominal: relating to the abdomen
- Pubic: relating to the groin
- Pelvic: relating to the pelvis, or bones of the hip
- Femoral: relating to the femur, or thigh bone
- Geniculate: relating to the knee
- Pedal: relating to the foot
- Palmar: relating to the palm of the hand
- Plantar: relating to the sole of the foot

Abdominopelvic Regions and Quadrants

The abdominopelvic region may be defined as the combination of the abdominal and the pelvic cavities. The region's upper border is the breasts and its lower border is the groin region. The region is divided into the following nine sections:

- Right hypochondriac: region below the cartilage of the ribs
- Epigastric: region above the stomach between the hypochondriac regions
- Left hypochondriac: region below the cartilage of the ribs
- Right lumbar: region of the waist
- Umbilical: region between the lumbar regions where the umbilicus, or belly button (navel), is located
- Left lumbar: region of the waist
- Right inguinal: region of the groin
- Hypogastric: region below the stomach between the inguinal regions
- Left inguinal: region of the groin

A simpler way to describe the abdominopelvic area would be to divide it into the following quadrants:

- Right upper quadrant (RUQ): Encompasses the right hypochondriac, right lumbar, epigastric, and umbilical regions.

- Right lower quadrant (RLQ): Encompasses the right lumbar, right inguinal, hypogastric, and umbilical regions.

- Left upper quadrant (LUQ): Encompasses the left hypochondriac, left lumbar, epigastric, and umbilical regions.

- Left lower quadrant (LLQ): Encompasses the left lumbar, left inguinal, hypogastric, and umbilical regions.

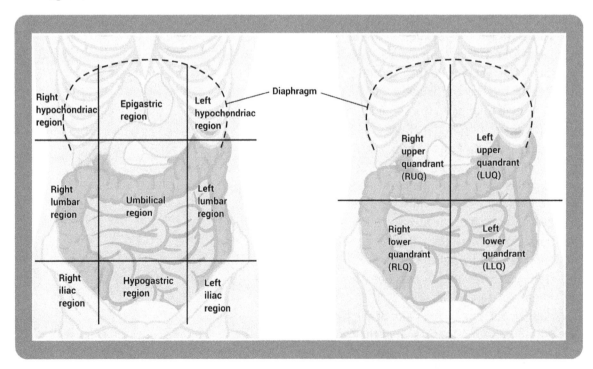

Cell Structure and Function
The cell is the main functional and structural component of all living organisms. Robert Hooke, an English scientist, coined the term "cell" in 1665. Hooke's discovery laid the groundwork for the cell theory, which is composed of three principals:

1. All organisms are composed of cells.

2. All existing cells are created from other living cells.

3. The cell is the most fundamental unit of life.

Organisms can be unicellular (composed of one cell) or multicellular (composed of many cells). All cells must be bounded by a cell membrane, be filled with cytoplasm of some sort, and be coded by a genetic sequence.

The cell membrane separates a cell's internal and external environments. It is a selectively permeable membrane, which usually only allows the passage of certain molecules by diffusion. Phospholipids and proteins are crucial components of all cell membranes. The cytoplasm is the cell's internal environment and is aqueous, or water-based. The genome represents the genetic material inside the cell that is passed on from generation to generation.

Prokaryotes and Eukaryotes
Prokaryotic cells are much smaller than eukaryotic cells. The majority of prokaryotes are unicellular, while the majority of eukaryotes are multicellular. Prokaryotic cells have no nucleus, and their genome is found in an area known as the nucleoid. They also do not have membrane-bound organelles, which are "little organs" that perform specific functions within a cell.

Eukaryotic cells have a proper nucleus containing the genome. They also have numerous membrane-bound organelles such as lysosomes, endoplasmic reticula (rough and smooth), Golgi complexes, and mitochondria. The majority of prokaryotic cells have cell walls, while most eukaryotic cells do not have cell walls. The DNA of prokaryotic cells is contained in a single circular chromosome, while the DNA of eukaryotic cells is contained in multiple linear chromosomes. Prokaryotic cells divide using binary fission, while eukaryotic cells divide using mitosis. Examples of prokaryotes are bacteria and archaea while examples of eukaryotes are animals and plants.

Nuclear Parts of a Cell
Nucleus (plural nuclei): Houses a cell's genetic material, deoxyribonucleic acid (DNA), which is used to form chromosomes. A single nucleus is the defining characteristic of eukaryotic cells. The nucleus of a cell controls gene expression. It ensures genetic material is transmitted from one generation to the next.

Chromosomes: Complex thread-like arrangements composed of DNA that is found in a cell's nucleus. Humans have 23 pairs of chromosomes for a total of 46.

Chromatin: An aggregate of genetic material consisting of DNA and proteins that forms chromosomes during cell division.

Nucleolus (plural nucleoli): The largest component of the nucleus of a eukaryotic cell. With no membrane, the primary function of the nucleolus is the production of ribosomes, which are crucial to the synthesis of proteins.

Cell Membranes

Cell membranes encircle the cell's cytoplasm, separating the intracellular environment from the extracellular environment. They are selectively permeable, which enables them to control molecular traffic entering and exiting cells. Cell membranes are made of a double layer of phospholipids studded with proteins. Cholesterol is also dispersed in the phospholipid bilayer of cell membranes to provide stability. The proteins in the phospholipid bilayer aid the transport of molecules across cell membranes.

Scientists use the term "fluid mosaic model" to refer to the arrangement of phospholipids and proteins in cell membranes. In that model, phospholipids have a head region and a tail region. The head region of the phospholipids is attracted to water (hydrophilic), while the tail region is repelled by it (hydrophobic). Because they are hydrophilic, the heads of the phospholipids are facing the water, pointing inside and outside of the cell. Because they are hydrophobic, the tails of the phospholipids are oriented inward between both head regions. This orientation constructs the phospholipid bilayer.

Cell membranes have the distinct trait of selective permeability. The fact that cell membranes are amphiphilic (having hydrophilic and hydrophobic zones) contributes to this trait. As a result, cell membranes are able to regulate the flow of molecules in and out of the cell.

Factors relating to molecules such as size, polarity, and solubility determine their likelihood of passage across cell membranes. Small molecules are able to diffuse easily across cell membranes compared to large molecules. Polarity refers to the charge present in a molecule. Polar molecules have regions, or poles, of positive and negative charge and are water soluble, while nonpolar molecules have no charge and are fat-soluble. Solubility refers to the ability of a substance, called a solute, to dissolve in a solvent. A soluble substance can be dissolved in a solvent, while an insoluble substance cannot be dissolved in a solvent. Nonpolar, fat-soluble substances have a much easier time passing through cell membranes compared to polar, water-soluble substances.

Passive Transport Mechanisms

Passive transport refers to the migration of molecules across a cell membrane that does not require energy. The three types of passive transport include simple diffusion, facilitated diffusion, and osmosis.

Simple diffusion relies on a concentration gradient, or differing quantities of molecules inside or outside of a cell. During simple diffusion, molecules move from an area of high concentration to an area of low concentration. Facilitated diffusion utilizes carrier proteins to transport molecules across a cell membrane. Osmosis refers to the transport of water across a selectively permeable membrane. During osmosis, water moves from a region of low solute concentration to a region of high solute concentration.

Active Transport Mechanisms

Active transport refers to the migration of molecules across a cell membrane that requires energy. It's a useful way to move molecules from an area of low concentration to an area of high concentration. Adenosine triphosphate (ATP), the currency of cellular energy, is needed to work against the concentration gradient.

Active transport can involve carrier proteins that cross the cell membrane to pump molecules and ions across the membrane, like in facilitated diffusion. The difference is that active transport uses the energy from ATP to drive this transport, as typically the ions or molecules are going against their concentration gradient. For example, glucose pumps in the kidney pump all of the glucose into the cells from the lumen of the nephron even though there is a higher concentration of glucose in the cell than in the lumen. This is because glucose is a precious food source and the body wants to conserve as much as possible. Pumps can either send a molecule in one direction, multiple molecules in the same direction (symports), or multiple molecules in different directions (antiports).

Active transport can also involve the movement of membrane-bound particles, either into a cell (endocytosis) or out of a cell (exocytosis). The three major forms of endocytosis are: pinocytosis, where the cell is *drinking* and intakes only small molecules; phagocytosis, where the cell is *eating* and intakes large particles or small organisms; and receptor-mediated endocytosis, where the cell's membrane splits off to form an internal vesicle as a response to molecules activating receptors on its surface. Exocytosis is the inverse of endocytosis, and the membranes of the vesicle join to that of the cell's surface while the molecules inside the vesicle are released outside. This is common in nervous and muscle tissue for the release of neurotransmitters and in endocrine cells for the release of hormones. The two major categories of exocytosis are excretion and secretion. Excretion is defined as the removal of waste from a cell. Secretion is defined as the transport of molecules from a cell such as hormones or enzymes.

Structure and Function of Cellular Organelles
Organelles are specialized structures that perform specific tasks in a cell. The term literally means "little organ." Most organelles are membrane bound and serve as sites for the production or degradation of chemicals. The following are organelles found in eukaryotic cells:

Nucleus: A cell's nucleus contains genetic information in the form of DNA. The nucleus is surrounded by the nuclear envelope. A single nucleus is the defining characteristic of eukaryotic cells. The nucleus is also the most important organelle of the cell. It contains the nucleolus, which manufactures ribosomes (another organelle) that are crucial in protein synthesis (also called gene expression).

Mitochondria: Mitochondria are oval-shaped and have a double membrane. The inner membrane has multiple folds called cristae. Mitochondria are responsible for the production of a cell's energy in the form of adenosine triphosphate (ATP). ATP is the principal energy transfer molecule in eukaryotic cells. Mitochondria also participate in cellular respiration.

Rough Endoplasmic Reticulum: The rough endoplasmic reticulum (RER) is composed of linked membranous sacs called cisternae with ribosomes attached to their external surfaces. The RER is responsible for the production of proteins that will eventually get shipped out of the cell.

Smooth Endoplasmic Reticulum: The smooth endoplasmic reticulum (SER) is composed of linked membranous sacs called cisternae without ribosomes, which distinguishes it from the RER. The SER's main function is the production of carbohydrates and lipids which can be created expressly for the cell or to modify the proteins from the RER that will eventually get shipped out of the cell.

Golgi Apparatus: The Golgi apparatus is located next to the SER. Its main function is the final modification, storage, and shipping of products (proteins, carbohydrates, and lipids) from the endoplasmic reticulum.

Lysosomes: Lysosomes are specialized vesicles that contain enzymes capable of digesting food, surplus organelles, and foreign invaders such as bacteria and viruses. They often destroy dead cells in order to recycle cellular components. Lysosomes are found only in animal cells.

Secretory Vesicles: Secretory vesicles transport and deliver molecules into or out of the cell via the cell membrane. Endocytosis refers to the movement of molecules into a cell via secretory vesicles. Exocytosis refers to the movement of molecules out of a cell via secretory vesicles.

Ribosomes: Ribosomes are not membrane bound. They are responsible for the production of proteins as specified from DNA instructions. Ribosomes can be free or bound.

Cilia and Flagella: Cilia are specialized hair-like projections on some eukaryotic cells that aid in movement, while flagella are long, whip-like projections that are used in the same capacity.

Here an illustration of the cell:

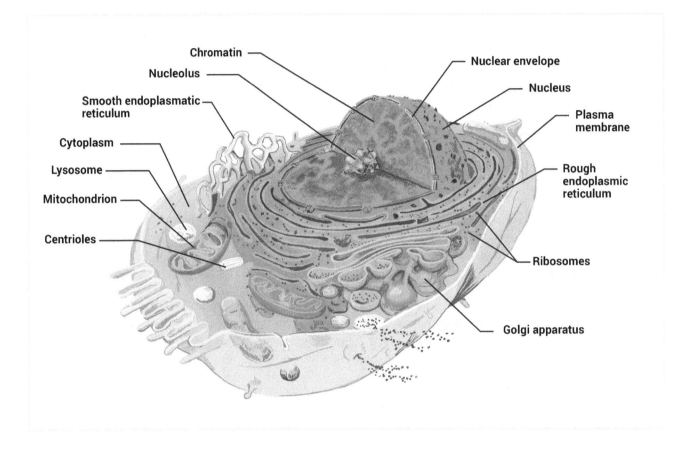

The following organelles are not found in animal cells:

Cell Walls: Cell walls can be found in plants, bacteria, and fungi, and are made of cellulose, peptidoglycan, and lignin according to the organism it is found around. Each of these materials is a type of sugar recognized as a structural carbohydrate. The carbohydrates are rigid structures located outside of the cell membrane. Cell walls function to protect the cell, help maintain a cell's shape, and provide structural support.

Vacuoles: Plant cells have central vacuoles, which are essentially a membrane surrounding a body of water. They may store nutrients or waste products. Since vacuoles are large, they also help to support the structure of plant cells.

Chloroplasts: Chloroplasts are membrane-bound organelles that perform photosynthesis. They contain structural units called thylakoids. Chlorophyll, a green pigment that circulates within the thylakoids, harnesses light energy (sunlight) and helps convert it into chemical energy (glucose).

Anatomy and Physiology of the Respiratory System

The respiratory system enables breathing and supports the energy-making process in our cells. The respiratory system transports an essential reactant, oxygen, to cells so that they can produce energy in their mitochondria via cellular respiration. The respiratory system also removes carbon dioxide, a waste product of cellular respiration.

This system is divided into the upper respiratory system and the lower respiratory system. The upper system comprises the nose, the nasal cavity and sinuses, and the pharynx. The lower respiratory system comprises the larynx (voice box), the trachea (windpipe), the small passageways leading to the lungs, and the lungs.

The pathway of oxygen to the bloodstream begins with the nose and the mouth. Upon inhalation, air enters the nose and mouth and passes into the sinuses where it gets warmed, filtered, and humidified. The throat, or the pharynx, allows the entry of both food and air; however, only air moves into the trachea, or windpipe, since the epiglottis covers the trachea during swallowing and prevents food from entering. The trachea contains mucus and cilia. The mucus traps many airborne pathogens while the cilia act as bristles that sweep the pathogens away toward the top of the trachea where they are either swallowed or coughed out.

The trachea itself has two vocal cords at the top which make up the larynx. At its bottom, the trachea forks into two major bronchi—one for each lung. These bronchi continue to branch into smaller and smaller bronchioles before terminating in grape-like air sacs called alveoli; these alveoli are surrounded by capillaries and provide the body with an enormous amount of surface area to exchange oxygen and carbon dioxide gases, in a process called external respiration.

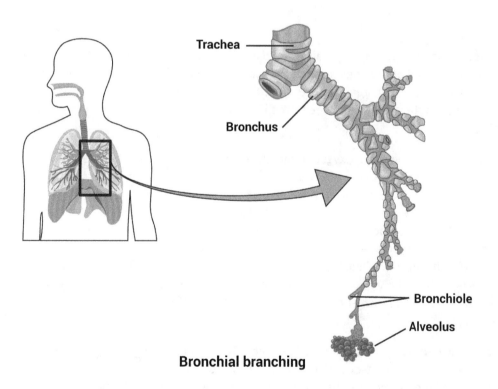

Bronchial branching

187

In total, the lungs contain about 1500 miles of airway passages. The right lung is divided into three lobes (superior, middle, and inferior), and the left lung is divided into two lobes (superior and inferior).

The left lung is smaller than the right lung, likely because it shares its space in the chest cavity with the heart.

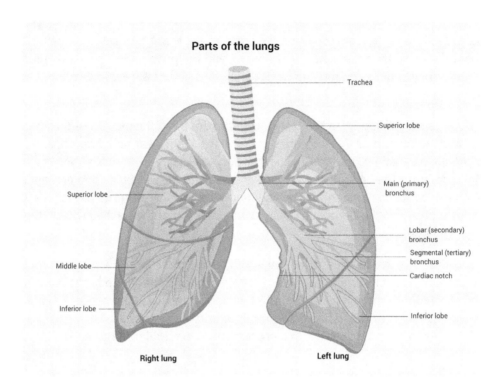

Parts of the lungs

Trachea

Superior lobe

Main (primary) bronchus

Lobar (secondary) bronchus

Segmental (tertiary) bronchus

Cardiac notch

Inferior lobe

Superior lobe

Middle lobe

Inferior lobe

Right lung

Left lung

A flat muscle underneath the lungs called the diaphragm controls breathing. When the diaphragm contracts, the volume of the chest cavity increases and indirectly decreases its air pressure. This decrease in air pressure creates a vacuum, and the lungs pull in air to fill the space. This difference in air pressure that pulls the air from outside of the body into the lungs in a process called negative pressure breathing.

Upon inhalation or inspiration, oxygen in the alveoli diffuses into the capillaries to be carried by blood to cells throughout the body, in a process called internal respiration. A protein called hemoglobin in red blood cells easily bonds with oxygen, removing it from the blood and allowing more oxygen to diffuse in. This protein allows the blood to take in 60 times more oxygen than the body could without it, and this explains how oxygen can become so concentrated in blood even though it is only 21% of the atmosphere. While oxygen diffuses from the alveoli into the capillaries, carbon dioxide diffuses from the capillaries into the alveoli. When the diaphragm relaxes, the elastic lungs snap back to their original shape; this decreases the volume of the chest cavity and increases the air pressure until it is back to normal. This increased air pressure pushes the carbon dioxide waste from the alveoli through exhalation or *expiration*.

The autonomic nervous system controls breathing. The medulla oblongata gets feedback regarding the carbon dioxide levels in the blood, and will send a message to the diaphragm that it is time for a contraction. While breathing can be voluntary, it is mostly under autonomic control.

Functions of the Respiratory System

The respiratory system has many functions. Most importantly, it provides a large area for gas exchange between the air and the circulating blood. It protects the delicate respiratory surfaces from environmental variations and defends them against pathogens. It is responsible for producing the sounds that the body makes for speaking and singing, as well as for non-verbal communication. It also helps regulate blood volume and blood pressure by releasing vasopressin, and it is a regulator of blood pH due to its control over carbon dioxide release, as the aqueous form of carbon dioxide is the chief buffering agent in blood.

Anatomy and Physiology of the Cardiovascular System

The cardiovascular system (also called the circulatory system) is a network of organs and tubes that transport blood, hormones, nutrients, oxygen, and other gases to cells and tissues throughout the body. It is also known as the cardiovascular system. The major components of the circulatory system are the blood vessels, blood, and heart.

Blood Vessels

In the circulatory system, blood vessels are responsible for transporting blood throughout the body. The three major types of blood vessels in the circulatory system are arteries, veins, and capillaries. Arteries carry blood from the heart to the rest of the body. Veins carry blood from the body to the heart. Capillaries connect arteries to veins and form networks that exchange materials between the blood and the cells.

In general, arteries are stronger and thicker than veins, as they withstand high pressures exerted by the blood as the heart pumps it through the body. Arteries control blood flow through either vasoconstriction (narrowing of the blood vessel's diameter) or vasodilation (widening of the blood vessel's diameter). The blood in veins is under much lower pressures, so veins have valves to prevent the backflow of blood.

Most of the exchange between the blood and tissues takes place through the capillaries. There are three types of capillaries: continuous, fenestrated, and sinusoidal.

Continuous capillaries are made up of epithelial cells tightly connected together. As a result, they limit the types of materials that pass into and out of the blood. Continuous capillaries are the most common type of capillary. Fenestrated capillaries have openings that allow materials to be freely exchanged between the blood and tissues. They are commonly found in the digestive, endocrine, and urinary systems. Sinusoidal capillaries have larger openings and allow proteins and blood cells through. They are found primarily in the liver, bone marrow, and spleen.

Blood

Blood is vital to the human body. It is a liquid connective tissue that serves as a transport system for supplying cells with nutrients and carrying away their wastes. The average adult human has five to six quarts of blood circulating through their body. Approximately 55% of blood is plasma (the fluid portion), and the remaining 45% is composed of solid cells and cell parts. There are three major types of blood cells:

- Red blood cells, or erythrocytes, transport oxygen throughout the body. They contain a protein called hemoglobin that allows them to carry oxygen. The iron in the hemoglobin gives the cells and the blood their red colors.

- White blood cells, or leukocytes, are responsible for fighting infectious diseases and maintaining the immune system. There are five types of white blood cells: neutrophils, lymphocytes, eosinophils, monocytes, and basophils.

- Platelets are cell fragments which play a central role in the blood clotting process.

All blood cells in adults are produced in the bone marrow—red blood cells from red marrow and white blood cells from yellow marrow.

Heart

The heart is a two-part, muscular pump that forcefully pushes blood throughout the human body. The human heart has four chambers—two upper atria and two lower ventricles, a pair on the left and a pair on the right. Anatomically, *left* and *right* correspond to the sides of the body that the patient themselves would refer to as left and right.

Four valves help to section off the chambers from one another. Between the right atrium and ventricle, the three flaps of the tricuspid valve keep blood from backflowing from the ventricle to the atrium, similar to how the two flaps of the mitral valve work between the left atrium and ventricle. As these two valves lie between an atrium and a ventricle, they are referred to as atrioventricular (AV) valves. The other two valves are semilunar (SL) and control blood flow into the two great arteries leaving the ventricles. The pulmonary valve connects the right ventricle to the pulmonary artery while the aortic valve connects the left ventricle to the aorta.

Use this image to better understand the components of the heart:

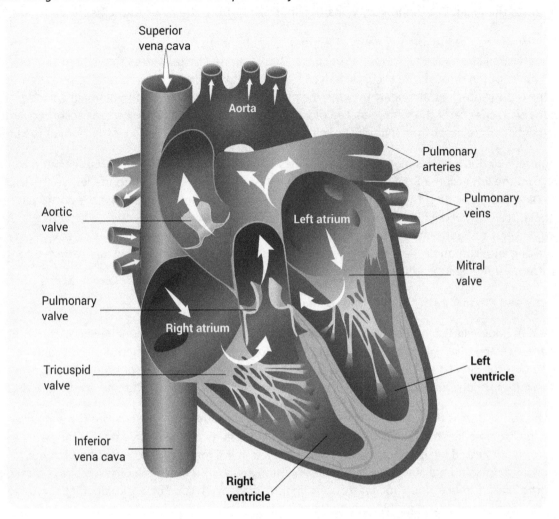

Cardiac Cycle
A cardiac cycle is one complete sequence of cardiac activity. The cardiac cycle represents the relaxation and contraction of the heart and can be divided into two phases: diastole and systole.

Diastole is the phase during which the heart relaxes and fills with blood. It gives rise to the diastolic blood pressure (DBP), which is the bottom number of a blood pressure reading. Systole is the phase during which the heart contracts and discharges blood. It gives rise to the systolic blood pressure (SBP), which is the top number of a blood pressure reading. The heart's electrical conduction system coordinates the cardiac cycle.

Types of Circulation
Five major blood vessels manage blood flow to and from the heart: the superior and inferior venae cavae, the aorta, the pulmonary artery, and the pulmonary vein.

The superior vena cava is a large vein that drains blood from the head and the upper body. The inferior vena cava is a large vein that drains blood from the lower body. The aorta is the largest artery in the human body and carries blood from the heart to body tissues. The pulmonary arteries carry blood from the heart to the lungs. The pulmonary veins transport blood from the lungs to the heart.

In the human body, there are two types of circulation: pulmonary circulation and systemic circulation. Pulmonary circulation supplies blood to the lungs. Deoxygenated blood enters the right atrium of the heart and is routed through the tricuspid valve into the right ventricle. Deoxygenated blood then travels from the right ventricle of the heart through the pulmonary valve and into the pulmonary arteries. The pulmonary arteries carry the deoxygenated blood to the lungs. In the lungs, oxygen is absorbed, and carbon dioxide is released. The pulmonary veins carry oxygenated blood to the left atrium of the heart.

Systemic circulation supplies blood to all other parts of the body, except the lungs. Oxygenated blood flows from the left atrium of the heart through the mitral, or bicuspid, valve into the left ventricle of the heart. Oxygenated blood is then routed from the left ventricle of the heart through the aortic valve and into the aorta. The aorta delivers blood to the systemic arteries, which supply the body tissues. In the tissues, oxygen and nutrients are exchanged for carbon dioxide and other wastes. The deoxygenated blood along with carbon dioxide and wastes enter the systemic veins, where they are returned to the right atrium of the heart via the superior and inferior vena cava.

Anatomy and Physiology of the Gastrointestinal System

The human body relies completely on the digestive system to meet its nutritional needs. After food and drink are ingested, the digestive system breaks them down into their component nutrients and absorbs them so that the circulatory system can transport them to other cells to use for growth, energy, and cell repair. These nutrients may be classified as proteins, lipids, carbohydrates, vitamins, and minerals.

The digestive system is thought of chiefly in two parts: the digestive tract (also called the alimentary tract or gastrointestinal tract) and the accessory digestive organs. The digestive tract is the pathway in which food is ingested, digested, absorbed, and excreted. It is composed of the mouth, pharynx, esophagus, stomach, small and large intestines, rectum, and anus. *Peristalsis*, or wave-like contractions of smooth muscle, moves food and wastes through the digestive tract. The accessory digestive organs are the salivary glands, liver, gallbladder, and pancreas.

<u>Mouth and Stomach</u>
The mouth is the entrance to the digestive system. Here, the mechanical and chemical digestion of the food begins. The food is chewed mechanically by the teeth and shaped into a *bolus* by the tongue so that it can be more easily swallowed by the esophagus. The food also becomes more watery and pliable with the addition of saliva secreted from the salivary glands, the largest of which are the parotid glands. The glands also secrete amylase in the saliva, an enzyme which begins chemical digestion and breakdown of the carbohydrates and sugars in the food.

The food then moves through the pharynx and down the muscular esophagus to the stomach.

The stomach is a large, muscular sac-like organ at the distal end of the esophagus. Here, the bolus is subjected to more mechanical and chemical digestion. As it passes through the stomach, it is physically squeezed and crushed while additional secretions turn it into a watery nutrient-filled liquid that exits into the small intestine as *chyme*.

The stomach secretes a great many substances into the *lumen* of the digestive tract. Some cells produce gastrin, a hormone that prompts other cells in the stomach to secrete a gastric acid composed mostly of hydrochloric acid (HCl). The HCl is at such a high concentration and low pH that it denatures most proteins and degrades a lot of organic matter. The stomach also secretes mucous to form a protective film that keeps the corrosive acid from dissolving its own cells. Gaps in this mucous layer can lead to peptic ulcers. Finally, the stomach also uses digestive enzymes like proteases and lipases to break down proteins and fats; although there are some gastric lipases here, the stomach is most known for breaking down proteins.

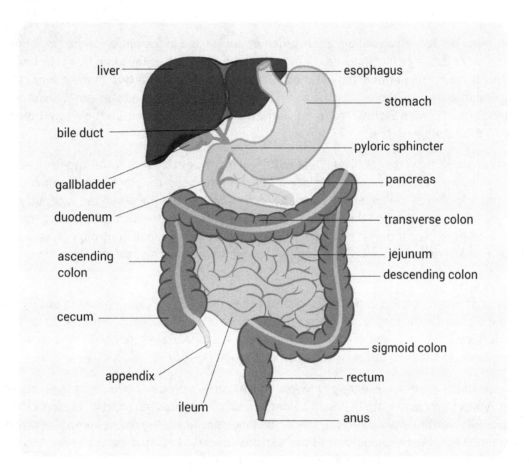

Small Intestine

The chyme from the stomach enters the first part of the small intestine, the *duodenum*, through the *pyloric sphincter*, and its extreme acidity is partly neutralized by sodium bicarbonate secreted along with mucous. The presence of chyme in the duodenum triggers the secretion of the hormones secretin and cholecystokinin (CCK). Secretin acts on the pancreas to dump more sodium bicarbonate into the small intestine so that the pH is kept at a reasonable level, while CCK acts on the gallbladder to release the *bile* that it has been storing. Bile is a substance produced by the liver and stored in the gallbladder which helps to *emulsify* or dissolve fats and lipids.

Because of the bile which aids in lipid absorption and the secreted lipases which break down fats, the duodenum is the chief site of fat digestion in the body. The duodenum also represents the last major site of chemical digestion in the digestive tract, as the other two sections of the small intestine (the *jejunum* and *ileum*) are instead heavily involved in absorption of nutrients.

The small intestine reaches 40 feet in length, and its cells are arranged in small finger-like projections called villi. This is due to its key role in the absorption of nearly all nutrients from the ingested and digested food, effectively transferring them from the lumen of the GI tract to the bloodstream where they travel to the cells which need them. These nutrients include simple sugars like glucose from carbohydrates, amino acids from proteins, emulsified fats, electrolytes like sodium and potassium, minerals like iron and zinc, and vitamins like D and B12. Vitamin B12's absorption, though it takes place in the intestines, is actually aided by *intrinsic factor* that was released into the chyme back in the stomach.

Large Intestine

The leftover parts of food which remain unabsorbed or undigested in the lumen of the small intestine next travel through the large intestine, which may also be referred to as the large bowel or colon. The large intestine is mainly responsible for water absorption. As the chyme at this stage no longer has anything useful that can be absorbed by the body, it is now referred to as *waste*, and it is stored in the large intestine until it can be excreted from the body. Removing the liquid from the waste transforms it from liquid to solid stool, or feces.

This waste first passes from the small intestine to the cecum, a pouch which forms the first part of the large intestine. In herbivores, it provides a place for bacteria to digest cellulose, but in humans most of it is vestigial and is known as the appendix. From the cecum, waste next travels up the ascending colon, across the transverse colon, down the descending colon, and through the sigmoid colon to the rectum. The rectum is responsible for the final storage of waste before being expelled through the anus. The anal canal is a small portion of the rectum leading through to the anus and the outside of the body.

Pancreas

The pancreas has endocrine and exocrine functions. The endocrine function involves releasing the hormones insulin, which decreases blood sugar (glucose) levels, and glucagon, which increases blood sugar (glucose) levels, directly into the bloodstream. Both hormones are produced in the islets of Langerhans, insulin in the beta cells and glucagon in the alpha cells.

The major part of the gland has exocrine function, which consists of acinar cells secreting inactive digestive enzymes (zymogens) into the main pancreatic duct. The main pancreatic duct joins the common bile duct, which empties into the small intestine (specifically the duodenum). The digestive enzymes are then activated and take part in the digestion of carbohydrates, proteins, and fats within chyme (the mixture of partially digested food and digestive juices).

Anatomy and Physiology of the Neuromuscular System

Nervous System

The human nervous system coordinates the body's response to stimuli from inside and outside the body. There are two major types of nervous system cells: neurons and neuroglia. Neurons are the workhorses of the nervous system and form a complex communication network that transmits electrical impulses termed action potentials, while neuroglia connect and support them.

Although some neurons monitor the senses, some control muscles, and some connect the brain to others, all neurons have four common characteristics:

- Dendrites: These receive electrical signals from other neurons across small gaps called *synapses*.
- Nerve cell body: This is the hub of processing and protein manufacture for the neuron.
- Axon: This transmits the signal from the cell body to other neurons.
- Terminals: These bridge the neuron to dendrites of other neurons and deliver the signal via chemical messengers called neurotransmitters.

Here is an illustration of this:

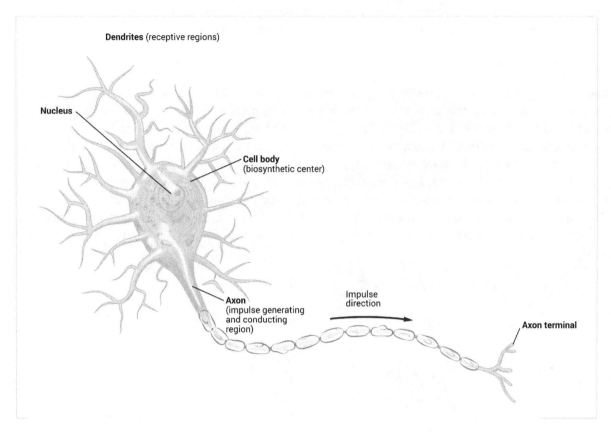

There are two major divisions of the nervous system: central and peripheral:

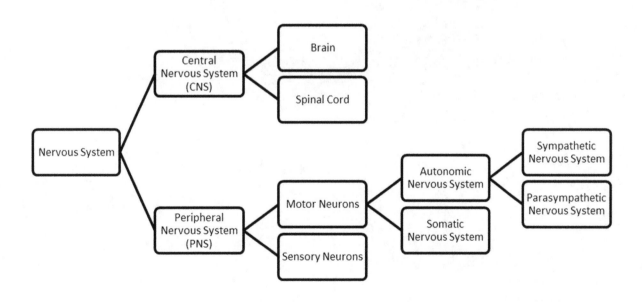

Central Nervous System

The central nervous system (CNS) consists of the brain and spinal cord. Three layers of membranes called the meninges cover and separate the CNS from the rest of the body.

The major divisions of the brain are the forebrain, the midbrain, and the hindbrain.

The forebrain consists of the cerebrum, the thalamus and hypothalamus, and the rest of the limbic system. The *cerebrum* is the largest part of the brain, and its most well-documented part is the outer cerebral cortex. The cerebrum is divided into right and left hemispheres, and each cerebral cortex hemisphere has four discrete areas, or lobes: frontal, temporal, parietal, and occipital. The frontal lobe governs duties such as voluntary movement, judgment, problem solving, and planning, while the other lobes are more sensory. The temporal lobe integrates hearing and language comprehension, the parietal lobe processes sensory input from the skin, and the occipital lobe functions to process visual input from the eyes. For completeness, the other two senses, smell and taste, are processed via the olfactory bulbs. The thalamus helps organize and coordinate all of this sensory input in a meaningful way for the brain to interpret.

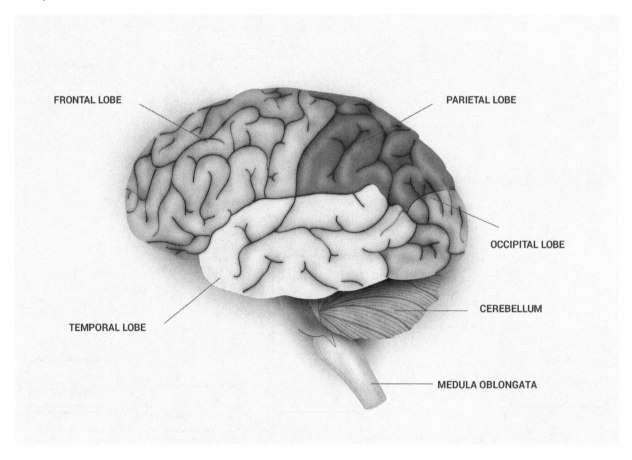

The hypothalamus controls the endocrine system and all of the hormones that govern long-term effects on the body. Each hemisphere of the limbic system includes a hippocampus (which plays a vital role in memory), an amygdala (which is involved with emotional responses like fear and anger), and other small bodies and nuclei associated with memory and pleasure.

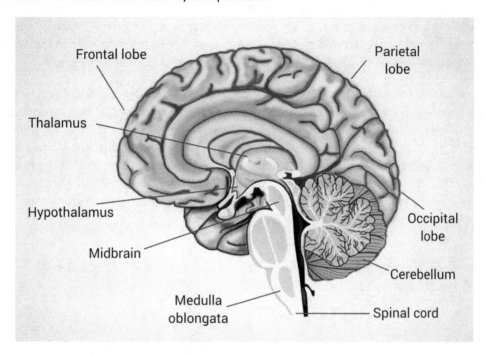

The midbrain is in charge of alertness, sleep/wake cycles, and temperature regulation, and it includes the substantia nigra which produces melatonin to regulate sleep patterns. The notable components of the hindbrain include the medulla oblongata and cerebellum. The medulla oblongata is located just above the spinal cord and is responsible for crucial involuntary functions such as breathing, heart rate, swallowing, and the regulation of blood pressure. Together with other parts of the hindbrain, the midbrain and medulla oblongata form the brain stem. The brain stem connects the spinal cord to the rest of the brain. To the rear of the brain stem sits the cerebellum which plays key roles in posture, balance, and muscular coordination. The spinal cord itself carries sensory information to the brain and motor information to the body, encapsulated by its protective bony spinal column.

Peripheral Nervous System
The peripheral nervous system (PNS) includes all nervous tissue besides the brain and spinal cord. The PNS consists of the sets of cranial and spinal nerves and relays information between the CNS and the rest of the body. The PNS has two divisions: the autonomic nervous system and the somatic nervous system.

Autonomic Nervous System
The autonomic nervous system (ANS) governs involuntary, or reflexive, body functions. Ultimately, the autonomic nervous system controls functions such as breathing, heart rate, digestion, body temperature, and blood pressure.

The ANS is split between parasympathetic nerves and sympathetic nerves. These two nerve types are antagonistic, and have opposite effects on the body. Parasympathetic nerves typically are useful when resting or during safe conditions and decrease heart rate, decrease inhalation speed, prepare digestion, and allow urination and excretion. Sympathetic nerves, on the other hand, become active when a person is under stress or excited, and they increase heart rate, increase breathing rates, and inhibit digestion, urination, and excretion.

Somatic Nervous System and the Reflex Arc
The somatic nervous system (SNS) governs the conscious, or voluntary, control of skeletal muscles and their corresponding body movements. The SNS contains afferent and efferent neurons. Afferent neurons carry sensory messages from the skeletal muscles, skin, or sensory organs to the CNS. Efferent neurons relay motor messages from the CNS to skeletal muscles, skin, or sensory organs.

The SNS also has a role in involuntary movements called reflexes. A reflex is defined as an involuntary response to a stimulus. They are transmitted via what is termed a *reflex arc*, where a stimulus is sensed by an affector and its afferent neuron, interpreted and rerouted by an interneuron, and delivered to effector muscles by an efferent neuron where they respond to the initial stimulus. A reflex is able to bypass the brain by being rerouted through the spinal cord; the interneuron decides the proper course of action rather than the brain. The reflex arc results in an instantaneous, involuntary response. For example, a physician tapping on the knee produces an involuntary knee jerk referred to as the patellar tendon reflex.

Muscular System
The muscular system is responsible for involuntary and voluntary movement of the body. There are three types of muscle: skeletal, cardiac, and smooth.

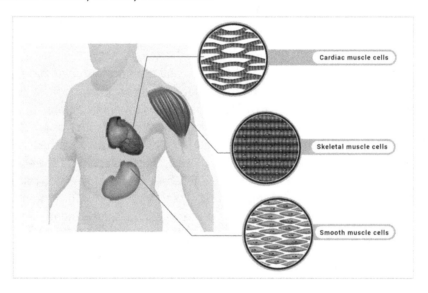

Skeletal Muscles
Skeletal muscles, or voluntary muscles, are attached to bones by tendons and are responsible for voluntary movement. The connecting tendons are made up of dense bands of connective tissue and have collagen fibers that firmly attach the muscle to the bone. Their fibers are actually woven into the coverings of the bone and muscle so that they can withstand pressure and tension. They usually work in opposing pairs like the bicep and tricep, for example.

Skeletal muscles are made of bundles of long fibers that are composed of cells with many nuclei due to their length. These fibers contain myofibrils, and myofibrils are made of alternating filaments. The thicker myosin filaments are in between the smaller actin filaments in a unit called a sarcomere, and the overlapping regions give the muscle their characteristic striated, or striped, appearance. Actin filaments are attached to exterior Z lines, myosin filaments are attached to a central M line, and when a muscle is at rest, there is a gap between the Z line and the myosin filaments. Only when the muscle contracts and the actin filaments slide over the myosin filaments does the myosin reach the Z line, as illustrated in the picture below. This sliding-filament model of muscle contraction is dependent on myosin molecules forming and breaking cross-bridges with actin in order to pull the actin filaments closer to the M line.

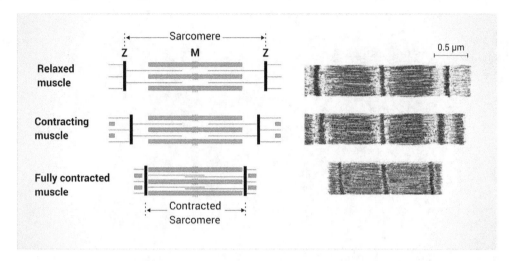

Skeletal muscles are controlled by the nervous system. Motor neurons connect to muscle fibers via neuromuscular junctions. Motor neurons must release the neurotransmitter acetylcholine which releases calcium ions to stimulate myosin cross-bridging and contraction. As the acetylcholine stops being released, the contraction ends.

Smooth Muscles
Smooth muscles are responsible for involuntary movement like food moving through the digestive tract and blood moving through vessels. They have only one nucleus and do not have striations because actin and myosin filaments do not have an organized arrangement like skeletal muscles do. Unlike skeletal muscle, these muscles don't require neuromuscular junctions. Instead, they operate via gap junctions which send impulses directly from cell to cell.

Use this image to understand muscles in the body:

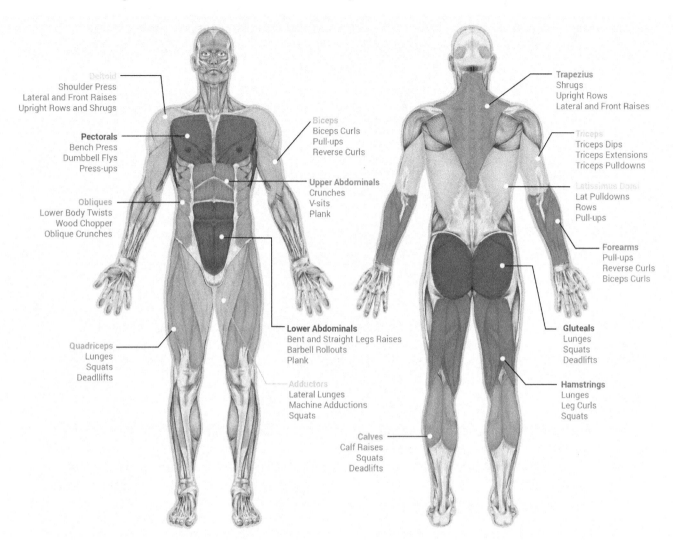

Deltoid
Shoulder Press
Lateral and Front Raises
Upright Rows and Shrugs

Pectorals
Bench Press
Dumbbell Flys
Press-ups

Obliques
Lower Body Twists
Wood Chopper
Oblique Crunches

Quadriceps
Lunges
Squats
Deadllifts

Biceps
Biceps Curls
Pull-ups
Reverse Curls

Upper Abdominals
Crunches
V-sits
Plank

Lower Abdominals
Bent and Straight Legs Raises
Barbell Rollouts
Plank

Adductors
Lateral Lunges
Machine Adductions
Squats

Calves
Calf Raises
Squats
Deadlifts

Trapezius
Shrugs
Upright Rows
Lateral and Front Raises

Triceps
Triceps Dips
Triceps Extensions
Triceps Pulldowns

Latissimus Dorsi
Lat Pulldowns
Rows
Pull-ups

Forearms
Pull-ups
Reverse Curls
Biceps Curls

Gluteals
Lunges
Squats
Deadlifts

Hamstrings
Lunges
Leg Curls
Squats

Cardiac Muscles
Cardiac muscle cells are found only in the heart where they control the heart's rhythm and blood pressure. Like skeletal muscle, cardiac muscle has striations, but cardiac muscle cells are smaller than skeletal muscle cells, so they typically have only one nucleus. Like smooth muscle, cardiac muscles do not require neurotransmitter release by motor neurons to function, and they instead operate via gap junctions.

Anatomy and Physiology of the Reproductive System

The reproductive system is responsible for producing, storing, nourishing, and transporting functional reproductive cells, or gametes, in the human body. It includes the reproductive organs, also known as gonads, the reproductive tract, the accessory glands and organs that secrete fluids into the reproductive tract, and the perineal structures, which are the external genitalia.

Reproduction involves the passing of genes from one generation to the next, and that is accomplished through haploid gametes. Gametes have gone through meiosis and have 23 chromosomes, half the normal number. The male gamete is sperm, and the female gamete is an egg or ovum. When a sperm fertilizes an egg, they create a zygote which is the first cell of a new organism. The zygote has a full set of 46 chromosomes because it received 23 from each parent. Because of sperm and egg development gene shuffling, sperm and egg chromosome sets are all different which results in the variety seen in humans.

Male Reproductive System

The entire male reproductive system is designed to generate sperm and produce semen that facilitate fertilization of eggs, the female gametes. The testes are the endocrine glands that secrete testosterone, a hormone that is important for secondary sex characteristics and sperm development, or spermatogenesis. Testosterone is in the androgen steroid-hormone family. The testes also produce and store 500 million spermatocytes, which are the male gametes, each day. Testes are housed in the scrotum which is a sac that hangs outside the body so that spermatogenesis occurs at cooler and optimal conditions.

The seminiferous tubules within the testes produce sperm and then they travel to epididymis where they are stored as they mature. Then, the sperm move to the ejaculatory duct via the vas deferens. The ejaculatory duct contains more than just sperm. The seminal vesicles secrete an alkaline substance that will help sperm survive in the acidic vagina. The prostate gland secretes enzymes bathed in a milky white fluid that is important for thinning semen after ejaculation to increase its likelihood of reaching the egg. The bulbourethral, or Cowper's, gland secretes an alkaline fluid that lubricates the urethra prior to ejaculation to neutralize any acidic urine residue.

The sperm along with all the exocrine secretions are collectively called semen. Their destination is the vagina and they can only get there if the penis is erect due to arousal and increased circulation. During sexual intercourse, ejaculation will forcefully expel the contents of the semen and effectively deliver the sperm to the egg. The muscular prostate gland is important for ejaculation. Each ejaculation releases 2 to 6 million sperm. Sperm has a whip-like flagellum tail that facilitates movement.

Female Reproductive System

The vagina is the passageway that sperm must travel through to reach an egg, the female gamete. Surrounding the vagina are the labia minor and labia major, both of which are folds that protect the urethra and the vaginal opening. The clitoris is rich in nerve-endings, making it sensitive and highly stimulated during sexual intercourse. It is above the vagina and urethra. An exocrine gland called the Bartholin's glands secretes a fluid during arousal that is important for lubrication.

The female gonads are the ovaries. Ovaries generally produce one immature gamete, an egg or oocyte, per month. They are also responsible for secreting the hormones estrogen and progesterone. Fertilization cannot happen unless the ejaculated sperm finds the egg, which are only available at certain times of the month. Eggs, or ova, develop in the ovaries in clusters surrounded by follicles, and after puberty, they are delivered to the uterus once a month via the fallopian tubes. The 28-day average journey of the egg to the uterus is called the menstrual cycle and it is highly regulated by the endocrine system. The regulatory hormones Gonadotropin releasing hormone (GnRH), luteinizing hormone (LH), and follicle-stimulating hormone (FSH) orchestrate the menstrual cycle. Ovarian hormones estrogen and progesterone are also important in timing as well as for vascularization of the uterus in preparation for pregnancy. Fertilization usually happens around ovulation, which is when the egg is inside the Fallopian tube. The resulting zygote travels down the tube and implants into the uterine wall. The uterus protects and nourishes the developing embryo for nine months until it is ready for the outside environment.

If the egg released is unfertilized, the uterine lining will slough off during menstruation. Should a fertilized egg, called a zygote, reach the uterus, it will embed itself into the uterine wall due to uterine vascularization that will deliver blood, nutrients, and antibodies to the developing embryo. The uterus is where the embryo will develop for the next nine months. Mammary glands are important female reproductive structures because they produce milk they provide for their young during lactation. Milk contains nutrients and antibodies that benefit the baby.

Anatomy and Physiology of the Integumentary System

The integumentary system includes skin, hair, nails, oil glands, and sweat glands. The largest organ of the integumentary system (and of the body), the skin, acts as a barrier and protects the body from mechanical impact, variations in temperature, microorganisms, chemicals, and UV radiation from the sun. It regulates body temperature, peripheral circulation, and excretes waste through sweat. It also contains a large network of nerve cells that relay changes in the external environment to the brain.

Layers of Skin
Skin consists of two layers, the surface epidermis and the inner dermis. The subcutaneous hypodermis is below the dermis and contains a layer of fat and connective tissue that are both important for insulation.

The whole epidermis is composed of epithelial cells that lack blood vessels. The outer epidermis is composed of dead cells which surround the living cells underneath. The most inner epidermal tissue is a single layer of cells called the stratum basale which is composed of rapidly dividing cells that push old cells to the skin's surface. When being pushed out, the cells' organelles disappear and they start producing a protein called keratin that eventually forms a tough waterproof layer. This outer layer sloughs off every four to five weeks. The melanocytes in the stratum basale produce the pigment melanin that absorbs UV rays and protects the skin. Skin also produces vitamin D if exposed to sunlight.

The dermis underneath the epidermis contains supporting collagen fibers peppered with nerves, blood vessels, hair follicles, sweat glands, oil glands, and smooth muscles.

Skin's Involvement in Temperature Homeostasis
The skin has a thermoregulatory role in the human body that is controlled by a negative feedback loop. The control center of temperature regulation is the hypothalamus in the brain. When the hypothalamus is alerted by receptors from the dermis, it secretes hormones that activate effectors to keep internal temperature at a set point of 98.6°F (37°C). If the environment is too cold, the hypothalamus will initiate a pathway that induces muscle shivering to release heat energy as well as constrict blood vessels to limit heat loss. In hot conditions, the hypothalamus will initiate a pathway that vasodilates blood vessels to increase heat loss and stimulate sweating for evaporative cooling. Evaporative cooling occurs when the hottest water particles evaporate and leave behind the coolest ones. This cools down the body.

Sebaceous Glands vs. Sweat Glands
The skin also contains oil glands, or sebaceous glands, and sweat glands that are exocrine because their substances are secreted through ducts. Endocrine glands secrete substances into the blood stream instead. Oil glands are attached to hair follicles. They secrete sebum, an oily substance that moisturizes

the skin, protecting it from water loss. Sebum also keeps the skin elastic. Also, sebum's slight acidity provides a chemical defense against bacterial and fungal infections.

Sweat glands not attached to hair follicles are called eccrine glands. They are all over the body and these are the ones responsible for thermoregulation. They also remove bodily waste by secreting water and electrolytes. Sweat glands attached to hair follicles are apocrine glands and there are not nearly as many. Apocrine glands are only active post-puberty. They secrete a thicker, viscous substance that is attractive to bacteria, leading to the unpleasant smell in armpits, feet, and the groin. They are stimulated during stress and arousal.

Anatomy and Physiology of the Endocrine System

The endocrine system is made up of the ductless tissues and glands that secrete hormones directly into the bloodstream. It is similar to the nervous system in that it controls various functions of the body, but it does so via secretion of hormones in the bloodstream as opposed to nerve impulses. The endocrine system is also different because its effects last longer than that of the nervous system. Nerve impulses are immediate while hormone responses can last for minutes or even days.

The endocrine system works closely with the nervous system to regulate the physiological activities of the other systems of the body in order to maintain homeostasis. Hormone secretions are controlled by tight feedback loops that are generally regulated by the hypothalamus, the bridge between the nervous and endocrine systems. The hypothalamus receives sensory input via the nervous system and responds by stimulating or inhibiting the pituitary gland which stimulates or inhibits several other glands. The tight control is due to hormone secretions.

Hormones are chemicals that bind to specific target cells. Each hormone will only bind to a target cell that has a specific receptor that has the correct shape. For example, testosterone will not attach to skin cells because skin cells have no receptor that recognizes testosterone.

There are two types of hormones: steroid and protein. Steroid hormones are lipid, nonpolar substances, and most are able to diffuse across cell membranes. Once they do, they bind to a receptor that initiates a signal transduction cascade that affects gene expression. Non-steroid hormones bind to receptors on cell membranes that also initiate a signal transduction cascade that affects enzyme activity and chemical reactions.

Major Endocrine Glands
Hypothalamus: This gland is a part of the brain. It connects the nervous system to the endocrine system because it receives sensory information through nerves and it sends instructions via hormones delivered to the pituitary.

Pituitary Gland: This gland is pea-sized and is found at the bottom of the hypothalamus. It has two lobes called the anterior and posterior lobes. It plays an important role in regulating other endocrine glands. For example, it secretes growth hormone which regulates growth. Other hormones that are released by this gland control the reproductive system, childbirth, nursing, blood osmolarity, and metabolism.

The hormones and glands respond to each other via feedback loops, and a typical feedback loop is illustrated in the following picture. The hypothalamus and pituitary gland are master controllers of most of the other glands.

Observe this flow chart:

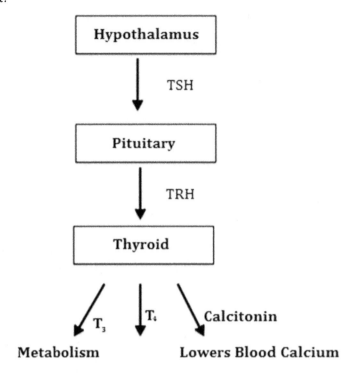

Thymus Gland: This gland is located in the chest cavity, embedded in connective tissue. It produces several hormones that are important for development and maintenance of T lymphocytes, which are important cells for immunity.

Adrenal Gland: One adrenal gland is attached to the top of each kidney. It produces epinephrine and norepinephrine which cause the "fight or flight" response in the face of danger or stress. These hormones raise heart rate, blood pressure, dilate bronchioles, and deliver blood to the muscles. All of these actions increase circulation and release glucose so that the body has an energy burst.

Pineal Gland: The pineal gland secretes melatonin, which is a hormone that regulates the body's circadian rhythms which are the natural wake-sleep cycles.

Testes and Ovaries: They secrete testosterone and both estrogen and progesterone, respectively. They are responsible for secondary sex characteristics, gamete development, and female hormones are important for embryonic development.

Thyroid Gland: This gland releases hormones like thyroxine and calcitonin. Thyroxine stimulates metabolism, and calcitonin monitors the amount of circulating calcium. Calcitonin signals the body to regulating calcium from bone reserves as well as kidney reabsorption of calcium.

Parathyroid Glands: These are four pea-sized glands located on the posterior surface of the thyroid. The main hormone that is secreted is called parathyroid hormone (PTH) which influences calcium levels like calcitonin, except it is antagonistic. PTH increases extracellular levels of calcium while calcitonin decreases it.

Pancreas: The pancreas is an organ that has both endocrine and exocrine functions. It functions outside of a typical feedback loop in that blood sugar seems to signal the pancreas itself. The endocrine functions are controlled by the pancreatic islets of Langerhans, which are groups of beta cells scattered throughout the gland that secrete insulin to lower blood sugar levels in the body. Neighboring alpha cells secrete glucagon to raise blood sugar. These complementary hormones keep blood sugar in check.

Anatomy and Physiology of the Genitourinary System

The urinary system is made up of the kidneys, ureters, urinary bladder, and the urethra. It is the system responsible for removing waste products and balancing water and electrolyte concentrations in the blood. The urinary system has many important functions related to waste excretion. It regulates the concentrations of sodium, potassium, chloride, calcium, and other ions in the filtrate by controlling the amount of each that is reabsorbed during filtration. The reabsorption or secretion of hydrogen ions and bicarbonate contributes to the maintenance of blood pH. Certain kidney cells can detect any reductions in blood volume and pressure. If that happens, they secrete renin which will activate a hormone that causes increased reabsorption of sodium ions and water, raising volume and pressure. Under hypoxic conditions, kidney cells will secrete erythropoietin in order to stimulate red blood cell production. It also synthesizes calcitriol, which is a hormone derivative of vitamin D3 that aids in calcium ion absorption by the intestinal epithelium.

Under normal circumstances, humans have two functioning kidneys in the lower back and on either side of the spinal cord. They are the main organs that are responsible for filtering waste products out of the blood and regulating blood water and electrolyte levels. Blood enters the kidney through the renal artery and urea and wastes are removed while water and the acidity/alkalinity of the blood is adjusted. Toxic substances and drugs are also filtered. Blood exits through the renal vein and the urine waste travels through the ureter to the bladder where it is stored until it is eliminated through the urethra.

The kidneys have an outer renal cortex and an inner renal medulla that contain millions of tiny filtering units called nephrons. Nephrons have two parts: a glomerulus, which is the filter, and a tubule. The glomerulus is a network of capillaries covered by the Bowman's capsule, which is the entrance to the tubule. As blood enters the kidneys via the renal artery, the glomerulus allows for fluid and waste products to pass through it and enter the tubule. Blood cells and large molecules, such as proteins, do not pass through and remain in the blood. The filtrate passes through the tubule, which has several parts. The proximal tubule comes first, and then the descending and ascending limbs of the loop of Henle dip into the medulla, followed by the distal tubule and collecting duct. The journey through the tubule involves a balancing act that regulates blood osmolarity, pH, and electrolytes exchange of materials between the tubule and the blood stream. The final product at the collecting tubule is called urine, and it is delivered to the bladder by the ureter. The most central part of the kidney is the renal pelvis, and it acts as a funnel by delivering the urine from the millions of the collecting tubules to the ureters. The filtered blood exits through the renal vein and is returned to circulation.

Here's a look at the genitourinary system:

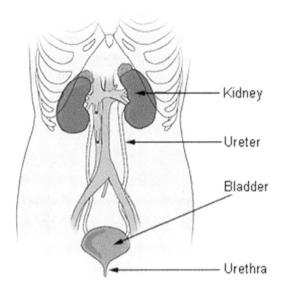

Here's a close up look at the kidney:

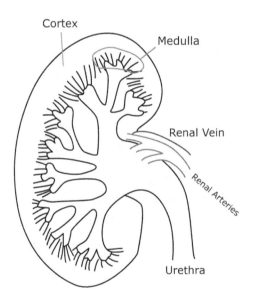

<u>Waste Excretion</u>
Once urine accumulates, it leaves the kidneys. The urine travels through the ureters into the urinary bladder, a muscular organ that is hollow and elastic. As more urine enters the urinary bladder, its walls stretch and become thinner so there is no significant difference in internal pressure. The urinary bladder stores the urine until the body is ready for urination, at which time the muscles contract and force the urine through the urethra and out of the body.

Anatomy and Physiology of the Immune System

The immune system is the body's defense against invading microorganisms (bacteria, viruses, fungi, and parasites) and other harmful, foreign substances. It is capable of limiting or preventing infection.

There are two general types of immunity: innate immunity and acquired immunity. Innate immunity uses physical and chemical barriers to block microorganism entry into the body. The biggest barrier is the skin; it forms a physical barrier that blocks microorganisms from entering underlying tissues. Mucous membranes in the digestive, respiratory, and urinary systems secrete mucus to block and remove invading microorganisms. Other natural defenses include saliva, tears, and stomach acids, which are all chemical barriers intended to block infection with microorganisms. Acid is inhospitable to pathogens, as are tears, mucus, and saliva which all contain a natural antibiotic called lysozyme. The respiratory passages contain microscopic cilia which are like bristles that sweep out pathogens. In addition, macrophages and other white blood cells can recognize and eliminate foreign objects through phagocytosis or toxic secretions.

Acquired immunity refers to a specific set of events used by the body to fight a particular infection. Essentially, the body accumulates and stores information about the nature of an invading microorganism. As a result, the body can mount a specific attack that is much more effective than innate immunity. It also provides a way for the body to prevent future infections by the same microorganism.

Acquired immunity is divided into a primary response and a secondary response. The primary immune response occurs the first time a particular microorganism enters the body, where macrophages engulf the microorganism and travel to the lymph nodes. In the lymph nodes, macrophages present the invader to helper T lymphocytes, which then activate humoral and cellular immunity. Humoral immunity refers to immunity resulting from antibody production by B lymphocytes. After being activated by helper T lymphocytes, B lymphocytes multiply and divide into plasma cells and memory cells. Plasma cells are B lymphocytes that produce immune proteins called antibodies, or immunoglobulins. Antibodies then bind the microorganism to flag it for destruction by other white blood cells. Cellular immunity refers to the immune response coordinated by T lymphocytes. After being activated by helper T lymphocytes, other T lymphocytes attack and kill cells that cause infection or disease.

The secondary immune response takes place during subsequent encounters with a known microorganism. Memory cells respond to the previously encountered microorganism by immediately producing antibodies. Memory cells are B lymphocytes that store information to produce antibodies. The secondary immune response is swift and powerful, because it eliminates the need for the time-consuming macrophage activation of the primary immune response. Suppressor T lymphocytes also take part to inhibit the immune response as an overactive immune response could cause damage to healthy cells.

Inflammation occurs if a pathogen evades the barriers and chemical defenses. It stimulates pain receptors, alerting the individual that something is wrong. It also elevates body temperature to speed up chemical reactions, although if a fever goes unchecked it can be dangerous due to the fact that extreme heat unfolds proteins. Histamine is secreted which dilates blood vessels and recruits white blood cells that destroy invaders non-specifically. The immune system is tied to the lymphatic system. The thymus, one of the lymphatic system organs, is the site of maturation of T-cells, a type of white blood cell. The lymphatic system is important in the inflammatory response because lymph vessels deliver leukocytes and collect debris that will be filtered in the lymph nodes and the spleen.

Antigen and Typical Immune Response

Should a pathogen evade barriers and survive through inflammation, an antigen-specific adaptive immune response will begin. Immune cells recognize these foreign particles by their antigens, which are their unique and identifying surface proteins. Drugs, toxins, and transplanted cells can also act as antigens. The body even recognizes its own cells as potential threats in autoimmune diseases.

When a macrophage engulfs a pathogen and presents its antigens, helper T cells recognize the signal and secrete cytokines to signal T lymphocytes and B lymphocytes so that they launch the cell-mediated and humoral response, respectively. The cell-mediated response occurs when the T lymphocytes kill infected cells by secreting cytotoxins. The humoral response occurs when B lymphocytes proliferate into plasma and memory cells. The plasma cells secrete antigen-specific antibodies which bind to the pathogens so that they cannot bind to host cells. Macrophages and other phagocytic cells called neutrophils engulf and degrade the antibody/pathogen complex. The memory cells remain in circulation and initiate a secondary immune response should the pathogen dare enter the host again.

Active and Passive Immunity

Acquired immunity occurs after the first antigen encounter. The first time the body mounts this immune response is called the primary immune response. Because the memory B cells store information about the antigen's structure, any subsequent immune response causes a secondary immune response which is much faster and substantially more antibodies are produced due to the presence of memory B cells. If the secondary immune response is strong and fast enough, it will fight off the pathogen before an individual becomes symptomatic. This is a natural means of acquiring immunity.

Vaccination is the process of inducing immunity. *Active immunization* refers to immunity gained by exposure to infectious microorganisms or viruses and can be *natural* or *artificial*. Natural immunization refers to an individual being exposed to an infectious organism as a part of daily life. For example, it was once common for parents to expose their children to childhood diseases such as measles or chicken pox. Artificial immunization refers to therapeutic exposure to an infectious organism as a way of protecting an individual from disease. Today, the medical community relies on artificial immunization as a way to induce immunity.

Vaccines are used for the development of active immunity. A vaccine contains a killed, weakened, or inactivated microorganism or virus that is administered through injection, by mouth, or by aerosol. Vaccinations are administered to prevent an infectious disease but do not always guarantee immunity. Due to circulating memory B cells after administration, the secondary response will fight off the pathogen should it be encountered again in many cases. Both illnesses and vaccinations cause active immunity.

Passive immunity refers to immunity gained by the introduction of antibodies. This introduction can also be natural or artificial. The process occurs when antibodies from the mother's bloodstream are passed on to the bloodstream of the developing fetus. Breast milk can also transmit antibodies to a baby. Babies are born with passive immunity, which provides protection against general infection for approximately the first six months of its life.

<u>Types of Leukocytes</u>

There are many leukocytes, or white blood cells, involved in both innate and adaptive immunity. All are developed in bone marrow. Many have been mentioned in the text above, but a comprehensive list is included here for reference.

- Monocytes are large phagocytic cells.
    - Macrophages engulf pathogens and present their antigen. Some circulate, but others reside in lymphatic organs like the spleen and lymph nodes.
    - Dendritic cells are also phagocytic and antigen-presenting.

- Granulocytes are cells that contain secretory granules.
    - Neutrophils are the most abundant white blood cell. They are circulating and aggressive phagocytic cells that are part of innate immunity. They also secrete substances that are toxic to pathogens.
    - Basophils and mast cells secrete histamine which stimulates the inflammatory response.
    - Eosinophils are found underneath mucous membranes and defend against multi-cellular parasites like worms. They have low phagocytic activity and primarily secrete destructive enzymes.
- T lymphocytes mature in the thymus.
    - Helper T cells recognize antigens presented by macrophages and dendritic cells and secrete cytokines that mount the humoral and cell-mediated immune response.
    - Killer T cells are cytotoxic cells involved in the cell-mediated response by recognizing and poisoning infected cells.
    - Suppressor T cells suppress the adaptive immune response when there is no threat to conserve resources and energy.
    - Memory T cells remain in circulation to aid in the secondary immune response.
- B lymphocytes mature in bone marrow.
    - Plasma B cells secrete antigen-specific antibodies when signaled by Helper T cells and are degraded after the immune response.
    - Memory B cells store antigen-specific antibody making instructions and remain circulating after the immune response is over.
- Natural killer cells are part of innate immunity and patrol and identify suspect-material. They respond by secreting cytotoxic substances.

Anatomy and Physiology of the Skeletal System

<u>Axial Skeleton and Appendicular Skeleton</u>

The skeletal system is composed of 206 bones interconnected by tough connective tissue called ligaments. The axial skeleton can be considered the north-south axis of the skeleton. It includes the spinal column, sternum, ribs, and skull. There are 80 bones in the axial skeleton, and 33 of them are vertebrae. The ribs make up 12 of the bones in the axial skeleton.

The remaining 126 bones are in the appendicular skeleton which contains bones of the appendages like the collarbone (clavicle), shoulders (scapula), arms, hands, hips, legs, and feet. The arm bones consist of the upper humerus with the radius and ulna that attach to the hands. The wrists, hands, and fingers are composed of the carpals, metacarpals, and phalanges, respectively. The femur attaches to the hips. The patella or kneecap connects the femur to the fibula and tibia. The ankles, feet, and toes are composed of the tarsals, metatarsals, and phalanges, respectively.

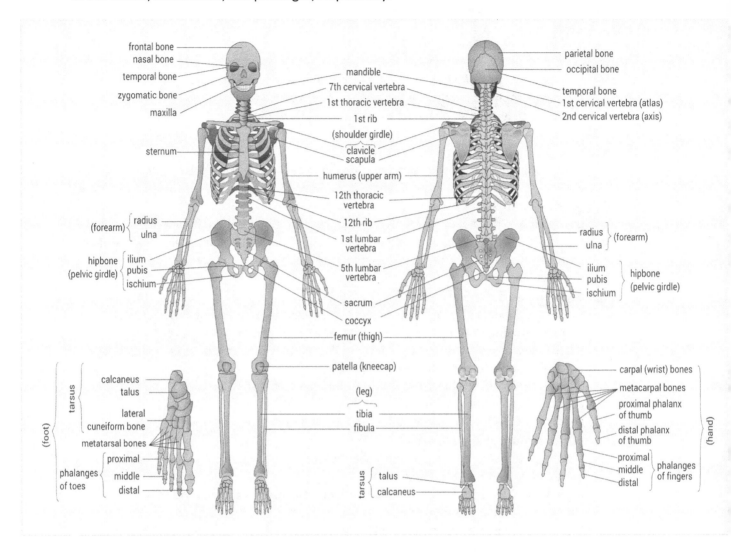

Functions of the Skeletal System

One of the skeletal system's most important functions is to protect vital internal organs. The skull protects the brain, the ribs protect the lungs and heart, the vertebrae protect the spinal column, and the pelvis protects the uterus and other reproductive organs. Red bone marrow produces red and white blood cells as well as platelets in a process known as hemopoiesis. The bones themselves store the essential minerals calcium and phosphorous. The organization of the skeleton allows us to stand upright and acts as a foundation for organs and tissues to attach and maintain their location. This is similar to how the wooden frame of a house has room partitions to designate the type of room and floors that furniture can attach to.

The skeletal system and the muscular system are literally interconnected and allow for voluntary movement. Strong connective tissues called tendons attach bones to muscles. Most muscles work in opposing pairs and act as levers. For example, flexing the biceps brings the arm bones together and flexing the triceps pushes them apart. Synovial joints are movable joints, and they are rich with cartilage, connective tissue, and synovial fluid which acts as a lubricant. The majority of joints are synovial joints, and they include hinge joints, like the one at the elbow, which allows for opening and closing.

The vertebrae are cartilaginous joints which have spaces between them filled with cushion-like discs that act as shock absorbers and glue that holds the vertebrae together. The reason for the tight packing of the vertebrae is to protect the spinal cord inside. This limits their movement, but because there are so many of them it allows the backbone to be flexible.

Fibrous joints like those in the skull have fibrous tissue between the bones and no cavity between them. These are fixed joints that are immobile.

Compact and Spongy Bone
Osteoclasts, osteoblasts, and osteocytes are the three types of bone cells. Osteoclasts break down old bone, osteoblasts make new bone, and osteocytes are the mature functional bone cells. Bone is constantly regenerating due to the osteoblasts/osteoclasts that line all types of bones and the blood vessels inside them. The cells all exist within a matrix of collagen fibers that provide resistance to tension and minerals that provide resistance to compression. Because of the collagen and mineral matrix, bones have ample reinforcement to collectively support the entire human body.

Bones can be classified as any of the following:

- Long bones include tube-like rods like the arm and leg bones.
- Short bones are tube-like rods that are smaller than long bones like the fingers and toes.
- Flat bones are thin and flat like the ribs and breastbone.
- Irregular bones like the vertebrae are compact and don't fit into the other categories.

The outer tissue of the bone is surrounded by connective tissue known as periosteum. It appears shiny, smooth, and white. It protects the bone, anchors the bone to the connective tissue that surrounds muscles, and links the bone to the circulatory and nervous system. Compact bone is underneath the periosteum and is made of a dense blend of tightly packed osteocytes. It serves as a mineral reservoir of calcium and phosphorous. Compact bones have a Haversian system that is composed of embedded blood vessels, lymph vessels, and nerve bundles that span the interior of the bone from one end to the other. Branching from the central canal to the surface of the bone are the canals of Volkmann which deliver materials to peripheral osteocytes. Concentric circles surround the central Haversian canal, and these lamallae have gaps between them called lacunae where osteocytes are embedded.

In contrast, spongy bone is very porous and more flexible than compact bone. It is at the ends of long bones and the central part of flat bones. It looks like a honeycomb, and the open spaces are connected by trabeculae which are beams of tissue that add support. They add strength without adding mass.

Cartilage is a very flexible connective tissue made of collagen and the flexible elastin. It has no blood vessels and obtains materials via diffusion. It is replaced by bone starting in infancy in a process called ossification.

Chemistry

Scientific Notation, the Metric System, and Temperature Scales

Scientific Notation
Scientific notation is the conversion of extremely small or large numbers into a format that is easier to comprehend and manipulate. It changes the number into a product of two separate numbers: a digit term and an exponential term.

Scientific notation = digit term x exponential term

To put a number into scientific notation, one should use the following steps:

- Move the decimal point to after the first non-zero number to find the digit number.
- Count how many places the decimal point was moved in step 1.
- Determine if the exponent is positive or negative.
- Create an exponential term using the information from steps 2 and 3.
- Combine the digit term and exponential term to get scientific notation.

For example, to put 0.0000098 into scientific notation, the decimal should be moved so that it lies between the last two numbers: 000009.8. This creates the digit number: *9.8*

Next, the number of places that the decimal point moved is determined; to get between the 9 and the 8, the decimal was moved six places to the right. It may be helpful to remember that a decimal moved to the right creates a negative exponent, and a decimal moved to the left creates a positive exponent. Because the decimal was moved six places to the right, the exponent is negative.

Now, the exponential term can be created by using the base 10 (this is *always* the base in scientific notation) and the number of places moved as the exponent, in this case: 10^{-6}

Finally, the digit term and the exponential term can be combined as a product. Therefore, the scientific notation for the number 0.0000098 is:

$$9.8 \times 10^{-6}$$

Standard vs. Metric Systems
The measuring system used today in the United States developed from the British units of measurement during colonial times. The most typically used units in this customary system are those used to measure weight, liquid volume, and length, whose common units are found below. In the customary system, the basic unit for measuring weight is the ounce (oz); there are 16 ounces (oz) in 1 pound (lb) and 2000 pounds in 1 ton. The basic unit for measuring liquid volume is the ounce (oz); 1 ounce is equal to 2 tablespoons (tbsp) or 6 teaspoons (tsp), and there are 8 ounces in 1 cup, 2 cups in 1 pint (pt), 2 pints in 1 quart (qt), and 4 quarts in 1 gallon (gal). For measurements of length, the inch (in) is the base unit; 12 inches make up 1 foot (ft), 3 feet make up 1 yard (yd), and 5280 feet make up 1 mile (mi). However, as there are only a set number of units in the customary system, with extremely large or extremely small amounts of material, the numbers can become awkward and difficult to compare.

Consider this chart:

Common Customary Measurements		
Length	**Weight**	**Capacity**
1 foot = 12 inches	1 pound = 16 ounces	1 cup = 8 fluid ounces
1 yard = 3 feet	1 ton = 2,000 pounds	1 pint = 2 cups
1 yard = 36 inches		1 quart = 2 pints
1 mile = 1,760 yards		1 quart = 4 cups
1 mile = 5,280 feet		1 gallon = 4 quarts
		1 gallon = 16 cups

Aside from the United States, most countries in the world have adopted the **metric system** embodied in the International System of Units (SI). The three main SI base units used in the metric system are the meter (m), the kilogram (kg), and the liter (L); meters measure length, kilograms measure mass, and liters measure volume.

These three units can use different prefixes, which indicate larger or smaller versions of the unit by powers of ten. This can be thought of as making a new unit which is sized by multiplying the original unit in size by a factor.

These prefixes and associated factors are:

Metric Prefixes			
Prefix	**Symbol**	**Multiplier**	**Exponential**
kilo	k	1,000	10^3
hecto	h	100	10^2
deca	da	10	10^1
no prefix		1	10^0
deci	d	0.1	10^{-1}
centi	c	0.01	10^{-2}
milli	m	0.001	10^{-3}

The correct prefix is then attached to the base. Some examples:

>   1 milliliter equals .001 liters.

>   1 kilogram equals 1,000 grams.

Some units of measure are represented as square or cubic units depending on the solution. For example, perimeter is measured in units, area is measured in square units, and volume is measured in cubic units.

Also, be sure to use the most appropriate unit for the thing being measured. A building's height might be measured in feet or meters while the length of a nail might be measured in inches or centimeters. Additionally, for SI units, the prefix should be chosen to provide the most succinct available value. For example, the mass of a bag of fruit would likely be measured in kilograms rather than grams or milligrams, and the length of a bacteria cell would likely be measured in micrometers rather than centimeters or kilometers.

<u>Temperature Scales</u>
There are three main temperature scales used in science. The scale most often used in the United States is the **Fahrenheit** scale. This scale is based on the measurement of water freezing at 32^0 F and water boiling at 212^0 F. The **Celsius** scale uses 0^0 C as the temperature for water freezing and 100^0 C for water boiling. The Celsius scale is the most widely used in the scientific community. The accepted measurement by the International System of Units (from the French Système international d'unités), or SI, for temperature is the Kelvin scale. This is the scale employed in thermodynamics, since its zero is the basis for absolute zero, or the unattainable temperature, when matter no longer exhibits degradation.

The conversions between the temperature scales are as follows:

^{0}Fahrenheit to ^{0}Celsius: $^0C = \frac{5}{9}(^0F - 32)$

^{0}Celsius to ^{0}Fahrenheit: $^0F = \frac{9}{5}(^0C) + 32$

^{0}Celsius to Kelvin: $K = {^0C} + 273.15$

Atomic Structure and the Periodic Table

<u>Atomic Structure</u>
The structure of an atom has two major components: the atomic nucleus and the atomic shells (also known as orbits). The **nucleus** is found in the center of an atom. The three major subatomic particles are protons, neutrons, and electrons and are found in the atomic nucleus and shells.

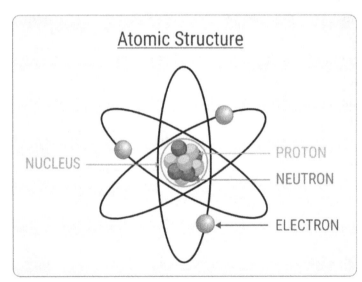

Atomic Structure

Protons are found in the atomic nucleus and are positively charged particles. The addition or removal of protons from an atom's nucleus creates an entirely different element. **Neutrons** are also found in the atomic nucleus and are neutral particles, meaning they have no net electrical charge. The addition or removal of neutrons from an atom's nucleus does not create a different element but instead creates a lighter or heavier form of that element called an isotope. **Electrons** are found orbiting in the atomic shells around the nucleus and are negatively charged particles. A proton or a neutron has nearly 2,000 times the mass of an electron.

Electrons orbit the nucleus in atomic shells, or electron clouds. For example, the first atomic shell can accommodate two electrons, the second atomic shell can hold a maximum of eight electrons, and the third atomic shell can house a maximum of eight electrons. The negatively charged electrons orbiting the nucleus are attracted to the positively charged protons in the nucleus via electromagnetic force. The attraction of opposite electrical charges gives rise to chemical bonds, which refers to the ways atoms are attached to each other.

The **atomic number** of an atom is determined by the number of protons within the nucleus. When a substance is composed of atoms that all have the same atomic number, it is called an **element**. Elements are arranged by atomic number and grouped by properties in the **Periodic table.**

An atom's **mass number** is determined by the sum of the total number of protons and neutrons in the atom. Most nuclei have a net neutral charge, and all atoms of one type have the same atomic number. However, there are some atoms of the same type that have a different mass number, due to an imbalance of neutrons. These are called **isotopes**. In isotopes, the atomic number, which is determined by the number of protons, is the same, but the mass number, which is determined by adding the protons and neutrons, is different due to the irregular number of neutrons.

Chemical Bonding
Chemical bonding typically results in the formation of a new substance, called a compound. Only the electrons in the outermost atomic shell are able to form chemical bonds. These electrons are known as **valence electrons**, and they are what determines the chemical properties of an atom.

Chemical bonding occurs between two or more atoms that are joined together. There are three types of chemical bonds: ionic, covalent, and metallic. The characteristics of the different bonds are determined by how electrons behave in a compound. **Lewis structures** were developed to help visualize the electrons in molecules; they are a method of writing a compound structure formula and including its electron composition. A Lewis symbol for an element consists of the element symbol and a dot for each valence electron. The dots are located on all four sides of the symbol, with a maximum of two dots per side, and eight dots, or electrons, total. The octet rule states that atoms tend to gain, lose, or share electrons until they have a total of eight valence electrons.

Ionic bonds are formed from the electrostatic attractions between oppositely charged atoms. They result from the transfer of electrons from a metal on the left side of the periodic table to a nonmetal on the right side. The metallic substance often has low ionization energy and will transfer an electron easily to the nonmetal, which has a high electron affinity. An example of this is the compound NaCl, which is sodium chloride or table salt, where the Na atom transfers an electron to the Cl atom. Due to strong bonding, ionic compounds have several distinct characteristics. They have high melting and boiling points and are brittle and crystalline. They are arranged in rigid, well-defined structures, which allow them to break apart along smooth, flat surfaces. The formation of ionic bonds is a reaction that is exothermic. In the opposite scenario, the energy it takes to break up a one mole quantity of an ionic compound is referred to as lattice energy, which is generally endothermic. The Lewis structure for NaCl is written as follows:

$$Na\cdot \ + \ :\overset{..}{\underset{..}{Cl}}\cdot \ \longrightarrow \ Na^+ \ + :\overset{..}{\underset{..}{Cl}}:^-$$

Covalent bonds are formed when two atoms share electrons, instead of transferring them as in ionic compounds. The atoms in covalent compounds have a balance of attraction and repulsion between their protons and electrons, which keeps them bonded together. Two atoms can be joined by single, double, or even triple covalent bonds. As the number of electrons that are shared increases, the length of the bond decreases. Covalent substances have low melting and boiling points and are poor conductors of heat and electricity.

The Lewis structure for Cl₂ is written as follows:

Lewis structure Cl₂

:Cl˙ + ˙Cl: ⟶ :Cl:Cl:

Metallic bonds are formed by electrons that move freely through metal. They are the product of the force of attraction between electrons and metal ions. The electrons are shared by many metal cations and act like glue that holds the metallic substance together, similar to the attraction between oppositely-charged atoms in ionic substances, except the electrons are more fluid and float around the bonded metals and form a sea of electrons. Metallic compounds have characteristic properties that include strength, conduction of heat and electricity, and malleability. They can conduct electricity by passing energy through the freely moving electrons, creating a **current**. These compounds also have high melting and boiling points. Lewis structures are not common for metallic structures because of the free-roaming ability of the electrons.

Periodic Table

The periodic table catalogues all of the elements known to man, currently 118. It is one of the most important references in the science of chemistry. Information that can be gathered from the periodic table includes the element's atomic number, atomic mass, and chemical symbol. The first periodic table was rendered by Mendeleev in the mid-1800s and was ordered according to increasing atomic mass. The modern periodic table is arranged in order of increasing atomic number. It is also arranged in horizontal rows known as **periods,** and vertical columns known as **families,** or **groups**. The periodic table contains seven periods and eighteen families. Elements in the periodic table can also be classified into three major groups: metals, metalloids, and nonmetals. **Metals** are concentrated on the left side of the periodic table, while **nonmetals** are found on the right side. **Metalloids** occupy the area between the metals and nonmetals.

Due to the fact the periodic table is ordered by increasing atomic number, the electron configurations of the elements show periodicity. As the atomic number increases, electrons gradually fill the shells of an atom. In general, the start of a new period corresponds to the first time an electron inhabits a new shell.

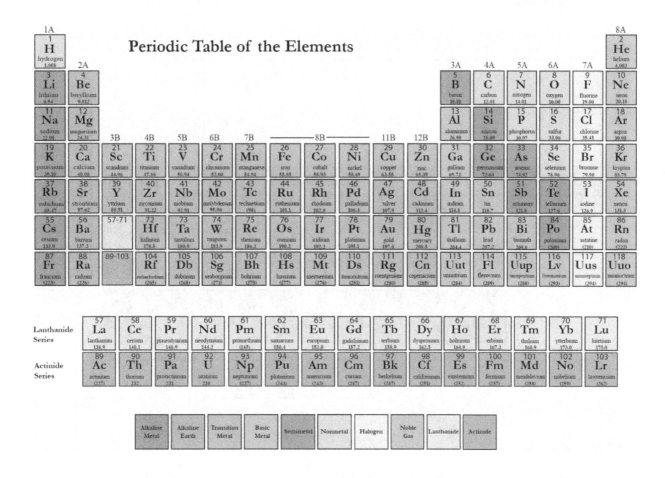

Other trends in the properties of elements in the periodic table are:

Atomic radius: One-half the distance between the nuclei of atoms of the same element.

Electronegativity: A measurement of the willingness of an atom to form a chemical bond.

Ionization energy: The amount of energy needed to remove an electron from a gas or ion.

Electron affinity: The ability of an atom to accept an electron.

Trends in the Periodic Table

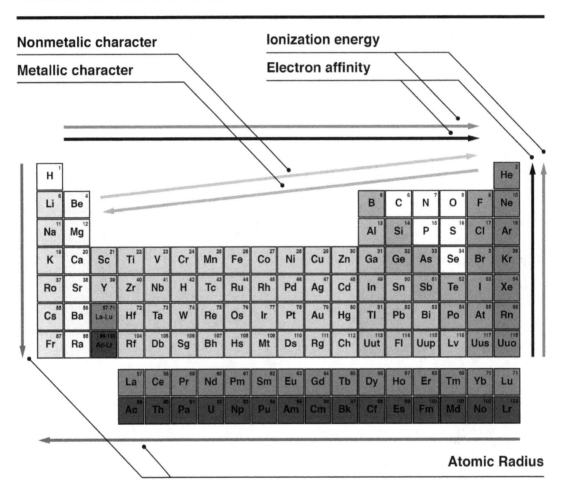

Chemical Equations

Chemical reactions are represented by **chemical equations**. The equations help to explain how the molecules change during the reaction. For example, when hydrogen gas (H_2) combines with oxygen gas (O_2), two molecules of water are formed. The equation is written as follows, where the "+" sign means *reacts with* and the "→" means *produces*:

$$2 H_2 + O_2 \rightarrow 2 H_2O$$

Two hydrogen molecules react with an oxygen molecule to produce two water molecules. In all chemical equations, the quantity of each element on the reactant side of the equation should equal the quantity of the same element on the product side of the equation due to the law of conservation of matter. If this is true, the equation is described as balanced. To figure out how many of each element there is on each side of the equation, the coefficient of the element should be multiplied by the subscript next to the element. Coefficients and subscripts are noted for quantities larger than one. The **coefficient** is the number located directly to the left of the element. The **subscript** is the small-sized number directly to the right of the element. In the equation above, on the left side, the coefficient of the hydrogen is two and the subscript is also two, which makes a total of four hydrogen atoms. Using the same method, there are two oxygen atoms. On the right side, the coefficient two is multiplied by the subscript in each element of the water molecule, making four hydrogen atoms and two oxygen atoms. This equation is balanced because there are four hydrogen atoms and two oxygen atoms on each side. The states of the reactants and products can also be written in the equation: gas (g), liquid (l), solid (s), and dissolved in water (aq). If they are included, they are noted in parentheses on the right side of each molecule in the equation.

Reaction Rates, Equilibrium, and Reversibility

Chemical reactions are conveyed using chemical equations. Chemical equations must be balanced with equivalent numbers of atoms for each type of element on each side of the equation. Antoine Lavoisier, a French chemist, was the first to propose the **Law of Conservation of Mass** for the purpose of balancing a chemical equation. The law states, "Matter is neither created nor destroyed during a chemical reaction."

The **reactants** are located on the left side of the arrow, while the **products** are located on the right side of the arrow. Coefficients are the numbers in front of the chemical formulas. Subscripts are the numbers to the lower right of chemical symbols in a formula. To tally atoms, one should multiply the formula's coefficient by the subscript of each chemical symbol. For example, the chemical equation $2 H_2 + O_2 \rightarrow 2H_2O$ is balanced. For H, the coefficient of 2 multiplied by the subscript 2 = 4 hydrogen atoms. For O, the coefficient of 1 multiplied by the subscript 2 = 2 oxygen atoms. Coefficients and subscripts of 1 are understood and never written.

Reaction Rates
The rate of a reaction is the measure of the change in concentration of the reactants or products over a certain period of time. Many factors affect how fast or slow a reaction occurs, such as concentration, pressure, or temperature. As the concentration of a reactant increases, the rate of the reaction also increases, because the frequency of collisions between elements increases. High-pressure situations for reactants that are gases cause the gas to compress and increase the frequency of gas molecule collisions, similar to solutions with higher concentrations. Reactions rates are then increased with the higher frequency of gas molecule collisions. Higher temperatures usually increase the rate of the reaction, adding more energy to the system with heat and increasing the frequency of molecular collisions.

Equilibrium
Equilibrium is described as the state of a system when no net changes occur. Chemical equilibrium occurs when opposing reactions occur at equal rates. In other words, the rate of reactants forming products is equal to the rate of the products breaking down into the reactants—the concentration of reactants and products in the system doesn't change. This happens in **reversible chemical reactions** as opposed to irreversible chemical reactions. In **irreversible chemical reactions**, the products cannot be changed back to reactants. Although the concentrations are not changing in equilibrium, the forward

and reverse reactions are likely still occurring. This type of equilibrium is called a **dynamic equilibrium**. In situations where all reactions have ceased, a **static equilibrium** is reached. Chemical equilibriums are also described as homogeneous or heterogeneous. **Homogeneous equilibrium** involves substances that are all in the same phase, while **heterogeneous equilibrium** means the substances are in different phases when equilibrium is reached. When a reaction reaches equilibrium, the conditions of the equilibrium are described by the following equation, based on the chemical equation $aA + bB \leftrightarrow cC + dD$:

Catalysts are substances that accelerate the speed of a chemical reaction. A catalyst remains unchanged throughout the course of a chemical reaction. In most cases, only small amounts of a catalyst are needed. Catalysts increase the rate of a chemical reaction by providing an alternate path requiring less activation energy. Activation energy refers to the amount of energy required for the initiation of a chemical reaction.

Catalysts can be homogeneous or heterogeneous. Catalysts in the same phase of matter as its reactants are homogeneous, while catalysts in a different phase than reactants are heterogeneous. It is important to remember catalysts are selective. They don't accelerate the speed of all chemical reactions, but catalysts do accelerate specific chemical reactions.

Solutions and Solution Concentrations

A homogeneous mixture, also called a **solution,** has uniform properties throughout a given sample. An example of a homogeneous solution is salt fully dissolved in warm water. In this case, any number of samples taken from the parent solution would be identical.

One **mole** is the amount of matter contained in 6.02×10^{23} of any object, such as atoms, ions, or molecules. It is a useful unit of measure for items in large quantities. This number is also known as **Avogadro's number**. One mole of ^{12}C atoms is equivalent to 6.02×10^{23} ^{12}C atoms. Avogadro's number is often written as an inverse mole, or as $6.02 \times 10^{23}/mol$.

Molarity is the concentration of a solution. It is based on the number of moles of solute in one liter of solution and is written as the capital letter M. A 1.0 molar solution, or 1.0 M solution, has one mole of solute per liter of solution. The molarity of a solution can be determined by calculating the number of moles of the solute and dividing it by the volume of the solution in liters. The resulting number is the mol/L or M for molarity of the solution.

Chemical Reactions

Chemical reactions are characterized by a chemical change in which the starting substances, or reactants, differ from the substances formed, or products. Chemical reactions may involve a change in color, the production of gas, the formation of a precipitate, or changes in heat content. The following are the five basic types of chemical reactions:

- **Decomposition Reactions:** A compound is broken down into smaller elements. For example, $2H_2O \rightarrow 2H_2 + O_2$. This is read as, "2 molecules of water decompose into 2 molecules of hydrogen and 1 molecule of oxygen."

- **Synthesis Reactions:** Two or more elements or compounds are joined together. For example, $2H_2 + O_2 \rightarrow 2H_2O$. This is read as, "2 molecules of hydrogen react with 1 molecule of oxygen to produce 2 molecules of water."

- **Single Displacement Reactions:** A single element or ion takes the place of another element in a compound. It is also known as a substitution reaction. For example, $Zn + 2\ HCl \rightarrow ZnCl_2 + H_2$. This is read as, "zinc reacts with 2 molecules of hydrochloric acid to produce one molecule of zinc chloride and one molecule of hydrogen." In other words, zinc replaces the hydrogen in hydrochloric acid.

- **Double Displacement Reactions:** Two elements or ions exchange a single element to form two different compounds, resulting in different combinations of cations and anions in the final compounds. It is also known as a metathesis reaction. For example, $H_2SO_4 + 2\ NaOH \rightarrow Na_2\ SO_4 + 2\ H_2O$

  - Special types of double displacement reactions include:

    - **Oxidation-Reduction (or Redox) Reactions:** Elements undergo a change in oxidation number. For example, $2\ S_2O_3^{2-}\ (aq) + I_2\ (aq) \rightarrow S_4O_6^{2-}\ (aq) + 2\ I^-\ (aq)$.

    - **Acid-Base Reactions:** Involves a reaction between an acid and a base, which produces a salt and water. For example, $HBr + NaOH \rightarrow NaBr + H_2O$.

    - **Combustion Reactions:** A hydrocarbon (a compound composed of only hydrogen and carbon) reacts with oxygen (O_2) to form carbon dioxide (CO_2) and water (H_2O). For example, $CH_4 + 2O_2 \rightarrow CO_2 + 2H_2O$.

Stoichiometry

Stoichiometry investigates the quantities of chemicals that are consumed and produced in chemical reactions. Chemical equations are made up of reactants and products; stoichiometry helps elucidate how the changes from reactants to products occur, as well as how to ensure the equation is balanced.

Chemical reactions are limited by the amount of starting material, or reactants, available to drive the process forward. The reactant that has the smallest amount of substance is called the limiting reactant. The **limiting reactant** is completely consumed by the end of the reaction. The other reactants are called **excess reactants**. For example, gasoline is used in a combustion reaction to make a car move and is the limiting reactant of the reaction. If the gasoline runs out, the combustion reaction can no longer take place, and the car stops.

The quantity of product that should be produced after using up all of the limiting reactant can be calculated and is called the **theoretical yield of the reaction**. Since the reactants do not always act as they should, the actual amount of resulting product is called the **actual yield**. The actual yield is divided by the theoretical yield and then multiplied by 100 to find the **percent yield** for the reaction.

Solution stoichiometry deals with quantities of solutes in chemical reactions that occur in solutions. The quantity of a solute in a solution can be calculated by multiplying the molarity of the solution by the volume. Similar to chemical equations involving simple elements, the number of moles of the elements that make up the solute should be equivalent on both sides of the equation.

When the concentration of a particular solute in a solution is unknown, a **titration** is used to determine that concentration. In a titration, the solution with the unknown solute is combined with a standard solution, which is a solution with a known solute concentration. The point at which the unknown solute has completely reacted with the known solute is called the **equivalence point**. Using the known information about the standard solution, including the concentration and volume, and the volume of the unknown solution, the concentration of the unknown solute is determined in a balanced equation. For example, in the case of combining acids and bases, the equivalence point is reached when the resulting solution is neutral. HCl, an acid, combines with NaOH, a base, to form water, which is neutral, and a solution of Cl^- ions and Na^+ ions. Before the equivalence point, there are an unequal number of cations and anions and the solution is not neutral.

Oxidation and Reduction

Oxidation and reduction reactions, also known as **redox reactions**, are those in which electrons are transferred from one element to another. Batteries and fuel cells are two energy-related technologies that utilize these reactions. When an atom, ion, or molecule loses its electrons and becomes more positively charged, it is described as being oxidized. When a substance gains electrons and becomes more negatively charged, it is reduced. In chemical reactions, if one element or molecule is oxidized, another must be reduced for the equation to be balanced. Although the transfer of electrons is obvious in some reactions where ions are formed, redox reactions also include those in which electrons are transferred but the products remain neutral.

Keep track of oxidation states or oxidation numbers to ensure the chemical equation is balanced. **Oxidation numbers** are assigned to each atom in a neutral substance or ion. For ions made up of a single atom, the oxidation number is equal to the charge of the ion. For atoms in their original elemental form, the oxidation number is always zero. Each hydrogen atom in an H_2 molecule, for example, has an oxidation number of zero. The sum of the oxidation numbers in a molecule should be equal to the overall charge of the molecule. If the molecule is a positively charged ion, the sum of the oxidation number should be equal to overall positive charge of the molecule. In ionic compounds that have a cation and anion joined, the sum of the oxidation numbers should equal zero.

All chemical equations must have the same number of elements on each side of the equation to be balanced. Redox reactions have an extra step of counting the electrons on both sides of the equation to be balanced. Separating redox reactions into oxidation reactions and reduction reactions is a simple way to account for all of the electrons involved. The individual equations are known as **half-reactions**. The number of electrons lost in the oxidation reaction must be equal to the number of electrons gained in the reduction reaction for the redox reaction to be balanced.

The oxidation of tin (Sn) by iron (Fe) can be balanced by the following half-reactions:

Oxidation: $Sn^{2+} \rightarrow Sn^{4+} + 2e^-$

Reduction: $2Fe^{3+} + 2e^- \rightarrow 2Fe^{2+}$

Complete redox reaction: $Sn^{2+} + 2Fe^{3+} \rightarrow Sn^{4+} + 2Fe^{2+}$

Acids and Bases

Acids and bases are defined in many different ways. An **acid** can be described as a substance that increases the concentration of H^+ ions when it is dissolved in water, as a proton donor in a chemical equation, or as an electron-pair acceptor. A **base** can be a substance that increases the concentration of OH^- ions when it is dissolved in water, accepts a proton in a chemical reaction, or is an electron-pair donor.

pH refers to the power or potential of hydrogen atoms and is used as a scale for a substance's acidity. In chemistry, pH represents the hydrogen ion concentration (written as $[H^+]$) in an aqueous, or watery, solution. The hydrogen ion concentration, $[H^+]$, is measured in moles of H^+ per liter of solution.

The pH scale is a logarithmic scale used to quantify how acidic or basic a substance is. pH is the negative logarithm of the hydrogen ion concentration: $pH = -\log [H^+]$. A one-unit change in pH correlates with a ten-fold change in hydrogen ion concentration. The pH scale typically ranges from zero to 14, although it is possible to have pHs outside of this range. Pure water has a pH of 7, which is considered **neutral**. pH values less than 7 are considered **acidic**, while pH values greater than 7 are considered **basic**, or **alkaline**.

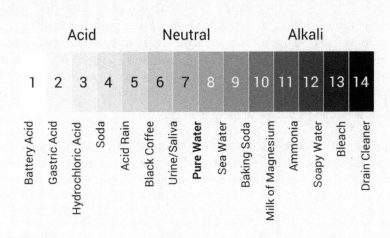

Generally speaking, an acid is a substance capable of donating hydrogen ions, while a base is a substance capable of accepting hydrogen ions. A **buffer** is a molecule that can act as either a hydrogen ion donor or acceptor. Buffers are crucial in the blood and body fluids and prevent the body's pH from fluctuating into dangerous territory. pH can be measured using a pH meter, test paper, or indicator sticks.

Water can act as either an acid or a base. When mixed with an acid, water can accept a proton and become an H_3O^+ ion. When mixed with a base, water can donate a proton and become an OH^- ion. Sometimes water molecules donate and accept protons from each other; this process is called **autoionization**. The chemical equation is written as follows: $H_2O + H_2O \rightarrow OH^- + H_3O^+$.

Acids and bases are characterized as strong, weak, or somewhere in between. Strong acids and bases completely or almost completely ionize in aqueous solution. The chemical reaction is driven completely forward, to the right side of the equation, where the acidic or basic ions are formed. Weak acids and bases do not completely disassociate in aqueous solution. They only partially ionize and the solution becomes a mixture of the acid or base, water, and the acidic or basic ions. Strong acids are complemented by weak bases, and vice versa. A **conjugate acid** is an ion that forms when its base pair gains a proton. For example, the conjugate acid NH_4^+ is formed from the base NH_3. The **conjugate base** that pairs with an acid is the ion that is formed when an acid loses a proton. NO_2^- is the conjugate base of the acid HNO_2.

Health

Health Promotion/Disease Prevention

Two of the most important aspects of providing exceptional nursing care are health promotion and disease prevention. Both are integral to ensuring the physical and psychological well-being of individuals, groups, and the community at large.

Health promotion can be loosely defined as the direct or indirect presentation of information, specifically designed to influence behaviors that are expected to result in positive health outcomes. When presented directly, the instruction may be in written form such as brochures, books, or articles in magazines or newspapers. Historically, these publications were typically available in physician's offices, clinics, and hospitals. For nurses, health promotion is no longer relegated to easily discarded brochures or pamphlets. With the introduction of the Internet, information targeting healthy activities can be found instantly after several keystrokes. Nursing interventions can be provided via webinars, face-to-face coaching sessions, telephonic care, and social media sites. These mediums allow the nurse to contact thousands of individuals at once and increase exposure.

Indirect presentation of healthy lifestyle choices often occurs through billboards, signage, or posters in physicians' offices, as well as strategic mention or product placement in movies and television shows. Increasing numbers of "reality TV" stars can be seen holding bottles of a specific brand of vitamins or diet pills, or leaving a restaurant noted for healthy dishes. Albeit not as successful as the direct-to-consumer approach, this allows for health promotion to sneak in the back doors of viewers' minds, slowly affecting their daily habits. Traditionally, nurses are not involved in this type of health promotion, but nurses can use this type of behavior when interacting with patients. Ensuring that hand washing posters are present in restrooms, display cases of vitamins and supplements in the office waiting area, and sponsorship or participation in local health fairs all support higher awareness.

In an effort to actively guide the prevention of disease, community health nurses employ numerous tactics. Each strategy is specific to a particular population to intervene at several stages of the disease process.

Primary prevention consists of the nursing strategies implemented to prevent the onset of a particular disease process. One well-known example of primary disease prevention is the "say no to drugs" movement. Nurses in this campaign can specifically target young children and teens to prevent their initial use of drugs with the use of buttons, posters, commercials, and rallies. Secondary prevention focuses on the early detection of disease and prevention of considerable damage from the disease process. Using the same example, "pill checks" at rave parties would represent secondary prevention. Nurses and often paraprofessionals attend parties with teens to test the pills of party goers. This is done onsite, in the presence of the user, explaining what is found in the pill and offering to discard it. Finally, tertiary prevention efforts with this same patient population would be nursing interventions implemented in drug treatment centers, clinics, and detox units in the hospital. These nurses work with the patients actively addicted to substances and collaborate to manage their disease.

Health Screening

Historically, nurses have been primarily responsible for conducting health screenings. Every biological system within the human body should be screened periodically to ensure that it is operating at optimal levels. At the start of every developmental stage, it is recommended that patients be screened and, if found deficient, treated and monitored for progress. Health screenings are suggested based on chronological age to guide both individual treatment and trends for developing community outreach. Armed with the data, nurses collaborate with patients, providers, and caregivers to formulate an effective treatment plan.

Nurses working within the community health sector also utilize health screenings to guide disease-prevention efforts on a larger scale. Nurse researchers can use the data to aide in the creation of medications and advertisement campaigns to target those individuals on the borderlines of a particular disease process. Further, community-health nurses can conduct health screenings to identify gaps in access to healthcare, barriers to care, and disease maintenance. Once the information is disseminated to surrounding healthcare providers, clinics, and local government officials, the community-health nurse can begin the dialogue to effect policy changes. More engagement with health fairs, educational seminars, and print and social media campaigns may also result from health screenings.

Overall, health screenings are an integral piece of the healthcare puzzle. As nurses, it is often necessary to discuss the importance of annual health-screening recommendations upon each patient encounter. If patients reject or accept the recommended testing, they become aware of any present risk factors. Nurses can probe for information as to their ambivalence. For example, while completing a depression screening, a nurse can determine if an individual is at risk for depression. A patient who scores higher on the questionnaire can reveal if the answers are an accurate representation of daily high-risk behavior, or situational in nature.

High Risk Behaviors

High-risk behaviors can be defined as actions that have a high probability of yielding a negative consequence. Nurses must develop a rapport with patients in an effort to create open communication so the patient will be more likely to reveal conduct that could have detrimental health outcomes. This technique can also encourage patients to ask questions about their risky behaviors. The nurse can then use the established rapport to discern if the patient's level of comfort and commitment to the behaviors is amenable to change.

One of the most effective methods of encouraging open communication with patients is motivational interviewing. Nurses use motivational interviewing to assess, collaborate, plan, and implement treatment with patients. There are five major components of motivational interviewing: express empathy, illustrate incongruity, manage resistance, encourage self-validation, and promote independence. The nurse can employ these steps when combatting ambivalence to change. For example, when working with a patient who is considering smoking cessation, begin with simple statements regarding the difficulties involved with quitting. This often results in the patient remarking about the number of attempts to quit, along with reasons why his or her prior attempts did not end in success. Next, draw from earlier statements concerning lifestyle choices, the patient's own reasons for quitting, and the potential for negative outcomes. In the next step, the nurse can tie the elements together, choosing carefully which area of resistance to target. What might the patient gain from quitting? What are the potential barriers to success from the patient's viewpoint? Asking these open-ended questions will help patients draw their own conclusions, validating the ability to self-navigate through possible obstacles. Once able to verbalize how the desired outcome could be achieved, the patient has managed to break through his or her own resistance, and the groundwork has been set for more internal dialogue.

Lifestyle Choices

Traditionally, nursing interventions are designed to target the lifestyle choices that affect disease processes. During every patient encounter, the nurse must ask open-ended questions in order to determine which interventions should be implemented. The acronym SMART (specific, measurable, attainable, relevant, and timely) is a concise reference for patients. When it is clearly what the main objective is, the likelihood of achieving that goal is increased.

When addressing multiple issues, chose one area with the highest likelihood of success to build momentum and patient confidence in the process. For example, when discussing diet, it is important for the nurse to first establish what the patient's current diet and exercise plan includes. This dialogue will open the door to likes, dislikes, preferred cooking methods, and diet history. As the discussion expands, inquire about budgetary constraints and actual access to healthy food options. Once eating habits are known, define daily scheduling conflicts that may become barriers to success. Create a contingency plan, with multiple options. Another major area of importance for lifestyle choices is exercise. Upon reviewing current diagnoses, medications, and any mobility or chronic pain concerns, the nurse can partner with the patient to formulate a reasonable plan. Set a specific goal on the type and duration of exercise; measure steps or activity as accurately as possible with a pedometer. Can they commit to exercise daily? What is an appropriate form of exercise? Maintain the stance of advocate and collaborator to preserve patients' autonomy and validate their experiences whenever possible.

Self-Care

The job of a nurse is physically, mentally, and emotionally stressful. The strain of moving and lifting patients, along with going from room to room constantly answering the needs of the patients for a long shift, can be physically exhausting. One must organize one's time, prioritize tasks, answer questions, and have countless conversations with the health care team and patients and their families, all of which can take a mental toll. Dealing with patients who are sick, in pain, suffering, and, in some cases, facing death, can drain a nurse's emotional reserves, which can quickly lead to burnout if left unaddressed. Being aware of this potential for overall fatigue is the first step to managing stress and maintaining one's own health.

It is important that a nurse knows how to cope with the effects of stress positively. *Negative coping mechanisms* include unhealthy eating habits and binging behavior, abusing substances such as alcohol and drugs, acting recklessly with one's own safety, and becoming abusive in personal relationships.

Positive coping mechanisms include finding an activity to engage in to unwind and relieve stress in a healthy way. Activities such as daily exercise, spending quality time with friends and family, cooking, yoga, biking, and hiking are all ways to deal with the stress of a demanding job in a healthy way.

The nurse should be careful not to work too many hours as well. It can be tempting to take on extra shifts continually to earn extra money for gifts, vacations, or simply to pay the bills and support a family. These extra shifts and long hours can put a nurse in a danger zone if they are using up too much mental, physical, and/or emotional energy. It is better to be well rested and have adequate mental and physical energy for a shift than to put the patient and oneself at risk for harm.

Being properly nourished, getting adequate exercise, and maintaining healthy sleep habits will all positively contribute to a nurse's health. The nurse's health is vital to helping their patients regain or maintain their own health and, thus, should be made a high priority. If one needs help learning healthy eating habits, meal planning, how to get involved in an exercise program or routine, or other methods of managing stress, many facilities have programs to help guide employees toward better health. There are a plethora of available online resources aimed at improving one's health as well.

Techniques of Physical Assessment

One of the most important skills that a nurse can possess is that of the physical assessment. Practically every area of nursing practice requires that a nurse have an accurate recall of normal physical functioning and be capable of observing areas of compromise. The nurse's awareness of baseline functioning for a patient within the specific age group and associated health concerns is essential. Physicians, nurse practitioners, and other healthcare providers routinely depend on the nurse's initial assessment of patients to guide their overall treatment of patients.

The initial assessment of a patient does not begin in the face-to-face interaction. As an expert, the nurse must start with any available historical data. Review prior history and physical records, diagnoses, medications, and treatment plans. Certain medications and disease processes can impact daily functioning and the nurse must consider this prior to patient interaction. Immediately upon introduction, the nurse must observe: gait, posture, and balance, skin tone, voice intonation, responsiveness, eye contact, hand grip with handshake, and general stature. While taking vital signs, assess mood, level of consciousness (LOC), orientation, short-term and long-term memory, bowel and urinary habits, and medication list. The aforementioned portions of the assessment can aide in the formulation of the rest of the clinical picture. It is also necessary to discuss daily habits, work schedule, social interactions, and physical activity. Those factors can influence adherence to suggested treatment plans. Once a full clinical picture falls into place, the nurse can utilize the findings to discuss interventions that would be helpful to the patient.

Physics

Nature of Motion

People have been studying the movement of objects since ancient times, sometimes prompted by curiosity, and sometimes by necessity. On Earth, items move according to specific guidelines and have motion that is fairly predictable. The measurement of an object's movement or change in position (x), over a change in time (t) is an object's **speed.** The average speed of an object is defined as the distance that the object travels divided by how long it takes the object to travel that distance. When the direction is included with the speed, it is referred to as the **velocity.** A "change in position" refers to the difference in location of an object's starting point and an object's ending point. In science, this change is represented by the Greek letter Delta, Δ.

$$velocity\ (v) = \frac{\Delta x}{\Delta t}$$

Distance is measured in meters, and time is measured in seconds. The standard scientific units for speed and velocity are meters/second (m/s), but units of miles/hour (mph) are also commonly used in America.

$$\frac{meters}{second} = \frac{m}{s}$$

Average velocity is calculated by averaging the beginning or initial velocity and the ending or final velocity of an object.

If a measurement includes its direction, it is called a **vector quantity**; otherwise, the measurement is called a **scalar quantity** and has only a numeric value without a particular direction. For example, speed is a scalar quantity while velocity is a vector quantity.

Acceleration

While an object's speed measures how fast the object's position will change in a certain amount of time, an object's **acceleration** measures how fast the object's speed will change in a certain amount of time. Acceleration can be thought of as the change in velocity or speed (Δv) divided by the change in the time (Δt).

$$acceleration\ (a) = \frac{\Delta v}{\Delta t}$$

Velocity is measured in meters/second and time is measured in seconds, so the standard unit for acceleration is meters / second2 (m/s2).

$$\frac{meters/second}{second} = \frac{meters}{second^2} = \frac{m}{s^2}$$

Acceleration is expressed by using both magnitude and direction, so it is a vector quantity like velocity. Acceleration is present when an object is slowing down, speeding up, or changing direction, since these represent instances where velocity is changing. This means that forces like friction and gravity accelerate objects and increase or decrease their velocities over time.

Projectile Motion

Projectile motion describes the way in which a projectile will move when the only force acting upon it is gravity. Since the force of Earth's gravity is nearly constant at sea level, its magnitude is approximated as a rate of 9.8 m/s2. For projectile motion problems, the projectile is assumed to travel a curved path to the ground and ignore air resistance, wind speed, and other such complications.

Projectile motion has two components: horizontal and vertical. Without air resistance, there is no horizontal acceleration, so the horizontal velocity won't change. However, the vertical velocity will change because of gravity's acceleration on the projectile. A sample parabolic curve of projectile motion is shown below.

Projectile Path for a Bullet Fired Horizontally from a Hill (Ignoring Air Resistance)

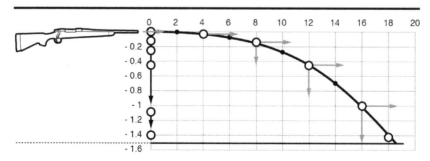

Horizontal distance (d_x) is defined as the relationship between velocity (v_x) and time (t), where x is the movement along the horizontal plane (x-axis).

$$d_x = v_x t$$

Because of the force of gravity, the vertical velocity and position is continuously changing and thus more complicated to calculate.

The following equations are different expressions of vertical motion:

$$v_f{}^2 = v_i{}^2 + 2ad$$

$$d = \frac{1}{2}at^2 + v_i t$$

$$v_f = v_i + at$$

These equations use v_f as the final velocity, v_i as the initial velocity, a as the acceleration, d as the horizontal distance traveled, and t as the time to describe functions of motion.

Newton's Laws of Motion

Sir Isaac Newton spent a great deal of time studying objects, forces, and how an object's motion responds to forces. Newton made great advancements by using mathematics to describe the motion of objects and to predict future motions of objects by applying his mathematical models to situations. Through his extensive research, Newton is credited for summarizing the basic laws of motion for objects here on Earth. These laws are as follows:

1. The law of inertia: An object in motion will remain in motion, unless acted upon by an outside force. An object at rest remains at rest, unless acted upon by an outside force. Simply put, **inertia** is the natural tendency of an object to continue along with what it is already doing; an outside force would have to act upon the object to make it change its course. This includes an object that is sitting still.

2. F = ma: The **force (F)** on an object is equal to the mass (m) multiplied by the acceleration (a) on that object. **Mass (m)** refers to the amount of a substance while acceleration (a) refers to a change in velocity over time.

- In the case of a projectile falling to Earth's surface, the acceleration is due to gravity.

- Multiplying an object's mass by its gravitational acceleration gives the special force that is called the object's **weight (W).** Note that weight is a force and is a vector quantity while mass is in kilograms and is a scalar quantity, as it has no acceleration.

- Forces are typically measured in Newtons (N), which are a derived SI unit equal to $1\frac{kg \cdot m}{s^2}$.

3. For every action, there is an equal and opposite reaction. This means that, if a book drops onto a desk, the book will exert a force on the desk due to hitting it, but the desk will also exert an equal force on the book in the opposite direction. This is what sometimes causes fallen objects to bounce once or twice after hitting the ground.

A clear understanding of force is crucial to using Newton's laws of motion. Forces are anything acting upon an object either in motion or at rest; this includes friction and gravity. These forces can push or pull on a mass, and they have a magnitude and a direction. Forces are represented by a **vector,** which is the arrow lined up along the direction of the force with its tip at the point of application. The magnitude of the force is represented by the length of the vector: Large forces have long vector lengths.

Friction

Friction is a resistance to movement that always imparts a negative acceleration to an object. Because it accelerates an object in the opposite direction than it wants to go, friction will cause moving objects to slow down and eventually stop. Frictional force depends on several factors including the texture of the two surfaces and the amount of contact force pushing the surfaces together. There are four types of friction: static, sliding, rolling, and fluid friction. **Static friction** occurs between stationary objects, while **sliding friction** occurs when solid objects slide over each other. **Rolling friction** happens when a solid object rolls over another solid object, and **fluid friction** is a friction caused by an object moving through a fluid or through fluid layers. These 'fluids' can be either a gas or a liquid, so this also includes air resistance.

Rotation

Rotating and spinning objects have a special type of movement. A spinning top can move across a table, demonstrating linear motion, but it can also spin in place, demonstrating angular motion. Just as a car moves from place to place by changing its location, its velocity, and its acceleration, so too can a rotating object change its orientation, its angular velocity, and its angular acceleration.

For linear movement, the first thing that is described is the object's displacement. The **displacement** of the object is how far it moves from its starting location; this linear change in location is usually represented by the symbol Δx. However, for the angular movement of a simple solid like a sphere, the distance that its surface travels isn't a good measure of its angular movement, since a large sphere would have to rotate a much smaller degree to move the same distance as a small sphere would. This angular distance is referred to as S, or the arc length.

A better measure of angular movement is the **angular displacement θ,** which is defined as the angle through which the object will rotate. Because there are a standard 360° in all circles, angular displacement can be used to compare angular movement between objects of different sizes, making it a much more versatile tool than the arc length. However, although a circle can be split up into 360 degrees, it can also be visualized as being split up into 2π **radians,** where radians is a unit similar to degrees that describes angles. The 2π is usually used in physics because a circle's circumference has a value of 2π times its radius, and radians is an easier unit to use than is degrees.

The angular displacement can be found by dividing the arc length that an object rotates through by the radius of the object's rotation. For example, if an object completes 1 full rotation, it has rotated through 360°. It has also traveled an arc length equal to its circumference, or $2\pi r$. Plugging this arc length S into the equation below, it can be seen that the angular displacement is 2π, which is correct since it is equal to the 360° as discussed previously.

$$angular\ displacement\ (\theta) = \frac{S}{r}$$

The angular speed or **angular velocity, w,** is the measure of how quickly the object is rotating, and w is defined as the angular displacement that is accomplished in a certain amount of time, as shown below.

$$angular\ speed\ (\omega) = \frac{\Delta\theta}{\Delta t}$$

Similar to linear velocity, angular velocity may accelerate due to external forces, and this angular acceleration is given by the variable α. Its equation, the change in angular velocity over a change in time, is given below.

$$angular\ acceleration\ (\alpha) = \frac{\Delta\omega}{\Delta t}$$

When objects are exhibiting circular motion, they also demonstrate the **conservation of angular momentum,** meaning that the angular momentum of a system is always constant, regardless of the placement of the mass. **Rotational inertia** can be affected by how far the mass of the object is placed with respect to the center of rotation (**axis of rotation**). The larger the distance between the mass and the center of rotation, the slower the rotational velocity. Conversely, if the mass is closer to the center of rotation, the rotational velocity increases. A change in one affects the other, thus conserving the angular momentum. This holds true if no external forces act upon the system.

Circular Motion

Circular motion is similar in many ways to linear (straight line) motion; however, there are a few additional points to note. In uniform circular motion, a spinning object is always linearly accelerating because it is always changing direction. The force causing this constant acceleration on or around an axis is called the **centripetal force,** and it is often associated with centripetal acceleration. Centripetal force always pulls toward the axis of rotation; this means that the force will always pull towards the center of the rotation circle. The relationship between the velocity (v) of an object and the radius (r) of the circle is centripetal acceleration, and the equation is as follows:

$$centripetal\ acceleration\ (a_c) = \frac{v^2}{r}$$

According to Newton's law, force is the combination of two factors, mass and acceleration. This is demonstrated by centripetal force. Centripetal force is shown mathematically by using the mass of an object (m), the velocity (v), and the radius (r).

$$centripetal\ force\ (F_c) = \frac{mv^2}{r}$$

Kinetic and Potential Energy

The two primary forms of energy are kinetic energy and potential energy. **Kinetic energy**, or KE, involves the energy of motion, and is easily found for Newtonian physics by an object's mass in kilograms and velocity in meters per second. Kinetic energy can be calculated using the following equation:

$$KE = \frac{1}{2}mv^2$$

Potential energy represents the energy possessed by an object by virtue of its position. In the classical example, an object's gravitational potential energy can be found as a simple function of its height or by what distance it drops. Potential energy, or PE, may be calculated using the following equation:

$$PE = mgh$$

Both kinetic energy and potential energy are scalar quantities measured in **Joules**. One Joule is the amount of energy that can push an object with 1 Newton of force for 1 meter, so it is also referred to as a Newton-meter. As mentioned previously, the **Law of Conservation of Energy** states that energy can neither be created nor destroyed. Therefore, potential and kinetic energy can be transformed into one another, depending on an object's speed and position.

Linear Momentum and Impulse

Motion creates something called **momentum.** This is a calculation of an object's mass multiplied by its velocity. Momentum can be described as the amount an object wants to continue moving along its current course. Momentum in a straight line is called linear momentum. Just as energy can be transferred and conserved, so too can momentum.

Changing the expression of Newton's second law of motion yields a new expression.

$$Force(F) = ma = m \times \frac{\Delta v}{\Delta t}$$

If both sides of the expression are multiplied by the change in time, the law produces the impulse equation.

$$F\Delta t = m\Delta v$$

This equation shows that the amount of force during a length of time creates an **impulse.** This means that if a force acts on an object during a given amount of time, it will have a determined impulse. However, if the same change in velocity happens over a longer amount of time, the required force is much smaller, due to the conservation of momentum.

$$p = mv$$

Linear momentum, p, is found by multiplying the mass of an object by its velocity. Since momentum, like mass and energy, is conserved, Newton's 2nd law can be restated for multiple objects. In this form, it can be used to understand the energy of objects that have interacted, since the conservation of momentum implies that the momentum before and after an interaction must be the same. This is best demonstrated in the case of elastic collision, where an object of mass m_1 with velocity v_1 collides with an object of mass m_2 with velocity v_2 and both object end with velocities v_1' and v_2', respectively.

$$m_1 v_1' + m_2 v_2' = m_1 v_1 + m_2 v_2$$

Universal Gravitation

Newton's **law of universal gravitation** addresses the universality of gravity. Gravity acts as a force at a distance and causes all bodies in the universe to attract each other.

The **force of gravity (F_g)** is proportional to the masses of two objects (m_1 and m_2) and inversely proportional to the square of the distance (r^2) between them. (G is the proportionality constant). This is shown in the following equation:

$$F_g = G\frac{m_1 m_2}{r^2}$$

All objects falling within the Earth's atmosphere are all affected by the force of gravity, so their rates of acceleration will be equal to 9.8 m/s^2, or gravity. Therefore, if two objects are dropped from the same height at the same time, they should hit the ground at the same time. This is irrespective of mass, since the previous kinetics equations don't include mass, so a bowling ball and a feather would theoretically fall at identical rates. Unfortunately, in the Earth's atmosphere, air resistance would slow the feather much more than the bowling ball, so the bowling ball would fall faster, but this effect can be minimized in a vacuum. In other words, without air resistance or other external forces acting on the objects, gravity will affect every object on the Earth with the same rate of acceleration.

Waves and Sound

Waves are periodic disturbances in a gas, liquid, or solid that are created as energy is transmitted. Each part of a wave has a different name and is used in different calculations. The four parts of a wave are the crest, the trough, the amplitude, and the wavelength. The **crest** is the highest point, while the **trough** is the lowest. The **amplitude** is the distance between a peak and the average of the wave; it is also the distance between a trough and the average of the wave, but an amplitude is always positive, since it is an absolute value. Finally, the distance between one wave and the exact same place on the next wave is the **wavelength.**

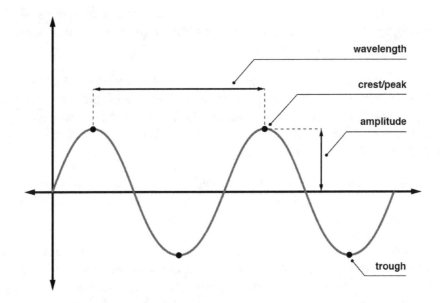

With amplitude and wavelength, it is possible to describe any wave, but an important question still remains unanswered: How fast is the wave traveling? A wave's speed can be shown as either its period or its frequency. A wave's period, T, is how long it takes for the wave to travel one wavelength, while a wave's frequency, f, is how many wavelengths are traveled in one second.

These are inversely related, so they are reciprocals of each other, as shown below.

$$f = \frac{1}{T} \text{ and } T = \frac{1}{f}$$

The largest categories of waves are electromagnetic waves and mechanical waves. **Electromagnetic waves can transmit energy through a vacuum and do not need a medium to travel through, examples of which are light, radio, microwaves, gamma rays, and other forms of electromagnetism. Mechanical waves** can only transmit energy through another form of matter called a medium. The particles of the medium are shifted as the wave moves through the medium and can be anything from solids to liquids to gasses. Examples of mechanical waves include auditory sounds heard by human ears in the air as well as percussive shocks like earthquakes.

There are two different forms of waves: transverse and longitudinal waves. **Transverse** waves are waves in which particles of the medium move in a direction perpendicular to the direction waves move, as in most electromagnetic waves. **Compression, or longitudinal, waves are waves in which the particles of the medium move in a direction parallel to the direction the waves move, as in most mechanical waves. A good example of a longitudinal wave is sound.** Waves travel within a medium at a speed that is determined by the wavelength (λ) and frequency (f) of the wave.

$$v = f\lambda$$

There is a proportional relationship between the amplitude of a wave and the potential energy in the wave. This means the taller the wave, the more stored energy it is transmitting.

Light

Light is an electromagnetic wave that is created by electric and magnetic interactions. Like other electromagnetic waves, light does not need a medium to travel. Light energy can be absorbed and changed into heat, reflected, or even transmitted.

A wave is reflected when it collides with a surface and bounces off, unharmed. The **law of reflection** shows that an **incident ray** (the wave that hits the surface) will bounce off the surface and become a reflected ray (the wave that leaves the surface). Because the wave doesn't lose any energy, the angle at which it hits the surface will be identical to the angle at which it leaves the surface, so the interaction produces identical waves. This is the definition of **reflection**.

On the other hand, a wave is refracted when a wave collides with a surface and bends, such as when the medium it is traveling through changes. Examples of **refraction** include the bending of light as it passes through a prism and sunlight passing through raindrops to create a rainbow.

To understand refraction, a 'normal' line is drawn perpendicular to the surface that the wave will hit. The angle created between the normal line and the incident ray is the angle of incidence, while the angle of reflection is the opposite and equal angle formed between the normal line and the reflected ray. The refraction of light depends on the varying speeds and densities of different media. As light passes through different media, the wave will bend toward or away from the normal line, depending on the material it is transitioning to.

Snell's law describes this behavior mathematically in the equation that follows:

$$n_1 \sin \theta_1 = n_2 \sin \theta_2$$

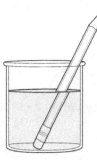

In this equation, n is the index of refraction and θ is the angle of refraction. The **index of refraction** determines the amount of light that bends or refracts when it encounters a medium. Materials that interact with and change the wave more will have higher indices of refraction, and any material's index of refraction can be found by the following equation.

$$n = \frac{c}{v_s}$$

Because the speed of light in a vacuum, c, is constant, it can be used to show how much a material will interact with a wave. The **refractive index, n,** shows how much the speed of light is changed when it travels through the material at a new velocity of v_s.

Optics

Spherical mirrors change the way light reflects. Lenses and curved mirrors are made to focus light in certain ways. There are several terms used to describe and define mirrors and lenses. The **principal axis** is a reference line that usually passes through the center of the curve of the mirror or lens. The **vertex, V,** is the point where the mirror is crossed by the principal axis. The sphere which contains the curve of the mirror has a center called the **center of curvature (C)**. The **focal point (F)** is halfway between the center of curvature and the vertex. The **focal length (f)** is measured by how far the focal point is from the mirror. The following graphic shows a visual representation of these terms in a concave mirror.

Consider this image:

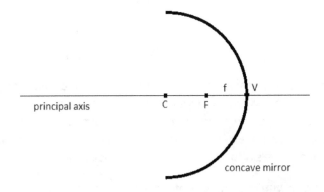

concave mirror

The focal lengths of concave mirrors are positive. Concave mirrors can produce images of various shapes and sizes as well as of different orientations based on the focal length of the mirror and the placement of the object. Convex mirrors differ from concave mirrors in that they have negative focal lengths. The other main difference is that convex mirrors always form images that are reduced in size and upright.

Lenses are pieces of transparent material molded to refract light rays to create an image. There are two types of lenses. Convex lenses, also called **converging lenses**, have positive focal lengths. Concave lenses, or **diverging lenses**, conversely have negative focal lengths. Images in convex lenses can look different depending on the focal length of the lens and where the object is located. Convex lenses only create images that are upright and smaller in size than the object.

Take a look at this image:

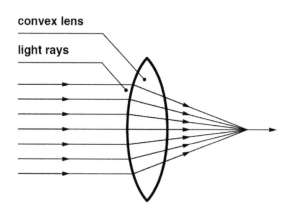

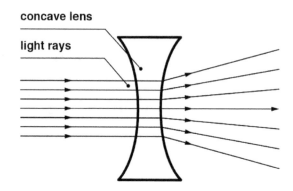

Atomic Structure

All known matter is made of atoms. Atoms have a nucleus composed of **protons** (with a positive charge) and **neutrons** (with no net charge), which is surrounded by a cloud of **electrons** (with negative charges). Since protons have a positive charge and neutrons have a neutral charge, an atom's nucleus typically has an overall positive electrical charge, but because electrons orbiting the nucleus have an overall negative charge, an atom with equal numbers of protons and electrons is considered stable.

The properties of an atom vary with the number of electrons and their arrangement in shells around the nucleus. Electrons are organized into distributions of subshells called **electron configurations**. Subshells fill from the inside (closest to the nucleus) to the outside and are lettered starting with "k." The strength of the bond between the nucleus and the electron is called the **binding energy**. The binding energy is stronger for those shells located closer to the nucleus.

The number of electrons in each shell can be determined using the following equation using n for the shell number:

$$2n^2$$

Nature of Electricity

The nature of electricity is based on the atoms of a given material, as objects develop electric charges when their atoms gain or lose electrons. The electrons that are in the furthest shell from an atom's nucleus are the most likely to interact, so they are specially termed valence electrons. If the electrons are tightly bound to their atoms, the material is an **insulator** because, like rubber, wood, and glass, the material prevents electrons from flowing freely. However, if the electrons are loosely bound to the atoms, the material is a **conductor** because, like iron and other metals, the electrons can flow freely throughout the material.

An atom can gain a charge by having greater or fewer electrons than protons, and any atom with a charge is referred to as an **ion**. If an ion has more electrons than protons, it has a negative charge and is an **anion**. If an atom has fewer electrons than protons, it has a positive charge and is a **cation**. It is important to note that opposite charges attract each other, while like charges repel each other. Interestingly, the repulsive force between two electrons is equivalent to the attractive force between an electron and a proton (only in different directions). Coulomb described these repellant and attractive forces between two objects in his namesake law. This electrical **Coulomb force, F,** is determined by multiplying the charges of the two objects, q_1 and q_2, by a constant, k, and dividing by the distance they are from one another squared, r^2.

$$F = \frac{kq_1q_2}{r^2}$$

If the force is negative, then the objects attract each other because q_1 and q_2 are of opposite charges. If the force is positive, then the objects repel each other because q_1 and q_2 are of the same charge.

An electric charge naturally produces an electric field around itself. Electric fields can vary in strength and magnitude depending on the type of charge (positive or negative) that generates the field. The nature of electric fields can be tested using a test charge. Mathematically, the magnitude of an electric field (E) can be found using the following equation:

$$E = \frac{F}{q_o}$$

Where F is the force a test charge would undergo, and q_o is the magnitude of the test charge. Electric fields are vector quantities; this means they have both a magnitude and a direction. In the case of electric fields, it is the convention to define the direction of the field vector as the way a positive test charge would move when positioned in the electric field, towards a negative charge and away from other positive charges.

An **electric circuit** is usually comprised of circuit elements joined by a wire or other object that allows an electric charge to move along the path without interruption—this moving electric charge is called an electric **current.** However, constant electric currents may only exist in a complete circuit if there is a voltage difference in the circuit. **Voltage** is literally the distance that a circuit's electrical force could move one electron, but voltage can be visualized as how much energy a certain part of the circuit has available to push around electrons. Electrons will flow from regions of higher voltage to regions of lower voltage, so it is the difference in voltages between two parts of a circuit that makes a current actually flow.

In other words, voltage difference is the difference in potential energy between two places measured in **volts (V),** while a circuit is a closed path through which electrons can flow. Because every atom has positive charges that pull on electrons and resist their flow, most real circuits have a **resistance** level, measured in **ohms**, which is described as the opposition to the flow of electric charge. The amount of current that can flow through a circuit depends on the voltage difference and how well the wire resists the flow of electricity. **Ohm's law** gives us the relationship between voltage (V), current in amperes (I), and resistance in ohms (R).

$$V = I \times R$$

Series Circuits (A) and Parallel Circuits (B)
Practical circuits have numerous loads which can be hooked up "in series" (A) or "in parallel" (B), as shown below.

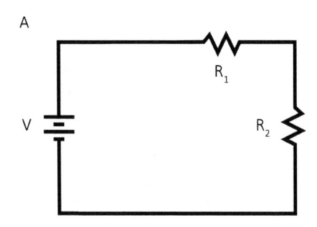

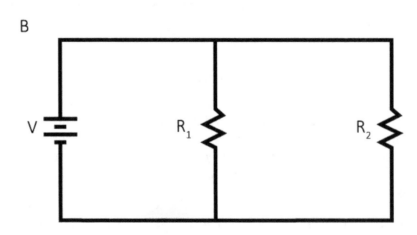

To determine the total voltage requirement for circuits with multiple component loads (in series or in parallel), it is necessary to find the equivalent resistance of the circuits.

Series circuits put resistors in a row or series so that current must flow from one to the other, while **parallel circuits** run resistors in parallel sections so that current can flow through one or the other. In a series circuit like the one in *A*, the voltage drops across each resistor, but the current is the same in all of them. The current must be the same across each resistor, as according to Ampere's law, the electrons in the current must continue flowing throughout the wire and not build up or disappear. In other words, the electrons going into the resistor must all go out so that the "flow in equals flow out."

The current through each resistor is the same, and the total voltage (*V*) equals the drop across R_1 plus the drop across R_2. The equivalent resistance is determined by solving Ohm's law for voltage:

$$V = V_1 + V_2 = IR_1 + IR_2 = I(R_1 + R_2) = IR_{eq}$$

Thus, in a series circuit, the equivalent resistance is equal to the sum of the component resistances, and this relation holds for any number of resistors in a series.

In a parallel circuit like the one in *(B)*, the voltage is the same across each resistor because each is attached directly to the power source and the ground. The electric current is divided between the loads depending on their resistances, since it can flow through either of them, but not both. If the resistance is the same in both loads, then the same amount of current passes through each one. If the resistance is different in each load, then more current passes through the load with the lower resistance, since energy takes the path of least resistance.

The **equivalent resistance (R_{eq})** of the parallel circuit is determined by solving Ohm's law for the current through each resistor, setting it equal to the total current (R_t), and remembering that the voltages are all the same:

$$I_t = \frac{V}{R_{eq}} = \frac{V}{R_1} + \frac{V}{R_2} \quad \textbf{or} \quad \frac{1}{R_{eq}} = \frac{1}{R_1} + \frac{1}{R_2} \quad \textbf{so} \quad R_{eq} = \frac{1}{\frac{1}{R_1} + \frac{1}{R_2}}$$

In a parallel circuit, the equivalent resistance is equal to one over the sum of the reciprocals of the component resistances.

Magnetism and Electricity

Magnetism can occur naturally in certain types of materials like iron, nickel, and cobalt. If two straight rods are made from iron, they will usually have a naturally negative end (pole) and a positive end (pole). These charged poles react just like any charged item: opposite charges attract and like charges repel. They will attract each other when set up positive to negative, but if one rod is turned around, the two rods will repel each other due to the alignment of negative to negative and positive to positive.

Magnetic fields can also be created and amplified by using an electric current. The force of attraction between two magnetic fields is measured in **Teslas**. The relationship between magnetic forces and electrical forces can be explored by sending an electric current through a stretch of wire, which creates an electromagnetic force around the wire from the charge of the current, as long as the flow of electricity is sustained. This magnetic force can also attract and repel other items with magnetic properties. Depending upon the strength of the current in the wire, a smaller or larger magnetic force can be generated around this wire. As soon as the current is cut off, the magnetic force also stops. When a magnetic field produces an electric current, this is called an **electromagnetic induction**.

Science Questions

1. Which statement about white blood cells is true?
   a. B cells are responsible for antibody production.
   b. White blood cells are made in the white/yellow cartilage before they enter the bloodstream.
   c. Platelets, a special class of white blood cell, function to clot blood and stop bleeding.
   d. The majority of white blood cells only activate during the age of puberty, which explains why children and the elderly are particularly susceptible to disease.

2. Which locations in the digestive system are sites of chemical digestion?
   I. Mouth
   II. Stomach
   III. Small Intestine

   a. II only
   b. III only
   c. II and III only
   d. I, II, and III

3. Which of the following are functions of the urinary system?
   I. Synthesizing calcitriol and secreting erythropoietin
   II. Regulating the concentrations of sodium, potassium, chloride, calcium, and other ions
   III. Reabsorbing or secreting hydrogen ions and bicarbonate
   IV. Detecting reductions in blood volume and pressure

   a. I, II, and III
   b. II and III
   c. II, III, and IV
   d. All of the above

4. Which of the following structures is unique to eukaryotic cells?
   a. Cell walls
   b. Nucleuses
   c. Cell membranes
   d. Vacuoles

5. Which is the cellular organelle used for digestion to recycle materials?
   a. The Golgi apparatus
   b. The lysosome
   c. The centrioles
   d. The mitochondria

6. A rock has a mass of 14.3 grams (g) and a volume of 5.4 cm^3, what is its density?
   a. 8.90 g/cm^3
   b. 0.38 g/cm^3
   c. 77.22 g/cm^3
   d. 2.65 g/cm^3

7. Why do arteries have valves?
   a. They have valves to maintain high blood pressure so that capillaries diffuse nutrients properly.
   b. Their valves are designed to prevent backflow due to their low blood pressure.
   c. They have valves due to a leftover trait from evolution that, like the appendix, are useless.
   d. They do not have valves, but veins do.

8. If the pressure in the pulmonary artery is increased above normal, which chamber of the heart will be affected first?
   a. The right atrium
   b. The left atrium
   c. The right ventricle
   d. The left ventricle

9. What is the purpose of sodium bicarbonate when released into the lumen of the small intestine?
   a. It works to chemically digest fats in the chyme.
   b. It decreases the pH of the chyme so as to prevent harm to the intestine.
   c. It works to chemically digest proteins in the chyme.
   d. It increases the pH of the chyme so as to prevent harm to the intestine.

10. Which of the following describes a reflex arc?
   a. The storage and recall of memory
   b. The maintenance of visual and auditory acuity
   c. The autoregulation of heart rate and blood pressure
   d. A stimulus and response controlled by the spinal cord

11. Describe the synthesis of the lagging strand of DNA.
   a. DNA polymerases synthesize DNA continuously after initially attaching to a primase.
   b. DNA polymerases synthesize DNA discontinuously in pieces called Okazaki fragments after initially attaching to primases.
   c. DNA polymerases synthesize DNA discontinuously in pieces called Okazaki fragments after initially attaching to RNA primers.
   d. DNA polymerases synthesize DNA discontinuously in pieces called Okazaki fragments which are joined together in the end by a DNA helicase.

12. Using anatomical terms, what is the relationship of the sternum relative to the deltoid?
   a. Medial
   b. Lateral
   c. Superficial
   d. Posterior

13. Ligaments connect what?
   a. Muscle to muscle
   b. Bone to bone
   c. Bone to muscle
   d. Muscle to tendon

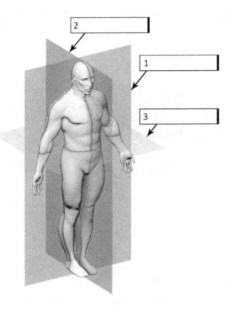

14. Identify the correct sequence of the 3 primary body planes as numbered 1, 2, and 3 in the above image.
    a. Plane 1 is coronal, plane 2 is sagittal, and plane 3 is transverse.
    b. Plane 1 is sagittal, plane 2 is coronal, and plane 3 is medial.
    c. Plane 1 is coronal, plane 2 is sagittal, and plane 3 is medial.
    d. Plane 1 is sagittal, plane 2 is coronal, and plane 3 is transverse.

15. Which of the following is NOT a major function of the respiratory system in humans?
    a. It provides a large surface area for gas exchange of oxygen and carbon dioxide.
    b. It helps regulate the blood's pH.
    c. It helps cushion the heart against jarring motions.
    d. It is responsible for vocalization.

16. Which of the following is NOT a function of the forebrain?
    a. To regulate blood pressure and heart rate
    b. To perceive and interpret emotional responses like fear and anger
    c. To perceive and interpret visual input from the eyes
    d. To integrate voluntary movement

17. What is the major difference between somatic and germline mutations?
    a. Somatic mutations usually benefit the individual while germline mutations usually harm them.
    b. Since germline mutations only affect one cell, they are less noticeable than the rapidly dividing somatic cells.
    c. Somatic mutations are not expressed for several generations, but germline mutations are expressed immediately.
    d. Germline mutations are usually inherited while somatic mutations will affect only the individual.

18. A child complains of heavy breathing even when relaxing. They are an otherwise healthy child with no history of respiratory problems. What might be the issue?

    a. Asthma

    b. Blood clot

    c. Hyperventilation

    d. Exercising too hard

19. Find the lowest coefficients that will balance the following combustion equation.

$$\_\_C_2H_{10} + \_\_O_2 \rightarrow \_\_H_2O + \_\_CO_2$$

    a. 1:5:5:2

    b. 4:10:20:8

    c. 2:9:10:4

    d. 2:5:10:4

20. What is the purpose of a catalyst?

    a. To increase a reaction's rate by increasing the activation energy

    b. To increase a reaction's rate by increasing the temperature

    c. To increase a reaction's rate by decreasing the activation energy

    d. To increase a reaction's rate by decreasing the temperature

21. Most catalysts found in biological systems are which of the following?

    a. Special lipids called cofactors.

    b. Special proteins called enzymes.

    c. Special lipids called enzymes.

    d. Special proteins called cofactors.

22. Which statement is true about the pH of a solution?

    a. A solution cannot have a pH less than 1.

    b. The more hydroxide ions in the solution, the higher the pH.

    c. If an acid has a pH of greater than 2, it is considered a weak base.

    d. A solution with a pH of 2 has ten times the amount of hydrogen ions than a solution with a power of 1.

23. Salts like sodium iodide (NaI) and potassium chloride (KCl) use what type of bond?

    a. Ionic bonds

    b. Disulfide bridges

    c. Covalent bonds

    d. London dispersion forces

24. Which of the following is unique to covalent bonds?

    a. Most covalent bonds are formed between the elements H, F, N, and O.

    b. Covalent bonds are dependent on forming dipoles.

    c. Bonding electrons are shared between two or more atoms.

    d. Molecules with covalent bonds tend to have a crystalline solid structure.

25. Which of the following describes a typical gas?
    a. Indefinite shape and indefinite volume
    b. Indefinite shape and definite volume
    c. Definite shape and definite volume
    d. Definite shape and indefinite volume

26. Which of the following areas of the body has the most sweat glands?
    a. Upper back
    b. Arms
    c. Feet
    d. Palms

27. A patient's body is not properly filtering blood. Which of the following body parts is most likely malfunctioning?
    a. Medulla
    B. Heart
    C. Nephrons
    D. Renal cortex

28. A pediatrician notes that an infant's cartilage is disappearing and being replaced by bone. What process has the doctor observed?
    a. Mineralization
    b. Ossification
    c. Osteoporosis
    d. Calcification

29. The epidermis is composed of what type of cells?
    a. Osteoclasts
    b. Connective
    c. Dendritic
    d. Epithelial

30. Which of the following is directly transcribed from DNA and represents the first step in protein building?
    a. siRNA
    b. rRNA
    c. mRNA
    d. tRNA

31. What information does a genotype give that a phenotype does not?
    a. The genotype necessarily includes the proteins coded for by its alleles.
    b. The genotype will always show an organism's recessive alleles.
    c. The genotype must include the organism's physical characteristics.
    d. The genotype shows what an organism's parents looked like.

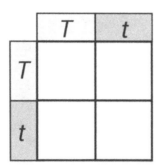

32. Which statement is supported by the Punnett square above, if "T" = Tall and "t" = short?
    a. Both parents are homozygous tall.
    b. 100% of the offspring will be tall because both parents are tall.
    c. There is a 25% chance that an offspring will be short.
    d. The short allele will soon die out.

33. Which of the following is a chief difference between evaporation and boiling?
    a. Liquids boil only at the surface while they evaporate equally throughout the liquid.
    b. Evaporating substances change from gas to liquid while boiling substances change from liquid to gas.
    c. Evaporation happens in nature while boiling is a manmade phenomenon.
    d. Evaporation can happen below a liquid's boiling point.

34. Which of the following CANNOT be found in a human cell's genes?
    a. Sequences of amino acids to be transcribed into mRNA
    b. Lethal recessive traits like sickle cell anemia
    c. Mutated DNA
    d. DNA that codes for proteins the cell doesn't use

35. Which of the following is a special property of water?
    a. Water easily flows through phospholipid bilayers.
    b. A water molecule's oxygen atom allows fish to breathe.
    c. Water is highly cohesive which explains its high melting point.
    d. Water can self-hydrolyze and decompose into hydrogen and oxygen.

36. What is an isotope? For any given element, it is an atom with which of the following?
    a. a different atomic number.
    b. a different number of protons.
    c. a different number of electrons.
    d. a different mass number.

37. What is the electrical charge of the nucleus?

a. A nucleus always has a positive charge.

b. A stable nucleus has a positive charge, but a radioactive nucleus may have no charge and instead be neutral.

c. A nucleus always has no charge and is instead neutral.

d. A stable nucleus has no charge and is instead neutral, but a radioactive nucleus may have a charge.

38. A student believes that there is an inverse relationship between sugar consumption and test scores. To test this hypothesis, he recruits several people to eat sugar, wait one hour, and take a short aptitude test afterwards. The student will compile the participants' sugar intake levels and test scores. How should the student conduct the experiment?

a. One round of testing, where each participant consumes a different level of sugar.

b. Two rounds of testing: The first, where each participant consumes a different level of sugar, and the second, where each participant consumes the same level as they did in Round 1.

c. Two rounds of testing: The first, where each participant consumes the same level of sugar as each other, and the second, where each participant consumes the same level of sugar as each other but at higher levels than in Round 1.

d. One round of testing, where each participant consumes the same level of sugar.

39. Which of the following creates sperm?

a. Prostate gland

b. Seminal vesicles

c. Scrotum

d. Seminiferous tubules

40. A researcher is exploring factors that contribute to the GPA of college students. While the sample is small, the researcher is trying to determine what the data shows. What can be reasoned from the table below?

Student	Maintains a Calendar?	Takes Notes?	GPA
A	sometimes	often	3.1
B	never	always	3.9
C	never	never	2.0
D	sometimes	often	2.7

a. No college students consistently maintain a calendar of events.

b. There is an inverse correlation between maintaining a calendar and GPA, and there is a positive correlation between taking notes and GPA.

c. There is a positive correlation between maintaining a calendar and GPA, and there is no correlation between taking notes and GPA.

d. There is no correlation between maintaining a calendar and GPA, and there is a positive correlation between taking notes and GPA.

41. A scientist is trying to determine how much poison will kill a rat the fastest. Which of the following statements is an example of an appropriate hypothesis?
    a. Rats that are given lots of poison seem to die quickly.
    b. Does the amount of poison affect how quickly the rat dies?
    c. The more poison a rat is given, the quicker it will die.
    d. Poison is fatal to rats.

42. In testing how quickly a rat dies by the amount of poison it eats, which of the following is the independent variable and which is the dependent variable?
    a. How quickly the rat dies is the independent variable; the amount of poison is the dependent variable.
    b. The amount of poison is the independent variable; how quickly the rat dies is the dependent variable.
    c. Whether the rat eats the poison is the independent variable; how quickly the rat dies is the dependent variable.
    d. The cage the rat is kept in is the independent variable; the amount of poison is the dependent variable.

43. Which of the following is a representation of a natural pattern or occurrence that's difficult or impossible to experience directly?
    a. A theory
    b. A model
    c. A law
    d. An observation

44. Which of the following is a standard or series of standards to which the results from an experiment are compared?
    a. A control
    b. A variable
    c. A constant
    d. Collected data

45. "This flower is dead; someone must have forgotten to water it." This statement is an example of which of the following?
    a. A classification
    b. An observation
    c. An inference
    d. A collection

46. Which of the following correctly displays 8,600,000,000,000 in scientific notation (to two significant figures)?
    a. 8.6×10^{12}
    b. 8.6×10^{-12}
    c. 8.6×10^{11}
    d. 8.60×10^{12}

47. The acceleration of a falling object due to gravity has been proven to be 9.8 m/s². A scientist drops a cactus four times and measures the acceleration with an accelerometer and gets the following results: 9.79 m/s², 9.81 m/s², 9.80 m/s², and 9.78 m/s². Which of the following accurately describes the measurements?

    a. They're both accurate and precise.

    b. They're accurate but not precise.

    c. They're precise but not accurate.

    d. They're neither accurate nor precise.

48. What is the molarity of a solution made by dissolving 4.0 grams of NaCl into enough water to make 120 mL of solution? The atomic mass of Na is 23.0 g/mol and Cl is 35.5 g/mol.

    a. 0.34 M

    b. 0.57 M

    c. 0.034 M

    d. 0.057 M

49. Considering a gas in a closed system, at a constant volume, what will happen to the temperature if the pressure is increased?

    a. The temperature will stay the same

    b. The temperature will decrease

    c. The temperature will increase

    d. It cannot be determined with the information given

50. What type of chemical reaction produces a salt?

    a. An oxidation reaction

    b. A neutralization reaction

    c. A synthesis reaction

    d. A decomposition reaction

51. What types of molecules can move through a cell membrane by passive transport?

    a. Complex sugars

    b. Non-lipid soluble molecules

    c. Oxygen

    d. Molecules moving from areas of low concentration to areas of high concentration

52. What is ONE feature that both prokaryotes and eukaryotes have in common?

    a. A plasma membrane

    b. A nucleus enclosed by a membrane

    c. Organelles

    d. A nucleoid

53. What is the LAST phase of mitosis?

    a. Prophase

    b. Telophase

    c. Anaphase

    d. Metaphase

54. How many daughter cells are formed from one parent cell during meiosis?
   a. One
   b. Two
   c. Three
   d. Four

55. Which level of protein structure is defined by the folds and coils of the protein's polypeptide backbone?
   a. Primary
   b. Secondary
   c. Tertiary
   d. Quaternary

56. What is the sensory threshold?
   a. The smallest amount of stimulus required for an individual to feel a sensation
   b. The amount of stimulus required for an individual to feel pain
   c. The amount of stimulus required to cause an individual to move away from the stimulus
   d. The place where the stimulus is coming from

57. How many neurons generally make up a sensory pathway?
   a. 1
   b. 2
   c. 3
   d. 4

58. In which part of the eye does visual processing begin?
   a. Cornea
   b. Optic nerve
   c. Retina
   d. Eyelid

59. What type of vessel carries oxygen-rich blood from the heart to other tissues of the body?
   a. Veins
   b. Intestines
   c. Bronchioles
   d. Arteries

60. The somatic nervous system is responsible for which of the following?
   a. Breathing
   b. Thought
   c. Movement
   d. Fear

61. The process of breaking large molecules into smaller molecules to provide energy is known as which of the following?
   a. Metabolism
   b. Bioenergetics
   c. Anabolism
   d. Catabolism

62. Which blood component is chiefly responsible for clotting?
    a. Platelets
    b. Red blood cells
    c. Antigens
    d. Plasma cells

63. Which is the first event to happen in a primary immune response?
    a. Macrophages phagocytose pathogens and present their antigens.
    b. Neutrophils aggregate and act as cytotoxic, nonspecific killers of pathogens.
    c. B lymphocytes make pathogen-specific antibodies.
    d. Helper T cells secrete interleukins to activate pathogen-fighting cells.

64. Where does sperm maturation take place in the male reproductive system?
    a. Seminal vesicles
    b. Prostate gland
    c. Epididymis
    d. Vas Deferens

65. Which of the following lists of joint types is in the correct order for increasing amounts of permitted motion (least mobile to most mobile)?
    a. Hinge, condyloid, saddle
    b. Saddle, hinge, condyloid
    c. Saddle, condyloid, hinge
    d. Hinge, saddle, condyloid

66. The function of synergists can best be described as which of the following?
    I. They assist primary movers in completing the specific movement
    II. They stabilize the point of origin and provide extra pull near the insertion
    III. They help prevent unwanted movement at a joint

    a. I, II
    b. I, III
    c. II, III
    d. All of the above

67. What makes bone resistant to shattering?
    a. The calcium salts deposited in the bone
    b. The collagen fibers
    c. The bone marrow and network of blood vessels
    d. The intricate balance of minerals and collagen fibers

68. How do organisms maintain homeostasis?
    a. They increase their body temperature, blood pH, and fluid balance.
    b. They undergo biochemical processes and absorb energy to increase entropy.
    c. They undergo biochemical processes to maintain the order of their external environment.
    d. They use free energy and matter via biochemical processes to work against entropy.

69. Which of the following correctly lists the four properties that all types of muscle tissue share?
    a. Contractile, excitable, elastic, extensible
    b. Contractile, voluntary, elastic, extensible
    c. Contractile, excitable, voluntary, extensible
    d. Contractile, excitable, elastic, voluntary

70. Which of the following about the autonomic nervous system (ANS) is true?
    a. It controls the reflex arc
    b. It contains motor (efferent) neurons
    c. It contains sensory (afferent) neurons
    d. It contains both parasympathetic nerves and sympathetic nerves

71. What is the function of the sinuses?
    a. To trap the many airborne pathogens
    b. To direct air down the trachea rather than the esophagus
    c. To warm, humidify, and filter air
    d. To sweep away pathogens and direct them toward the top of the trachea

72. Which of the following structures acts like a funnel by delivering the urine from the millions of the collecting tubules to the ureters?
    a. The renal pelvis
    b. The renal cortex
    c. The renal medulla
    d. Bowman's capsule

73. Which of the following is the body cavity that contains the urinary bladder, urethra, and ureters?
    a. The thoracic cavity
    b. The pelvic cavity
    c. The abdominal cavity
    d. The spinal cavity

74. Which of the following best defines the term *amphoteric*?
    a. A substance that conducts electricity due to ionization when dissolved in a solvent
    b. A substance that can act as an acid or a base depending on the properties of the solute
    c. A substance that, according to the Brønsted-Lowry Acid-Base Theory, is a proton-donor
    d. A substance that donates its proton and forms its conjugate base in a neutralization reaction

75. Which of the following touch receptors respond to light touch and slower vibrations?
    a. Merkel's discs
    b. Pacinian corpuscles
    c. Meissner's corpuscles
    d. Ruffini endings

76. Nociceptors detect which of the following?
    a. Deep pressure
    b. Vibration
    c. Pain
    d. Temperature

77. A cluster of capillaries that functions as the main filter of the blood entering the kidney is known as which of the following?
    a. The Bowman's capsule
    b. The Loop of Henle
    c. The glomerulus
    d. The nephron

78. What is an alteration in the normal gene sequence called?
    a. DNA mutation
    b. Gene migration
    c. Polygenetic inheritance
    d. Incomplete dominance

79. Blood type is a trait determined by multiple alleles, and two of them are co-dominant: I^A codes for A blood and I^B codes for B blood. i codes for O blood and is recessive to both. If an A heterozygote individual and an O individual have a child, what is the probably that the child will have A blood?
    a. 25%
    b. 50%
    c. 75%
    d. 100%

80. Which of the choices below are the reproductive cells produced by meiosis?
    a. Genes
    b. Alleles
    c. Chromatids
    d. Gametes

Answer Explanations

1. A: When activated, B cells create antibodies against specific antigens. White blood cells are generated in yellow bone marrow, not cartilage. Platelets are not a type of white blood cell and are typically cell fragments produced by megakaryocytes. White blood cells are active throughout nearly all of one's life, and have not been shown to specially activate or deactivate because of life events like puberty or menopause.

2. D: Mechanical digestion is physical digestion of food and tearing it into smaller pieces using force. This occurs in the stomach and mouth. Chemical digestion involves chemically changing the food and breaking it down into small organic compounds that can be utilized by the cell to build molecules. The salivary glands in the mouth secrete amylase that breaks down starch, which begins chemical digestion. The stomach contains enzymes such as pepsinogen/pepsin and gastric lipase, which chemically digest protein and fats, respectively. The small intestine continues to digest protein using the enzymes trypsin and chymotrypsin. It also digests fats with the help of bile from the liver and lipase from the pancreas. These organs act as exocrine glands because they secrete substances through a duct. Carbohydrates are digested in the small intestine with the help of pancreatic amylase, gut bacterial flora and fauna, and brush border enzymes like lactose. Brush border enzymes are contained in the towel-like microvilli in the small intestine that soak up nutrients.

3. D: The urinary system has many functions, the primary of which is removing waste products and balancing water and electrolyte concentrations in the blood. It also plays a key role in regulating ion concentrations, such as sodium, potassium, chloride, and calcium, in the filtrate. The urinary system helps maintain blood pH by reabsorbing or secreting hydrogen ions and bicarbonate as necessary. Certain kidney cells can detect reductions in blood volume and pressure and then can secrete renin to activate a hormone that causes increased reabsorption of sodium ions and water. This serves to raise blood volume and pressure. Kidney cells secrete erythropoietin under hypoxic conditions to stimulate red blood cell production. They also synthesize calcitriol, a hormone derivative of vitamin D3, which aids in calcium ion absorption by the intestinal epithelium.

4. B: The structure exclusively found in eukaryotic cells is the nucleus. Animal, plant, fungi, and protist cells are all eukaryotic. DNA is contained within the nucleus of eukaryotic cells, and they also have membrane-bound organelles that perform complex intracellular metabolic activities. Prokaryotic cells (archae and bacteria) do not have a nucleus or other membrane-bound organelles and are less complex than eukaryotic cells.

5. B: The cell structure responsible for cellular storage, digestion and waste removal is the lysosome. Lysosomes are like recycle bins. They are filled with digestive enzymes that facilitate catabolic reactions to regenerate monomers. The Golgi apparatus is designed to tag, package, and ship out proteins destined for other cells or locations. The centrioles typically play a large role only in cell division when they ratchet the chromosomes from the mitotic plate to the poles of the cell. The mitochondria are involved in energy production and are the powerhouses of the cell.

6. D: Density is found by dividing mass by volume:

$$density = \frac{mass}{volume}$$

The unit for mass (in this case grams) and the units for volume (in this case cm^3) need to be combined together. They're combined as grams over volume since that's how they were set up in the equation:

$$d = \frac{14.3 \; g}{5.4 \; cm^3} = 2.65 \; g/cm^3$$

7. D: Veins have valves, but arteries do not. Valves in veins are designed to prevent backflow, since they are the furthest blood vessels from the pumping action of the heart and steadily increase in volume (which decreases the available pressure). Capillaries diffuse nutrients properly because of their thin walls and high surface area and are not particularly dependent on positive pressure.

8. C: The blood leaves the right ventricle through a semi-lunar valve and goes through the pulmonary artery to the lungs. Any increase in pressure in the artery will eventually affect the contractibility of the right ventricle. Blood enters the right atrium from the superior and inferior venae cava veins, and blood leaves the right atrium through the tricuspid valve to the right ventricle. Blood enters the left atrium from the pulmonary veins carrying oxygenated blood from the lungs. Blood flows from the left atrium to the left ventricle through the mitral valve and leaves the left ventricle through a semi-lunar valve to enter the aorta.

9. D: Sodium bicarbonate, a very effective base, has the chief function to increase the pH of the chyme. Chyme leaving the stomach has a very low pH, due to the high amounts of acid that are used to digest and break down food. If this is not neutralized, the walls of the small intestine will be damaged and may form ulcers. Sodium bicarb is produced by the pancreas and released in response to pyloric stimulation so that it can neutralize the acid. It has little to no digestive effect.

10. D: A reflex arc is a simple nerve pathway involving a stimulus, a synapse, and a response that is controlled by the spinal cord—not the brain. The knee-jerk reflex is an example of a reflex arc. The stimulus is the hammer touching the tendon, reaching the synapse in the spinal cord by an afferent pathway. The response is the resulting muscle contraction reaching the muscle by an efferent pathway. None of the remaining processes is a simple reflex. Memories are processed and stored in the hippocampus in the limbic system. The visual center is located in the occipital lobe, while auditory processing occurs in the temporal lobe. The sympathetic and parasympathetic divisions of the autonomic nervous system control heart and blood pressure.

11. C: The lagging strand of DNA falls behind the leading strand because of its discontinuous synthesis. DNA helicase unzips the DNA helices so that synthesis can take place, and RNA primers are created by the RNA primase for the polymerases to attach to and build from. The lagging strand is synthesizing DNA in a direction that is hard for the polymerase to build, so multiple primers are laid down so that the entire length of DNA can be synthesized simultaneously, piecemeal. These short pieces of DNA being synthesized are known as Okazaki fragments and are joined together by DNA ligase.

12. A: The sternum is medial to the deltoid because it is much closer (typically right on) the midline of the body, while the deltoid is lateral at the shoulder cap. Superficial means that a structure is closer to the body surface and posterior means that it falls behind something else. For example, skin is superficial to bone and the kidneys are posterior to the rectus abdominus.

13. B: Ligaments connect bone to bone. Tendons connect muscle to bone. Both are made of dense, fibrous connective tissue (primary Type 1 collagen) to give strength. However, tendons are more organized, especially in the long axis direction like muscle fibers themselves, and they have more collagen. This arrangement makes more sense because muscles have specific orientations of their fibers, so they contract in somewhat predictable directions. Ligaments are less organized and more of a woven pattern because bone connections are not as organized as bundles or muscle fibers, so ligaments must have strength in multiple directions to protect against injury.

14. A: The three primary body planes are coronal, sagittal, and transverse. The coronal or frontal plane, named for the plane in which a corona or halo might appear in old paintings, divides the body vertically into front and back sections. The sagittal plane, named for the path an arrow might take when shot at the body, divides the body vertically into right and left sections. The transverse plane divides the body horizontally into upper or superior and lower or inferior sections. There is no medial plane, per se. The anatomical direction medial simply references a location close or closer to the center of the body than another location.

15. C: Although the lungs may provide some cushioning for the heart when the body is violently struck, this is not a major function of the respiratory system. Its most notable function is that of gas exchange for oxygen and carbon dioxide, but it also plays a vital role in the regulation of blood pH. The aqueous form of carbon dioxide, carbonic acid, is a major pH buffer of the blood, and the respiratory system directly controls how much carbon dioxide stays and is released from the blood through respiration. The respiratory system also enables vocalization and forms the basis for the mode of speech and language used by most humans.

16. A: The forebrain contains the cerebrum, the thalamus, the hypothalamus, and the limbic system. The limbic system is chiefly responsible for the perception of emotions through the amygdale, while the cerebrum interprets sensory input and generates movement. Specifically, the occipital lobe receives visual input, and the primary motor cortex in the frontal lobe is the controller of voluntary movement. The hindbrain, specifically the medulla oblongata and brain stem, control and regulate blood pressure and heart rate.

17. D: Germline mutations in eggs and sperm are permanent, can be on the chromosomal level, and will be inherited by offspring. Somatic mutations cannot affect eggs and sperm, and therefore are not inherited by offspring. Mutations of either kind are rarely beneficial to the individual, but do not necessarily harm them. Germline cells divide much more rapidly than do somatic cells, and a mutation in a sex cell would promulgate and affect many thousands of its daughter cells.

18. A: It is most likely asthma. Any of the answer choices listed can cause heavy breathing. A blood clot in the lung (*B*) could cause this, but this would be very uncommon for a child. Choices *C* and *D* can both be ruled out because the question mentions that it occurs even when the patient is relaxing. Hyperventilation is usually caused by a panic attack or some sort of physical activity. Asthma often develops during childhood. It would stand to reason then that the child may have not yet been diagnosed. While asthma attacks can be caused by exercise they can also occur when a person is not exerting themselves.

19. C: 2:9:10:4. These are the coefficients that follow the law of conservation of matter. The coefficient times the subscript of each element should be the same on both sides of the equation.

256

20. C: A catalyst functions to increase reaction rates by decreasing the activation energy required for a reaction to take place. Inhibitors would increase the activation energy or otherwise stop the reactants from reacting. Although increasing the temperature usually increases a reaction's rate, this is not true in all cases, and most catalysts do not function in this manner.

21. B: Biological catalysts are termed *enzymes*, which are proteins with conformations that specifically manipulate reactants into positions which decrease the reaction's activation energy. Lipids do not usually affect reactions, and cofactors, while they can aid or be necessary to the proper functioning of enzymes, do not make up the majority of biological catalysts.

22. B: Substances with higher amounts of hydrogen ions will have lower pHs, while substances with higher amounts of hydroxide ions will have higher pHs. Choice *A* is incorrect because it is possible to have an extremely strong acid with a pH less than 1, as long as its molarity of hydrogen ions is greater than 1. Choice *C* is false because a weak base is determined by having a pH lower than some value, not higher. Substances with pHs greater than 2 include anything from neutral water to extremely caustic lye. Choice *D* is false because a solution with a pH of 2 has ten times fewer hydrogen ions than a solution of pH 1.

23. A: Salts are formed from compounds that use ionic bonds. Disulfide bridges are special bonds in protein synthesis which hold the protein in their secondary and tertiary structures. Covalent bonds are strong bonds formed through the sharing of electrons between atoms and are typically found in organic molecules like carbohydrates and lipids. London dispersion forces are fleeting, momentary bonds which occur between atoms that have instantaneous dipoles but quickly disintegrate.

24. C: As in the last question, covalent bonds are special because they share electrons between multiple atoms. Most covalent bonds are formed between the elements H, F, N, O, S, and C, while hydrogen bonds are formed nearly exclusively between H and either O, N, or F. Covalent bonds may inadvertently form dipoles, but this does not necessarily happen. With similarly electronegative atoms like carbon and hydrogen, dipoles do not form, for instance. Crystal solids are typically formed by substances with ionic bonds like the salts sodium iodide and potassium chloride.

25. A: Gases like air will move and expand to fill their container, so they are considered to have an indefinite shape and indefinite volume. Liquids like water will move and flow freely, so their shapes change constantly, but do not change volume or density on their own. Solids change neither shape nor volume without external forces acting on them, so they have definite shapes and volumes.

26. A: The upper back has the one of the high densities of sweat glands of any area on the body. While palms, arms, and feet are often thought of as sweaty areas, they have relatively low amounts of sweat glands compared to other parts of the body. Remember that one of the purposes of sweat is thermoregulation, or controlling the temperature of the body. Regulating the temperature of one's core is more important than adjusting the temperature of one's extremities.

27. C: Nephrons are responsible for filtering blood. When functioning properly they allow blood cells and nutrients to go back into the bloodstream while sending waste to the bladder. However, nephrons can fail at doing this, particularly when blood flood to the kidneys is limited. The medulla (also called the renal medulla) (*A*) and the renal cortex (*D*) are both parts of the kidney but are not specifically responsible for filtering blood. The medulla is in the inner part of the kidney and contains the nephrons. The renal cortex is the outer part of the kidney. The heart (*B*) is responsible for pumping blood throughout the body rather than filtering it.

28. B: Ossification is the process by which cartilage, a soft, flexible substance is replaced by bone throughout the body. All humans regardless of age have cartilage, but cartilage in some areas goes away to make way for bones.

29. D: The outermost layer of the skin, the epidermis, consists of epithelial cells. This layer of skin is dead, as it has no blood vessels. Osteoclasts are cells that make up bones. Notice the prefix *Osteo-* which means bone. Connective tissue macrophage cells can be found in a variety of places, and dendritic cells are part of the lymphatic system.

30. C: mRNA is directly transcribed from DNA before being taken to the cytoplasm and translated by rRNA into a protein. tRNA transfers amino acids from the cytoplasm to the rRNA for use in building these proteins. siRNA is a special type of RNA which interferes with other strands of mRNA typically by causing them to get degraded by the cell rather than translated into protein.

31. B: Since the genotype is a depiction of the specific alleles that an organism's genes code for, it includes recessive genes that may or may not be otherwise expressed. The genotype does not have to name the proteins that its alleles code for; indeed, some of them may be unknown. The phenotype is the physical, visual manifestations of a gene, not the genotype. The genotype does not necessarily include any information about the organism's physical characters. Although some information about an organism's parents can be obtained from its genotype, its genotype does not actually show the parents' phenotypes.

32. C: One in four offspring (or 25%) will be short, so all four offspring cannot be tall. Although both of the parents are tall, they are hybrid or heterozygous tall, not homozygous. The mother's phenotype is for tall, not short. A Punnett square cannot determine if a short allele will die out. Although it may seem intuitive that the short allele will be expressed by lower numbers of the population than the tall allele, it still appears in 75% of the offspring (although its effects are masked in 2/3 of those). Besides, conditions could favor the recessive allele and kill off the tall offspring.

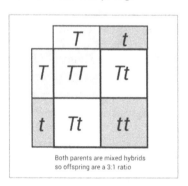

Both parents are mixed hybrids
so offspring are a 3:1 ratio

33. D: Evaporation takes place at the surface of a fluid while boiling takes place throughout the fluid. The liquid will boil when it reaches its boiling or vaporization temperature, but evaporation can happen due to a liquid's volatility. Volatile substances often coexist as a liquid and as a gas, depending on the pressure forced on them. The phase change from gas to liquid is condensation, and both evaporation and boiling take place in nature.

34. A: Human genes are strictly DNA and do not include proteins or amino acids. A human's genome and collection of genes will include even their recessive traits, mutations, and unused DNA.

35. C: Water's polarity lends it to be extremely cohesive and adhesive; this cohesion keeps its atoms very close together. Because of this, it takes a large amount of energy to melt and boil its solid and liquid forms. Phospholipid bilayers are made of nonpolar lipids and water, a polar liquid, cannot flow through it. Cell membranes use proteins called aquaporins to solve this issue and let water flow in and out. Fish breathe by capturing dissolved oxygen through their gills. Water can self-ionize, wherein it decomposes into a hydrogen ion (H^+) and a hydroxide ion (OH^-), but it cannot self-hydrolyze.

36. D: An isotope of an element has an atomic number equal to its number of protons, but a different mass number because of the additional neutrons. Even though there are differences in the nucleus, the behavior and properties of isotopes of a given element are identical. Atoms with different atomic numbers also have different numbers of protons and are different elements, so they cannot be isotopes.

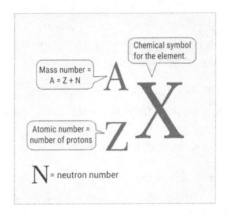

37. A: The neutrons and protons make up the nucleus of the atom. The nucleus is positively charged due to the presence of the protons. The negatively charged electrons are attracted to the positively charged nucleus by the electrostatic or Coulomb force; however, the electrons are not contained in the nucleus. The positively charged protons create the positive charge in the nucleus, and the neutrons are electrically neutral, so they have no effect. Radioactivity does not directly have a bearing on the charge of the nucleus.

38. C: To gather accurate data, the student must be able compare a participant's test score from round 1 with their test score from round 2. The differing levels of intellect among the participants means that comparing participants' test scores to those of other participants would be inaccurate. This requirement excludes choices A and D, which involve only one round of testing. The experiment must also involve different levels of sugar consumption from round 1 to round 2. In this way, the effects of different levels of sugar consumption can be seen on the same subjects. Thus, B is incorrect because the experiment provides for no variation of sugar consumption. C is the correct answer because it allows the student to compare each participant's test score from round 1 with their test score from round 2 after different level of sugar consumption.

39. D: The seminiferous tubules are responsible for sperm production. Had *testicles* been an answer choice, it would also have been correct since it houses the seminiferous tubules. The prostate gland (*A*) secretes enzymes that help nourish sperm after creation. The seminal vesicles (*B*) secrete some of the components of semen. The scrotum (*C*) is the pouch holding the testicles.

40. D: Based on this table, it can be reasoned that there is not a correlation between maintaining a calendar and GPA, since Student B never maintains a calendar but has the highest GPA of the cohort. Furthermore, it can be reasoned that there is a positive correlation between taking notes and GPA since the more notes a student takes, the higher the GPA they have Thus, Choice *D* is the correct answer. Choice *A* offers an absolute that cannot be proven based on this study; thus, it is incorrect. Choices B and C are incorrect because they have at least one incorrect correlation.

41. C: A hypothesis is a statement that makes a prediction between two variables. The two variables here are the amount of poison and how quickly the rat dies. Choice *C* states that the more poison a rat is given, the more quickly it will die, which is a prediction. Choice *A* is incorrect because it's simply an observation. Choice *B* is incorrect because it's a question posed by the observation but makes no predictions. Choice *D* is incorrect because it's simply a fact.

42. B: The independent variable is the variable manipulated and the dependent variable is the result of the changes in the independent variable. Choice *B* is correct because the amount of poison is the variable that is changed, and the speed of rat death is the result of the changes in the amount of poison administered. Choice *A* is incorrect because that answer states the opposite. Choice *C* is false because the scientist isn't attempting to determine whether the rat will die *if* it eats poison; the scientist is testing how quickly the rat will die depending on *how much* poison it eats. Choice *D* is incorrect because the cage isn't manipulated in any way and has nothing to do with the hypothesis.

43. B: Models are representations of concepts that are impossible to experience directly, such as the 3D representation of DNA, so Choice *B* is correct. Choice *A* is incorrect because theories simply explain why things happen. Choice *C* is incorrect because laws describe how things happen. Choice *D* is false because an observation analyzes situations using human senses.

44. A: A control is the component or group of the experimental design that isn't manipulated—it's the standard against which the resultant findings are compared, so Choice *A* is correct. A variable is an element of the experiment that is able to be manipulated, making Choice *B* false. A constant is a condition of the experiment outside of the hypothesis that remains unchanged in order to isolate the changes in the variables; therefore, Choice *C* is incorrect. Choice *D* is false because collected data are simply recordings of the observed phenomena that result from the experiment.

45. C: An inference is a logical prediction of a why an event occurred based on previous experiences or education. The person in this example knows that plants need water to survive; therefore, the prediction that someone forgot to water the plant is a reasonable inference, hence Choice *C* is correct. A classification is the grouping of events or objects into categories, so Choice *A* is false. An observation analyzes situations using human senses, so Choice *B* is false. Choice *D* is incorrect because collecting is the act of gathering data for analysis.

46. A: The decimal point for this value is located after the final zero. Because the decimal is moved 12 places to the left in order to get it between the *8* and the *6*, then the resulting exponent is positive, so Choice *A* is the correct answer. Choice *B* is false because the decimal has been moved in the wrong direction. Choice *C* is incorrect because the decimal has been moved an incorrect number of times. Choice *D* is false because this value is written to three significant figures, not two.

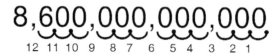

47. B: The set of results is close to the actual value of the acceleration due to gravity, making the results accurate. However, there is a different value recorded every time, so the results aren't precise, which makes Choice *B* the correct answer.

48. B: To solve this, the number of moles of NaCl needs to be calculated:

First, to find the mass of NaCl, the mass of each of the molecule's atoms is added together as follows:

$$23.0g\ (Na) + 35.5g\ (Cl) = 58.8g\ NaCl$$

Next, the given mass of the substance is multiplied by one mole per total mass of the substance:

$$4.0g\ NaCl \times (1\ mol\ NaCl/58.5g\ NaCl) = 0.068\ mol\ NaCl$$

Finally, the moles are divided by the number of liters of the solution to find the molarity:

$$(0.068\ mol\ NaCl)/(0.120L) = 0.57\ M\ NaCl$$

Choice A incorporates a miscalculation for the molar mass of NaCl, and Choices C and D both incorporate a miscalculation by not converting mL into liters (L), so they are incorrect by a factor of 10.

49. C: According to the *ideal gas law* (*PV = nRT*), if volume is constant, the temperature is directly related to the pressure in a system. Therefore, if the pressure increases, the temperature will increase in direct proportion. Choice A would not be possible, since the system is closed and a change is occurring, so the temperature will change. Choice B incorrectly exhibits an inverse relationship between pressure and temperature, or *P = 1/T*. Choice D is incorrect because even without actual values for the variables, the relationship and proportions can be determined.

50. B: A solid produced during a reaction is called a *precipitate.* In a neutralization reaction, the products (an acid and a base) react to form a salt and water. Choice A, an oxidation reaction, involves the transfer of an electron. Choice C, a synthesis reaction, involves the joining of two molecules to form a single molecule. Choice D, a decomposition reaction, involves the separation of a molecule into two other molecules.

51. C: Molecules that are soluble in lipids, like fats, sterols, and vitamins (A, D, E and K), for example, are able to move in and out of a cell using passive transport. Water and oxygen are also able to move in and out of the cell without the use of cellular energy. Complex sugars and non-lipid soluble molecules are too large to move through the cell membrane without relying on active transport mechanisms. Molecules naturally move from areas of high concentration to those of lower concentration. It requires active transport to move molecules in the opposite direction, as suggested by Choice D.

52. A: Both types of cells are enclosed by a cell membrane, which is selectively permeable. Selective permeability means essentially that it is a gatekeeper, allowing certain molecules and ions in and out, and keeping unwanted ones at bay, at least until they are ready for use. Prokaryotes contain a nucleoid and do not have organelles; eukaryotes contain a nucleus enclosed by a membrane, as well as organelles.

53. B: During telophase, two nuclei form at each end of the cell and nuclear envelopes begin to form around each nucleus. The nucleoli reappear, and the chromosomes become less compact. The microtubules are broken down by the cell, and mitosis is complete. The process begins with prophase as the mitotic spindles begin to form from centrosomes. Prometaphase follows, with the breakdown of the nuclear envelope and the further condensing of the chromosomes. Next, metaphase occurs when the microtubules are stretched across the cell and the chromosomes align at the metaphase plate. Finally, in the last step before telophase, anaphase occurs as the sister chromatids break apart and form chromosomes.

54. D: Meiosis has the same phases as mitosis, except that they occur twice—once in meiosis I and once in meiosis II. During meiosis I, the cell splits into two. Each cell contains two sets of chromosomes. Next, during meiosis II, the two intermediate daughter cells divide again, producing four total haploid cells that each contain one set of chromosomes.

55. B: The secondary structure of a protein refers to the folds and coils that are formed by hydrogen bonding between the slightly charged atoms of the polypeptide backbone. The primary structure is the sequence of amino acids, similar to the letters in a long word. The tertiary structure is the overall shape of the molecule that results from the interactions between the side chains that are linked to the polypeptide backbone. The quaternary structure is the complete protein structure that occurs when a protein is made up of two or more polypeptide chains.

56. A: The sensory threshold is the smallest amount of stimulus that is required for an individual to experience one of the senses. For example, during a hearing test, the sensory threshold would be the quietest sound that a person could detect. This threshold is an important indicator of whether a person's senses are working within a normal range.

57. C: Generally, all sensory pathways that extend from the sensory receptor to the brain are composed of three long neurons called the primary, secondary, and tertiary neurons. The primary one stretches from the sensory receptor to the dorsal root ganglion of the spinal nerve; the secondary one stretches from the cell body of the primary neuron to the spinal cord or the brain stem; the tertiary one stretches from the cell body of the secondary one into the thalamus. Each type of sense, such as touch, hearing, and vision, has a different pathway designed specifically for that sensation.

58. C: Visual processing begins in the retina. When an individual sees an image, it is taken in through the cornea and lens and then transmitted upside down onto the retina. The cells in the retina process what is being seen and then send signals to the ganglion cells, whose axons make up the optic nerve. The optic nerve cells connect the retina to the brain, which is where the processing of the visual information is completed and the images are returned to their proper orientation.

59. D: Arteries carry oxygen-rich blood from the heart to the other tissues of the body. Veins carry oxygen-poor blood back to the heart. Intestines carry digested food through the body. Bronchioles are passageways that carry air from the nose and mouth to the lungs.

60. C: The somatic nervous system is the voluntary nervous system, responsible for voluntary movement. It includes nerves that transmit signals from the brain to the muscles of the body. Breathing is controlled by the autonomic nervous system. Thought and fear are complex processes that occur in the brain, which is part of the central nervous system.

61. D: Catabolism is the process of breaking large molecules into smaller molecules to release energy for work. Carbohydrates and fats are catabolized to provide energy for exercise and daily activities. Anabolism synthesizes larger molecules from smaller constituent building blocks. Bioenergetics and metabolism are more general terms involving overall energy production and usage.

62. A: Platelets are the blood components responsible for clotting. There are between 150,000 and 450,000 platelets in healthy blood. When a clot forms, platelets adhere to the injured area of the vessel and promote a molecular cascade that results in adherence of more platelets. Ultimately, the platelet aggregation results in recruitment of a protein called fibrin, which adds structure to the clot. Too many platelets can cause clotting disorders. Not enough leads to bleeding disorders.

63. A: Choice B might be an attractive answer choice, but neutrophils are part of the innate immune system and are not considered part of the primary immune response. The first event that happens in a primary immune response is that macrophages ingest pathogens and display their antigens. Then, they secrete interleukin 1 to recruit helper T cells. Once helper T cells are activated, they secrete interleukin 2 to simulate plasma B and killer T cell production. Only then can plasma B make the pathogen specific antibodies.

64. C: The epididymis stores sperm and is a coiled tube located near the testes. The immature sperm that enters the epididymis from the testes migrates through the 20-foot long epididymis tube in about two weeks, where viable sperm are concentrated at the end. The vas deferens is a tube that transports mature sperm from the epididymis to the urethra. Seminal vesicles are pouches attached that add fructose to the ejaculate to provide energy for sperm. The prostate gland excretes fluid that makes up about a third of semen released during ejaculation. The fluid reduces semen viscosity and contains enzymes that aid in sperm functioning; both effects increase sperm motility and ultimate success.

65. A: All three joint types given are synovial joints, allowing for a fair amount of movement (compared with fibrous and cartilaginous joints). Of the three given, hinge joints, such as the elbow, permit the least motion because they are uniaxial and permit movement in only one plane. Saddle joints and condyloid joints both have reciprocating surfaces that mate with one another and allow a variety of motions in numerous planes, but saddle joints, such as the thumb carpal metacarpal joint allow more motion than condyloid joints. In saddle joints, two concave surfaces articulate, and in a condyloid joint, such as the wrist, a concave surface articulates with a convex surface, allowing motion in mainly two planes.

66. D: All of the above. Synergists are responsible for helping the primary movers or agonists carry out their specific movements. Synergists can help stabilize the point of origin of a muscle or provide extra pull near the insertion; in this sense, they can be considered "fixators." Some synergists can help prevent undesired movement at a joint. For example, for elbow flexion, the brachialis is a synergist to the biceps.

67. D: Bony matrix is an intricate lattice of collagen fibers and mineral salts, particularly calcium and phosphorus. The mineral salts are strong but brittle, and the collagen fibers are weak but flexible, so the combination of the two makes bone resistant to shattering and able to withstand the normal forces applied to it.

68. D: The natural tendency in the universe is to increase entropy and disorder, so organisms undergo biochemical processes and use free energy and matter to stabilize their internal environment against this changing external environment in a process called homeostasis. Organisms strive to maintain physiologic factors such as body temperature, blood pH, and fluid balance in equilibrium or around a set point. Choice A is incorrect because homeostasis in organisms involves trying to maintain internal conditions around their set point, which doesn't always involve increasing body temperature, blood pH, and fluid balance; the organism may need to work to decrease these values. Choice B is incorrect because maintaining homeostasis expends energy; it does not absorb it. Choice C is incorrect because homeostasis involves maintaining order in the organism's internal, not external, environment.

69. A: All three types of muscle tissue (skeletal, cardiac, and smooth) share four important properties: They are contractile, meaning they can shorten and pull on connective tissue; excitable, meaning they respond to stimuli; elastic, meaning they rebound to their original length after a contraction; and extensible, meaning they can be stretched repeatedly, but maintain the ability to contract. While skeletal muscle is under voluntary control, both cardiac and smooth muscle are involuntary.

70. D: The autonomic nervous system (ANS), a division of the PNS controls involuntary functions such as breathing, heart rate, blood pressure, digestion, and body temperature via the antagonistic parasympathetic and sympathetic nerves. Choices A, B, and C are incorrect because they describe characteristics of the somatic nervous system, which is the other division of the PNS. It controls skeletal muscles via afferent and efferent neurons. Afferent neurons carry sensory messages from skeletal muscles, skin, or sensory organs to the CNS, while efferent neurons relay motor messages from the CNS to skeletal muscles, skin, or sensory organs. While skeletal muscle movement is under voluntary control, the somatic nervous system also plays a role in the involuntary reflex arc.

71. C: The sinuses function to warm, filter, and humidify air that is inhaled. Choice A is incorrect because mucus traps airborne pathogens. Choice B is incorrect because the epiglottis is the structure in the pharynx that covers the trachea during swallowing to prevent food from entering it. Lastly, Choice D, sweeping away pathogens and directing them toward the top of the trachea, is the function of cilia. Respiratory structures, such as the nasal passages and trachea, are lined with mucus and cilia.

72. A: The renal pelvis acts like funnel by delivering the urine from the millions of the collecting tubules to the ureters. It is the most central part of the kidney. The renal cortex is the outer layer of the kidney, while the renal medulla is the inner layer. The renal medulla contains the functional units of the kidneys—nephrons—which function to filter the blood. Choice D, Bowman's capsule, is the name for the structure that covers the glomeruli.

73. B: The pelvic cavity is the area formed by the bones of the hip. Housed in that space are the urinary bladder, urethra, ureters, anus, and rectum. This hollow space also contains the uterus in females. The other body cavities listed contain other organs not specified in the question.

74. B: An amphoteric substance can act as an acid or a base depending on the properties of the solute. Water is a common example and because of its amphoteric property, it serves as a universal solvent. Choice A is incorrect because it describes electrolytes. Choices C and D are incorrect because they both describe an acid.

75. C: The body has a variety of touch receptors that detect tactile information, which gets carried via general somatic afferents and general visceral afferents to the CNS. Meissner's corpuscles respond to light touch and slower vibrations. Choice A is incorrect because Merkel's discs respond to sustained pressure. Choice B is incorrect because Pacinian corpuscles detect rapid vibration and in the skin and fascia, and Choice D is incorrect because Ruffini endings detect deep touch and tension in the skin and fascia.

76. C: Nociceptor are a type of touch receptor that detect pain. They relay this information to the CNS via afferent nerves. Efferent nerves then carry motor signals back, which may cause muscle contractions that move the body part away from the source of the pain. For example, if a person places his or her hand on a hot stove, nociceptors detect the painful burning sensation. Then they relay this information up to the brain, where a response signal travels down the efferent nerves that control the muscles of the shoulder, arm, forearm, and/or hand to retract the hand from the hot stove. Choice *A* is incorrect because that is mainly the function of Ruffini endings. Choice *B* describes the function of several mechanoreceptors such as Meissner's corpuscles, Pacinian corpuscles, and Merkel's discs. Lastly, thermoreceptors detect changes in pressure, so Choice *D* is incorrect.

77. C: A cluster of capillaries that functions as the main filter of the blood entering the kidney is known as the glomerulus, so Choice *C* is correct. The Bowman's capsule surrounds the glomerulus and receives fluid and solutes from it; therefore, Choice *A* is incorrect. The loop of Henle is a part of the kidney tubule where water and nutrients are reabsorbed, so *B* is false. The nephron is the unit containing all of these anatomical features, making Choice *D* incorrect as well.

78. A: An alteration in the normal gene sequence is called a DNA point mutation. Mutations can be harmful, neutral, or even beneficial. Sometimes, as seen in natural selection, a genetic mutation can improve fitness, providing an adaptation that will aid in survival. DNA mutations can happen as a result of environmental damage, for example, from radiation or chemicals. Mutations can also happen during cell replication, as a result of incorrect pairing of complementary nucleotides by DNA polymerase. There are also chromosomal mutations as well, where entire segments of chromosomes can be deleted, inverted, duplicated, or sent or received from a different chromosome.

79. B: 50%. According to the Punnett square, the child has a 2 out of 4 chance of having A-type blood, since the dominant allele I^A is present in two of the four possible offspring. The O-type blood allele is masked by the A-type blood allele since it is recessive.

I^A i	ii
I^A i	ii

80. D: Reproductive cells are referred to as gametes: egg (female) and sperm (male). These cells have only 1 set of 23 chromosomes and are haploid so that when they combine during fertilization, the zygote has the correct diploid number, 46. Reproductive cell division is called meiosis, which is different from mitosis, the type of division process for body (somatic) cells.

Dear PAX Test Taker,

We would like to start by thanking you for purchasing this study guide for your PAX exam. We hope that we exceeded your expectations.

Our goal in creating this study guide was to cover all of the topics that you will see on the test. We also strove to make our practice questions as similar as possible to what you will encounter on test day. With that being said, if you found something that you feel was not up to your standards, please send us an email and let us know.

We would also like to let you know about other books in our catalog that may interest you.

TEAS 6

This can be found on amazon.com/dp/162845427X

HESI A2

Amazon.com/dp/1628456019

CEN

Amazon.com/dp/1628454768

CNOR

Amazon.com/dp/162845556X

We have study guides in a wide variety of fields. If the one you are looking for isn't listed above, then try searching for it on Amazon or send us an email.

Thanks Again and Happy Testing!
Product Development Team
info@studyguideteam.com

Interested in buying more than 10 copies of our product? Contact us about bulk discounts:

bulkorders@studyguideteam.com

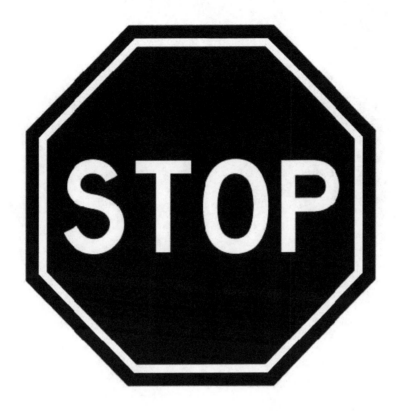

FREE Test Taking Tips DVD Offer

To help us better serve you, we have developed a Test Taking Tips DVD that we would like to give you for FREE. **This DVD covers world-class test taking tips that you can use to be even more successful when you are taking your test.**

All that we ask is that you email us your feedback about your study guide. Please let us know what you thought about it – whether that is good, bad or indifferent.

To get your **FREE Test Taking Tips DVD**, email freedvd@studyguideteam.com with "FREE DVD" in the subject line and the following information in the body of the email:

>   a. The title of your study guide.

>   b. Your product rating on a scale of 1-5, with 5 being the highest rating.

>   c. Your feedback about the study guide. What did you think of it?

>   d. Your full name and shipping address to send your free DVD.

If you have any questions or concerns, please don't hesitate to contact us at freedvd@studyguideteam.com.

Thanks again!

CPSIA information can be obtained
at www.ICGtesting.com
Printed in the USA
BVHW011911180419
545933BV00007B/157/P